HAY FEVER

THE COMPLETE GUIDE

By the same authors

Asthma: The Complete Guide to Integrative Therapies

Food Allergies and Food Intolerance:
The Complete Guide to Their Identification and Treatment

HAY FEVER

THE COMPLETE GUIDE

Find Relief from Allergies to Pollens, Molds, Pets, Dust Mites, and More

JONATHAN BROSTOFF, M.D. and LINDA GAMLIN

Healing Arts Press
Rochester, Vermont

Healing Arts Press
One Park Street
Rochester, Vermont 05767
www.InnerTraditions.com

Healing Arts Press is a division of Inner Traditions International

Library of Congress Cataloging-in-Publication Data
Brostoff, Jonathan.
    Hay fever : the complete guide : find relief from allergies to pollens, molds, pets, dust, and more / Jonathan Brostoff and Linda Gamlin.
        p. cm.
    Rev. ed. of : The complete guide to hayfever. London : Bloomsbury, 1993.
    Includes index.
    ISBN 0-89281-988-X
    1. Hay fever—Popular works. I. Brostoff, Jonathan. Complete guide to hayfever.
II. Gamlin, Linda. III. Title.

RC590 .B764 2002
616.2'02—dc21   2001059379

Printed and bound in the United States at Lake Book Manufacturing, Inc.

10 9 8 7 6 5 4 3 2 1

Text design by Mary Anne Hurhula and Priscilla Baker
This book was typeset in Granjon, with Agenda as a display font

CONTENTS

ACKNOWLEDGMENTS

Many people have given freely of their time in helping us with the research for this book, and we are immensely grateful to them. We would particularly like to thank Dr. A. Armentia-Medina, Mina Barge, Dr. Diana Bass, Peter Bateman, Dr. Ian Burgess, David Burnie, Sheila Burnie, Stuart Collier, Dr. Matthew Colloff, Dr. Roland Davies, Dr. Eugenio Dominguez-Vilches, Dr. Keith Eaton, Dr. Michael Emanuel, Dr. Nils Eriksson, Dr. Penny Fitzharris, Dr. William Frankland, Dr. Tony Ganderton, Dr. Richard Godfrey, Derek Hall, Dr. R. J. Harris, Professor John Heslop-Harrison, Dr. Stephen Holgate, Andrew Jones, Dr. Richard Lawson, Dr. George Lewith, Dr. Colin Little, Dr. Christina Luczynska, Dr. Jonathan Maberly, Dr. Len McEwen, Quintin McKenzie, Dr. Charlie McSharry, Dr. John Mansfield, Dr. Bruce Mitchell, Dr. John Morrison-Smith, Dr. Harry Morrow-Brown, Dr. Masaharu Muranaka, Gerard Nelson, Shigeki Ohyama, Professor Eldryd Parry, Dr. John Pettitt, Pavel Pietrzak, Professor Tom Platts-Mills, Morrika Rae, Dr. Kyllikki Remes, Dr. Tim Rich, Mohammed Saleem, Ludmilla Semenova-Ducksbury, Dr. Bonnie Sibbald, Don Skelton, Simon Small, Dr. Ian Smith, Dr. David Strachan, Lynne Strugnell, Colin Taylor, Dr. Morton Teich, Dr. Gilles Vincent, Dr. Victoria von Witt, Dr. Tony Walter, Dr. Alan Wheeler, Professor Bruno Wüthrich, and Professor V. Zavazal.

Finally, we would like to thank Fraser May for his excellent work on the illustrations and Lee Juvan for all her effort, dedication, and enthusiasm in preparing this edition for North America.

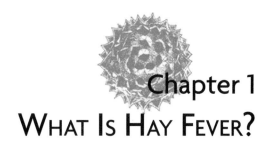

Chapter 1
WHAT IS HAY FEVER?

Sex causes hay fever. Most people are surprised to discover this, because they had no idea that plants, whose lives seem fairly dull and uneventful, actually engage in sex. But the fact is that they do, and that the sexual exploits of plants set millions of people sneezing and sniffing every year. (Very occasionally, the sexual exploits of human beings spark off hay fever–like symptoms in the participants, or an attack of asthma, or both. This unusual reaction is discussed in chapter 13.)

Plant sex is no different from sex between animals, in that it involves an interaction between male and female. But being rooted firmly to the ground makes it difficult for plants to pursue their mate, so they do it all at a distance, in a detached and dispassionate fashion that is rather like artificial insemination. Mating takes place without any meeting. Pollen—a fine powder that is the plants' equivalent of semen—is dispatched from one plant to another while the plants themselves stay put. A tiny pinch of pollen dust contains thousands of microscopic pollen grains, and each of these carries inside it a potent male cell, equivalent to the sperm cell of an animal.

For plants such as roses and buttercups, the pollen is transported by a six-legged artificial inseminator—a bee, butterfly, or other insect. The plant depends on the insect pollinator, which is lured into its flowers by a free meal of syrupy liquid—nectar. As the insect feeds, it brushes against the pollen-producing organs, called anthers, and inadvertently collects pollen on its head or body. At the next flower, some of this pollen brushes on to the female parts of the flower. Assuming the two flowers are compatible, the pollen will fertilize the egg cells in the flower, and each of these will develop into a seed.

As a way of improving the efficiency of this system, most flowers have both male and female parts—they are hermaphrodites—so they can dispatch pollen to other plants and receive it as well. In the majority of plants, there are special mechanisms that prevent them from fertilizing themselves.

BEES OR BREEZE? THE POLLINATION OPTIONS

Pollination by insects was used by the very earliest flowering plants, which were evolving their first colorful petals and sugary nectar as the dinosaurs plodded by, more than 100 million years ago. Those early flowers were something like modern-day magnolias and were probably pollinated by small beetles.

In time, some flowering plants developed other ways of being pollinated. Insects, as it turned out, had certain drawbacks. They did not fly far enough to pollinate plants that were widely scattered, and they were fussy about the weather—if it was too cold, they stayed at home. A few plants developed larger flowers and more nectar, attracting active warm-blooded animals such as bats and small birds to act as their pollinators. But this worked only in certain parts of the tropics, where there were flowers available all year round to keep these large and hungry pollinators well fed.

What other options were available for a plant that needed to dispense with insect pollinators? There was only one realistic possibility: the wind. Many flowering plants gradually evolved in this direction, notably the grasses, all of which are wind-pollinated. In time they lost the showy, colorful petals that had been used to attract insects. They also stopped producing nectar to feed the insects and sweet scents to beguile them.

All these measures saved the plants a great deal of energy, so dispensing with insects was worthwhile. However, there was one huge disadvantage to set against these energy savings—an insect carries pollen straight to other flowers, while the wind simply blows it anywhere.

The solution that evolution came up with was to saturate the air with pollen—to release millions of pollen grains from every flower. Among modern plants the champion pollen producer, the giant ragweed, can generate a million pollen grains in a day, a staggering rate of production that brings misery to ragweed-sensitive patients.

As wind pollination evolved, natural selection also favored pollen grains that were extremely light in weight, so as not to settle rapidly but to remain suspended on the breeze for hours. This greatly increases the chance of the right pollen grain reaching the right flower. Unfortunately, it also maximizes the chance of it reaching the nose of a hay fever victim.

In a sense, by developing wind pollination in flowering plants, the forces of evolution were just reinventing the wheel. A separate group of plants, an older and more primitive group, had been using wind pollination for millions of years; in fact, they had never tried any other method. These were the coniferous trees such as pines, firs, and spruces, which still grow in many parts of

WHAT DOES HAY FEVER MEAN?

The term "hay fever" can be used in two different ways. The most common meaning, and the one used in this book, is an allergic reaction to pollen—any sort of pollen.

However, when the word was coined in the 19th century by the general public (and later taken up, rather reluctantly, by the medical profession), it was intended to mean an unusual reaction to hay. Since hay is a mixture of grass and wildflowers, and it is the grass pollen that causes the symptoms in this mixture, "hay fever," strictly speaking, means a reaction to grass pollen. A few doctors and researchers still use the word in this restrictive sense. This is particularly true in Britain and northern Europe, where in any case allergy to pollen means allergy to grass pollen for the great majority of sufferers.

For those using "hay fever" in this restrictive sense, another word is needed to cover pollen allergy generally. The word "pollinosis" (or "pollenosis") is sometimes used, but this has not caught on as widely as "hay fever," even though it is far more scholarly and precise.

A third possibility, sometimes used by doctors, is seasonal allergic rhinitis or SAR. Apart from being excessively long-winded, this term is rather confusing, since it lumps pollen allergy together with seasonal mold-spore allergy while excluding perennial mold-spore allergy.

the world today. Their pollen is produced in such huge amounts that, close to a pine forest, it can form a slick of yellow scum on the surface of puddles. But despite their abundance, conifer pollens are not common culprits in hay fever.

FEAR OF FLOWERS?

The differences between insect-pollinated and wind-pollinated flowers are not just a matter of academic interest—they are very important to anyone with hay fever. Pollen grains that are carried by insects are slightly sticky to ensure that they become attached to their insect pollinator. This also makes them stick to each other, so they form clusters of pollen grains that are then easily visible. (You may see the pollen among the petals of flowers or stuck to the "fur" on a bee.) By contrast, the pollen of grasses and most other wind-pollinated plants is virtually invisible because it comes in minute, separate grains that disperse rapidly. On a sunny day, if you watch a nettle flower or a birch catkin that is catching the sun but is positioned against a dark background, you may just see a puff of pollen escaping, but you have to look very carefully because it disperses in seconds.

Being relatively large, heavy, and sticky, the pollen grains of insect-pollinated plants do not become airborne easily, and only small amounts are inhaled. Such flowers are far less likely to cause hay fever than wind-pollinated flowers, because the amount of pollen in the air is insufficient to sensitize most people.

The sorts of flowers that are picked and placed in vases are almost all insect-pollinated: the scents and showy petals that appeal to us are exactly those that evolved to attract insects. Virtually any large-petaled flower, from a daisy to an orchid, falls into this category.

Some people make the mistake of thinking that such flowers—pretty, scented, conspicuous flowers—cause their hay fever. They can even develop floriphobia, a deadly fear of flowers! In fact, it is the plants you scarcely notice, the self-effacing ones with tiny, dull green flowers, that are really to blame. Likewise, it is the pollen you *cannot see* that is likely to be causing your hay fever. The golden powder produced by garden flowers is probably harmless to you.

So much for the public misconception about insect-pollinated flowers. *But there is a widespread medical misconception about them too.* This is that insect-pollinated flowers *never* cause hay fever, and that none of their pollen becomes airborne. This view is equally mistaken, yet it is the firm belief of many doctors. A study in Britain found pollen from dandelions, buttercups, and elderberries all floating in the air, along with pollen from plants of the carrot, cabbage, and rose families. Scientists in India found that 12 percent of airborne pollen was from insect-pollinated plants. When two American researchers set out to find well-verified cases of hay fever to insect-pollinated plants, they came up with hundreds of case reports involving more than 40 different species of plant.

There are two main situations in which insect-pollinated plants produce hay fever. The first involves those unfortunate, highly sensitive individuals who can become allergic to a pollen even though the amounts in the air are small. The second occurs when people are exposed to huge quantities of a particular insect-dispersed pollen, either at work or around the home.

The first situation produces some rare cases of allergy to plants such as honeysuckle, hydrangea, rose, sweet pea, and dahlia. Usually, these patients are highly prone to allergy and react to other pollens as well, but occasionally there is just one offender and it is an insect-pollinated plant. **Cross-reactions** between related plants may be important here. For example, ragweed belongs to the same botanical family (the Compositae or Asteraceae) as dandelions. Children who are ragweed-sensitive may suffer a bad attack of hay fever after rolling in grass that is full of flowering dandelions. This is uncommon, but several cases have been reported in areas where ragweed hay fever is rife. (In other parts of the world, such as Britain, where dandelion is equally common but ragweed is rare, children roll among the dandelions with impunity—sensitivity to dandelion pollen is unknown.)

The second situation, when people are exposed to large numbers of a particular insect-pollinated plant, produces far more cases of hay fever because it is not just those who are highly prone to allergy who succumb.

In some regions of Russia, fields of golden sunflowers stretch as far as the eye can see, and there are many cases of allergy to sunflower pollen. Wherever a large area of farmland is devoted to a particular insect-pollinated crop, the potential for sensitization may be present. Big orchards of apples, cherries, or plums can produce hay fever in a few of the local residents, while in California, Florida, and Israel—all major producers of oranges—sensitivity to orange pollen is found. (In this case, an interesting discovery has been made about how the pollen becomes airborne: overladen bees flying away from the orange trees drop some of their pollen on the way back to the hive.)

Could the same be happening with oil-seed rape, the oil and fodder crop that is adding squares of brilliant yellow to our landscape? Its pollen is found in the air around rape fields, and many people believe they suffer hay fever when close to these fields. Whether this is really a response to oil-seed rape itself is still under discussion. Nor is it certain whether the rape pollen or some other substance given off by the plants is to blame (see page 117).

Those whose work brings them into close daily contact with a particular insect-pollinated plant—plant breeders, farmworkers, flower growers, and florists, for example—also encounter enough pollen to increase their risk of hay fever. Chrysanthemums are a common problem for florists, and mimosa (which may be pollinated by insects or wind) causes a lot of hay fever among commercial flower growers in Italy. Farmers and farm laborers who grow alfalfa, lucerne, or clover may be exposed to the pollen all year round because it remains in the dried fodder that they feed to their animals during the winter months. Hay fever in response to these pollens has been reported from many parts of the United States and from South Africa.

A study of gardeners, plant specialists, and nursery workers in Germany discovered eight cases of hay fever to cyclamen, three to begonias, and one to lilies. A weeping undertaker at a funeral may be one of an unusually sentimental nature, but it is also possible that his red, watery eyes are a response to the Easter lilies about the casket. They cause one of the more esoteric forms of occupational hay fever.

Plant breeders are a particularly vulnerable group of workers because their job involves actually handling pollen, as they cross-pollinate one plant with another. One plant breeder found that he had to repeatedly change the

THE CONIFER PUZZLE

All conifers are wind-pollinated, yet they cause hay fever far less often than wind-pollinated flowering plants. In Scandinavia, where forests of spruce and pine cover vast areas (and where the pollen cloud is so dense that it can blow across the North Sea to Britain), it is not these trees that generally cause hay fever. The guilty trees are the delicate little birches that grow among the conifers or along the forest edges: birches belong to the flowering plant group. Only a tiny minority of Scandinavians are sensitive to pine pollen.

There are occasional reports of pine hay fever from some Mediterranean countries and from North America, but again these are relatively rare, with very few people being affected. The only true pine that produces hay fever to any appreciable extent is the eastern white pine of New England, and even this affects only 10 percent of those with spring hay fever. As for spruces, firs, larches, and cedars, hay fever in response to these trees is unknown. The same is true of yews. The possible reasons for the lack of hay fever in response to these conifers will be discussed later in this chapter.

There are some notable exceptions to the rule about conifers, however. Certain types *do* cause hay fever, particularly the cypresses and junipers (a group of closely related conifers), the white cypress pine (which is not a true pine at all, but a native Australian conifer), and the Japanese red cedar (a relative of the American redwoods). Other trees in the redwood family, such as the bald cypress, may sometimes cause hay fever.

Of these, the only one to cause a major outbreak of hay fever—the sort of widespread outbreak that grasses, ragweeds, or other flowering plants can produce—is the Japanese red cedar. This has, in the past 40 years, produced a dramatic hay fever epidemic in Japan. There is some intriguing research from California, which suggests that people of Asiatic origin are more likely than Caucasians to react allergically to conifer pollen—cypresses and junipers in this case—but their **allergens** (see page 10) are similar to those of Japanese red cedar. This ethnic difference may help to explain the unprecedented scale of the Japanese epidemic, although other factors undoubtedly play a part.

Sometimes people are aware of being affected by pine pollen, although medical tests show no real allergic reaction to it. This seems to be particularly true in New Zealand and Australia, where introduced pines have been planted for timber. The most plausible explanation for this is that the sheer volume of pine pollen in the air, and its relatively large size, may make it an irritant to the nose. (A grain of pine pollen is more than twice the size of other airborne pollens, and should not, by rights, become airborne at all, but it has two large air bladders that keep it buoyant.) Another possible cause of the symptoms is an irritant chemical, called benzoic acid, that is released by some pine pollen.

type of crop he worked on because he became sensitive to almost any plant after a year or two. Having started as a carrot breeder, he was forced to move on to beans, then to cabbages, and then to a succession of other crops. (All these crops are insect-pollinated.) Research programs already begun had to be conducted at long distance using assistants because he could no longer enter the glasshouses where the offending crops were growing.

In conclusion, then, how should you proceed if your hay fever seems to be brought on by sniffing a rose, although your doctor says this is nonsense? First, consider the other possibilities. The most likely explanation is that you are sensitive to grass or some other wind-pollinated plant that pollinates at the same time as roses are in flower. When sniffing a rose, you may inhale a little rose pollen that acts as an irritant and aggravates, or precipitates, the reaction to grass. Once hay fever has set in, the membranes of the nose become oversensitive and can be affected by all kinds of minor irritants. Even the scent of the rose (or other flowers) can rank among those irritants and apparently trigger an attack of hay fever (see "Vasomotor Rhinitis" in chapter 13). In these cases, the rose is just an innocent bystander, and floriphobia is an inappropriate reaction. Ask the doctor for a skin-prick test to the common windborne pollens, and this may reveal the culprit.

A true sensitivity to the rose (or other insect-pollinated plant) is far less likely, but it is possible. Unfortunately, neither skin-prick tests nor allergy shots (see chapter 9) are likely to be available, since extracts of such pollen are not found commercially. But an enterprising allergist should be able to produce "home-made" extracts, for either diagnosis or treatment. The standard drug treatments are just the same as for wind-pollinated plants, so you do not necessarily need to be sure which plant is causing your symptoms.

THE RACE TO POLLINATE

So far, we have considered how pollen gets from one plant to another, but we have not looked at what happens to the pollen on arrival at its destination. This is crucial, because knowing how pollen grains "behave" in normal circumstances can help us to understand what causes hay fever. A pollen grain that lands in the nose goes through a sequence of actions, which in the right place would help it to father a seed. In your nose or eyes, it is doing the right thing but in the wrong place.

The right place to be for a pollen grain is on the **stigma** of another flower. The stigma protrudes from the center of most flowers and is the only entrance-way to a hidden cavity, deep inside the flower, that contains the egg cell. However, it is not an open entrance. The pollen has to work to get its male cell through the stigma to the egg, and this is the key to its "behavior" when it reaches a stigma—or a nose.

In wind-pollinated flowers, the stigma is often feathery to maximize its chance of catching any pollen floating past in the air, and slightly moist, so that pollen tends to stick to it. The moisture of the stigma tells the pollen grain that it has hit its target.

From that moment, the pollen grain is in a hurry. Only one pollen grain can fertilize each egg cell, and there may be other pollen grains elsewhere on the stigma racing to be the first there.

Microscopes reveal pollen grains as incredibly beautiful little objects, with intricately sculpted surfaces. Like most things in nature, this exquisite piece of decoration actually serves a purpose, playing a part in the race for fertilization, as we shall see.

The egg cell, which is the prize for the winner of that race, is safely enclosed by a solid mass of green tissue. The only way to reach the egg cell is to penetrate the stigma, forcing a way through the apparently solid tissue. To achieve this, and to get there before competing pollen grains, the pollen grain has to react promptly.

Within a few seconds of landing on the stigma, the pollen grain discharges

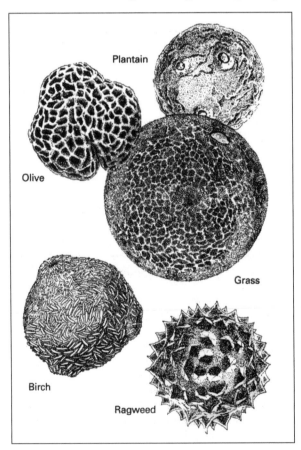

Pollen Grains

chemicals, specific types of **proteins** that are characteristic of the plant species. And this is where the intricately sculpted pollen coat comes in. The proteins to be discharged first are held in the crevices of the pollen grain's outer coat, lightly sealed in by a fatty layer, ready for a quick release. These first proteins act as chemical passwords, revealing the identity of the pollen to the receiving plant. Only if the pollen comes from the right sort of plant will the stigma allow it to compete for the egg.

If it passes this fast test, the pollen grain's next task is to penetrate the stigma by literally growing into it. To achieve this it produces more chemicals, special types of protein known as **enzymes,** that can chemically "chew" holes in the fabric of the stigma. Hot on the heels of these enzymes comes a special cell that grows out of the pollen grain, and continues to grow, very fast and straight, pushing its way through the enzyme-damaged tissue of the stigma toward the egg cell. If successful, this pioneering cell creates a tunnel leading from the pollen grain straight down the stigma to the egg cell. Known as the pollen tube, this is the highway to fertilization for the male cell, which now emerges from the pollen grain to make its triumphal journey to the egg.

Only a few lucky pollen grains will achieve such fulfillment. The vast majority are doomed to a brief and pointless existence, floating about on the wind and landing nowhere in particular. Some of these end their days caught on the inner membranes that line the human nose: the nose exists in order to filter air before it gets to the lungs, and pollen grains are among the particles that it removes.

Unfortunately, most pollen grains cannot tell the difference between a nose and a stigma. Both are moist, and the pollen grain that lands in a nose reacts just as if it had landed on a stigma—it promptly discharges the proteins from its outer coat, followed by a battery of other chemicals, including those enzymes whose rightful job is to penetrate the stigma.

This could be part of the reason that pollen provokes such a powerful reaction from some human noses—its behavior, as "interpreted" by the human body, is highly suspect. Hay fever is, in effect, an attack on pollen by the body's defensive system, or **immune system,** whose proper role is to protect the body from infection. To the immune system, a small particle that lands in the nose and immediately discharges proteins from its surface could very well be a living invader, such as a bacterium, intent on penetrating the body. The pollen's behavior is actually quite harmless, but it could seem suspiciously like that of a parasitic intruder, and so trigger a violent immune reaction.

Although many other substances cause an allergic reaction in some noses (substances as diverse as mold spores and dried-up cat saliva), none can match pollen in the sheer numbers of people affected. Pollen provokes more allergies than any other substance and this could well be due to the apparently aggressive behavior of the pollen grain on landing in the nose. However, as we shall see in chapter 4, pollen was disregarded by the immune system of most human beings before 1800, and hay fever has become common only during the 20th century. Somehow, the noses of our ancestors could distinguish pollen from parasites.

How did they do it and why have things changed? These are questions that chapter 4 will consider.

KNOW YOUR ENEMY—HOW THE IMMUNE SYSTEM DOES IT

The immune system will be explained in greater detail in chapter 3, but one crucial fact should be mentioned here. If the immune system is to fight off a parasite or any other disease-causing microbe, it must be able to recognize that microbe. More important, it must distinguish it from the body's own cells and from the many harmless substances it encounters. It generally does so by recognizing particular chemicals carried on the invader's surface.

These are chemicals with individual and highly recognizable features, the chemical equivalent of a distinctive aquiline nose, a mole on the chin, or unusually bushy eyebrows—features that make a particular face quite unmistakable. These distinctive recognition features are called **epitopes,** and the chemicals that carry them are known as **antigens.**

Hay fever is an **allergy,** a particularly violent type of immune reaction that is mistakenly directed against a harmless item such as pollen, dust, or food. (There will be more on allergies in chapter 3.) Allergic reactions affect only certain people, and they are different from other immune reactions in many ways, but in one respect they are the same—they depend on the body specifically recognizing particular antigens. In this case, however, the antigens are often referred to as **allergens,** to emphasize the fact that they help to cause allergies.

It takes a special sort of chemical to act as an allergen, and only a tiny minority of proteins fit the bill, which is some small comfort for those prone to allergy. Medical researchers believe that the shape and chemical details of the proteins play a part in determining which ones act as allergens, but they are still trying to discover exactly what it is that makes them special.

THE THREE FACTORS IN HAY FEVER

So far, we have identified three characteristics that can make pollen into a hay fever provoker: being spread by the wind, discharging its proteins rapidly in the nose, and having allergenic proteins.

UNDERSTANDING PROTEINS

The majority of antigens are made of **protein,** a word that is worth explaining because it is so widely misunderstood. Most people think of protein as something they must have in their diet. This is entirely correct, but there is much more to proteins than that. They are a wonderfully diverse group of chemicals that are the mainstay of all living bodies. They allow animals to move about (muscle proteins), they make up the skin, hair, and nails (keratin), carry oxygen in the blood (hemoglobin), and support and shape every organ of the body.

Most important, they get things done, chemically speaking. The proteins known as **enzymes** act as catalysts in the body, chemical entrepreneurs that turn one substance into another, build things up if they are needed, and break them down if they are not. Without enzymes, there would be no life, and plants use them just as much as animals do.

In the case of hay fever, proteins are of prime interest as **allergens,** the provokers of allergic reactions. Such reactions are the work of the **immune system,** which exists to defend the body against disease.

Because proteins are highly individual and distinctive chemicals, they are particularly useful to the body's immune system, acting as markers or "identity badges." For example, the proteins on the outer coat of a *Salmonella* bacterium are very different from those on the coat of a harmless bacterium living normally in the gut, and the immune system uses these proteins to tell the difference. A cell in the nose that is infected with influenza virus has typical influenza proteins on its surface that are not normally there, and the immune system responds to these by destroying the infected cell. In both these cases the proteins are acting as **antigens**—molecules that stimulate the immune system. An allergen is simply an antigen that provokes allergic reactions by the body, rather than any other type of immune reaction.

The last of these factors is undoubtedly the most crucial. Of the quarter of a million flowering plants, it is only a small minority—as few as 1 percent—that contain allergenic proteins. And within those offending pollen grains, there are often only two or three proteins that act as major allergens out of the 20 to 40 proteins that they release into the nose.

The first factor, being spread by the wind, is also important, as we have already seen. Pollen that is carried by insects rarely causes hay fever, except in situations where people are exposed to unusually large amounts every day. Even among wind-pollinated plants, however, there are some that fail to produce hay fever because their pollen does not travel far enough or remain airborne for long enough. Corn (or sweet corn) is a good example. Although it is wind-pollinated, and has allergenic proteins like most members of the grass family, corn is not often a cause of hay fever. This is probably because its pollen grains are relatively large and do not travel far in the air. The enormous stigmas of the corn flower—the silky "tassels" that extend from the top of the corncob—are probably so efficient in picking up pollen grains that dense clouds of pollen in the air are unnecessary.

The remaining factor of the three is the seemingly "aggressive" behavior of pollen grains in rapidly discharging proteins when they encounter a moist surface, such as the lining of the nose. It is likely that, combined with allergenic proteins, this characteristic makes pollen a powerful challenge to the immune system. Some pollen grains do not behave in this way, notably those of pines, which have a thick, waxy covering and a built-in delay that prevents them from starting to grow a pollen tube immediately. Their reticent attitude toward releasing proteins may help to make these pollen grains less allergenic, but other factors probably play a large part as well, particularly the nature of their proteins.

SNEEZE-FREE GRASSES

Since most plants are both male and female, they could, in theory, fertilize themselves. A few plants have in fact become self-pollinators, producing pollen but keeping it within the flower, where it pollinates the same flower's egg cells. Although some of this pollen does escape inadvertently, there is not a great deal of it floating about in the air, and it is therefore unlikely to produce hay fever.

Several cereal crops are among the self-pollinators, including wheat, barley, oats, and rice. Since these are grasses (like all cereal crops), those who are allergic to grass pollen might expect to react badly to fields of these crops. They can relax, however, in the knowledge that self-pollinators release very little pollen unless there is substantial disturbance to the plants, which can break open the flowers. Only the most sensitive individuals, or those who work closely with such plants, are likely to react.

Not all cereal crops are self-pollinating. Rye cross-pollinates, as does millet. Corn is cross-pollinating, but the pollen causes relatively few problems. Sorghum is largely self-pollinated, but can release great amounts of pollen. Sugarcane, another grass, is a cross-pollinator and allergenic, but in many areas where it is grown (e.g., the Caribbean islands) it is harvested before it flowers.

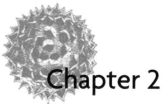

Chapter 2
THE SYMPTOMS OF HAY FEVER

One of the greatest honors of a successful medical career is to have a disease named after you. For many years the medical profession used the term "Bostock's catarrh" for hay fever, in memory of John Bostock, a London physician who, in 1819, reported the strange case of a patient with "a periodical affection of the eyes and chest." The patient was Bostock himself, and he attributed his symptoms (which were highly unusual in those days) to the heat and sunshine of summer.

His failure to identify the real cause lost Bostock his chance for medical immortality. By the 1820s, a fair number of the public were similarly afflicted, mainly those of the upper classes, and they became convinced that the new disease was "produced by the effluvium from new hay." To suffer from this novel disease was a sign of good breeding; it became something of a fad, and the public, or the newspapers perhaps, thought up the term "hay fever." Doctors of the day rejected the explanation, deplored the fashionable nature of the disease, and disliked the name. But it happened that the public was right about hay while Bostock and his colleagues were wrong, so the name "hay fever" stuck.

Although many doctors now use "pollinosis" for this disease (see the box "What Does Hay Fever Mean?" in chapter 1), the term "hay fever" is not entirely inappropriate because some patients actually do feel feverish and sweat easily during the pollen season. However, their temperature is usually normal and feverishness is not the most typical symptom of hay fever: the major reactions to pollen occur in the nose and eyes.

An attack of hay fever often begins with an unpleasant, itchy sensation in the mouth, nose, throat, and eyes. This is a sign that the allergic reaction to the pollen (described more fully in chapter 3) has begun. Shortly after this, symptoms begin in the nose, with volleys of sneezes, a runny nose, or a completely blocked nose.

Sneezing is a natural reflex that serves to remove bothersome particles from the nose by expelling them violently. The production of large amounts of mucus serves a similar end—it is intended to flush the unwanted items out of the nose. The fact that the symptoms persist suggests that neither response is of much use in expelling pollen, probably because each new breath brings in a fresh supply. Thus, the sneezing and the runny nose are part of a frustrated and futile effort to eject pollen from the nose.

A blocked nose occurs for different reasons. In this case, the degree of **inflammation** in the nose is so great that the delicate membranes swell up and block the air passages. "Inflammation" is a term used to describe the reaction that occurs whenever there is an intense immune response in a particular area of the body. This reaction is usually characterized by swelling and redness (hence "in flames"). Inflammation in the nose produces no obvious redness, but the swelling is very apparent to those who find that they can no longer breathe with their mouth closed!

A blocked nose can make it difficult to sleep, and constant breathing through the mouth may lead to dryness of the tongue and throat. For some hay fever sufferers, there is also a loss of the sense of smell. (This seemingly trivial symptom can prove fatal if there is something ablaze in the kitchen and you are watching television, oblivious to the smell. Fitting smoke detectors in the home is a good idea for anyone whose sense of smell is lost, either permanently or temporarily.)

SYMPTOMS IN THE EYE

Hay fever often involves the eyes just as much as the nose, and it is the eye symptoms that can help to distinguish it from the common cold, and to some extent from allergies to other airborne substances such as mold spores and house dust. Given the way air flows around the body, particles of different sizes and shapes move around us in different ways and settle out of the air at different points on the body's surface. The size of pollen grains makes them especially likely to flow close to the eye as we walk or run about, and to stick to its moist surface.

When the eyes react allergically to pollen, they first tend to water copiously. In the normal, healthy eye, tear fluid is secreted all the time and flows across the surface of the eye, then drains away down a tiny tube, called the tear duct, that leads from the inner corner of the eye to the nose. In doing so, it sweeps away dust and bacteria, keeping the eye clean and disease-free. The reaction to pollen during the hay fever season is simply an exaggerated version of this normal cleansing process.

One of the consequences of a blocked nose, or a nose that is producing a

HELPING CHILDREN WITH HAY FEVER

Philip developed hay fever very early in life, when he was only six years old. His parents were aware that he sneezed a lot in the summer and always had a runny nose, but they had no idea that there was anything wrong with his eyes as well.

When Philip was referred to a consultant allergist by his family doctor, the allergist noticed that Philip blinked a great deal. The family had always put this down to shyness. As well as a nose spray, the allergist prescribed eye drops for Philip, containing a drug that prevents the allergic reaction from occurring. After using the drops for a while, Philip reported that his eyes felt "not so itchy," although he had never mentioned that there

was anything wrong with them before. His blinking decreased noticeably.

Philip is not unusual in suffering symptoms in the eye. An allergic reaction to pollen often involves the eyes, although most people think of hay fever as mainly affecting the nose. Just occasionally, patients have symptoms in the eye alone.

As Philip showed, small children may not always think to tell an adult exactly what is wrong with them, or they may not know how to describe their symptoms clearly. Parents and doctors alike need to question children carefully and sometimes observe them closely (as this allergist did) in order to find out exactly what is wrong with them.

great deal of watery mucus, is that the tear duct runs into a dead end or an already flooded channel. Either way, the tear fluid cannot seep away, so an overflow occurs at the top of the tear duct. Since there may well be more tears from the eye anyway, the overflow can become a steady stream of tears down the face. The effect is similar to a heavy storm on a house whose drainpipes are already choked with leaves.

Watery eyes, however, are only a minor symptom. In some people there is also **conjunctivitis,** inflammation of the outer surface of the eyeball, the **conjunctiva.** The effect is to produce soreness, redness, and severe itching of the eyes. *Occasionally conjunctivitis is the only sign of hay fever, with no symptoms in the nose at all.*

Anyone who wears contact lenses and also suffers from hay fever is likely to find the lenses especially uncomfortable during the pollen season. Some people have to revert to glasses for a few weeks at the height of the season. However, certain types of lenses, or certain cleaning solutions, may be aggravating the sore eyes, and a change may make it possible to keep wearing lenses all year round. A good optician should be able to advise you on this point. Bear in mind that glasses can help to keep pollen out of the eyes (see "Protecting Your Eyes from Pollen" in chapter 8), so abandoning lenses for a while may have a double benefit.

Some people are unfortunate enough to suffer far more serious eye problems, ranging from swollen eyelids to very severe inflammation in the eye that can lead to blistering or ulceration. Needless to say, severe inflammation requires prompt medical treatment, as there is a risk of blindness.

NO NOSE IS AN ISLAND UNTO ITSELF

If your nose is inflamed and unhappy, the chances are that it will affect some other organ. The nose, after all, is connected to the mouth, the lungs, the ears, and the sinuses. Its malaise can spread to all these organs.

The Sinuses

The sinuses are air-filled cavities within the bones of the skull that serve no other purpose than to make it a lighter burden for the neck to bear. No cavity in the body can afford to be unprotected, so the sinuses are lined with delicate membranes that connect up with those lining the nose. The membranes are there to supply blood and immune cells to the sinus cavities.

Because these cavities are rather isolated, peaceful culs-de-sac that usually remain free of infection or inflammation, most people are unaware that they even exist. When they do become infected or inflamed, however, they can cause a gnawing pain in the face that makes the location of the sinuses all too apparent. And if the problem does not clear up of its own accord, but requires medical attention, their relative inaccessibility within the skull becomes something of a disadvantage because they are not open to direct treatment. An antibiotic taken by mouth, which is carried to the membranes of the sinus cavities in the blood, is the usual form of treatment.

Most cases of **sinusitis** stem from an infection that begins in the nose and spreads outward. However, allergic reactions in the nose can also spread to the sinuses, producing a headache over the eyes if the frontal sinuses are involved or an aching in the cheeks if the maxillary sinuses are affected.

There is one very simple treatment that is worth trying for sinusitis. First, take in a deep breath. Then hold your nose, shut your mouth, and blow hard. This creates high pressure in the nasal cavity, which may open up the blocked passages to the sinus cavities.

Children with allergies to pollen or dust mites (see chapter 12), or both, are sometimes afflicted with recurrent bouts of sinusitis. Often these children are treated with a course of antibiotics each time, and the antibiotics achieve some partial success, suggesting that an infection is playing its part in the symptoms. However, experience in allergy clinics shows that when these children's allergies are dealt with, their regular bouts of sinusitis often disappear. It cannot be

THE OVER-DOSED CHILD

Children with recurrent attacks of sinusitis have often been given repeated courses of antibiotics by their doctor. Tackling their allergy problems can relieve the sinusitis, but the children may still be generally unwell. Common symptoms are tiredness, colic, and a pale face with dark rings under the eyes. They may also have itchiness around the anus. These symptoms seem to be a result of the antibiotics, which have disturbed the **gut flora**, the beneficial bacteria that are normally found in a healthy person's intestine. It is probably an overgrowth of yeasts (one-celled fungi) in the gut that causes the problem—these yeasts are present in everyone, but their numbers are kept in check by the bacteria present. Children with these symptoms are often helped by a course of the antifungal drug nystatin. This is a very safe drug with virtually no side effects.

good to dose children with antibiotics regularly and unnecessarily, so if allergy treatment can remove the symptoms instead, this is surely preferable. For more information on effective treatment of chronic sinusitis, please see *Asthma* by Jonathan Brostoff, M.D., and Linda Gamlin (Healing Arts Press, 2000).

The Ear

Most people discover their **Eustachian tube** in an airplane. It is a small piece of plumbing that functions perfectly well until you ascend to or descend from high altitude.

The Eustachian tube runs from the middle ear (the chamber behind the eardrum) down to the nasal cavity. The function of this tube is to drain any fluid from the ear and to allow air to get from the nose into the middle ear. This ensures that the air pressure in the middle ear is equalized with that outside the eardrum. If the pressure is higher on one side than the other, the eardrum bulges away from the high pressure, causing intense pain. Normally this does not occur, because every time you swallow or yawn the Eustachian tube is opened wide and air can rush into the middle ear from the nose or out from the middle ear through the nose.

When you go up in an airplane, however, the pressure in the cabin falls slightly, and this affects the outer part of the ear immediately. The middle ear has to "catch up" by expelling air through the nose, thus lowering its pressure. As the plane descends, the reverse process is needed. Chewing gum or sucking on hard candy speeds up the process, as the repeated swallowing opens the Eustachian tube every few seconds. Falling asleep during ascent or descent can result in severe earache, as swallowing occurs much less frequently and the pressure gets little chance to equalize.

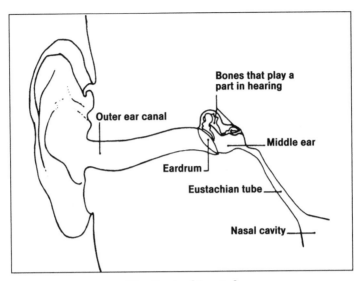

The Eustachian tube

So much for the Eustachian tube in flight; how does it react in hay fever? Problems arise when the buildup of mucus in the nose is so great that it works its way up into the Eustachian tube and blocks it off. Air can no longer get into the middle ear, so pressure cannot be equalized, which may cause "popping" or a "stuffy feeling" in the ears, or mild earache. A few people notice that their hearing is not quite as good as usual. For hay fever sufferers, the symptoms are unlikely to get any worse than this, but a few children with hay fever suffer from glue ear (see the box on page 175) as a secondary effect. Usually this occurs when they have other allergies as well, to substances such as house dust, that are present all year round.

Itching in the ears is another unpleasant symptom, and it is of little comfort to most sufferers to discover that it is probably illusory! There is no allergic reaction in the ears themselves to produce itching. It seems to arise because the nerves leading from the nose to the brain run alongside those leading from the ears. If the interconnections between these particular nerves are less than perfect, there could be a "crossed wire" on the way to the brain, with the result that an itchy sensation in the nose can be attributed, by the brain, to itchiness in the inner ear. (Occasionally, intense itchiness in the ears is the only symptom of rhinitis, apart from a slightly runny nose. Such patients usually turn out to be allergic to dust mites, but they may need a skin-prick test—see chapter 6—to be sure.)

The Lungs and Airways

One simple way in which the nose can affect the airways is through **postnasal drip.** The mucus in the nose builds up to such an extent that some trickles from the back of the nose down the throat and into the **trachea,** the tube that leads to the lungs. This mucus has to be coughed up later, which is why some hay fever sufferers find that they constantly need to clear their throats. The mucus does not generally cause any serious problems, but occasionally the sheer quantity of it being coughed up and then swallowed can upset the stomach. Other people find that they get a sore throat from postnasal drip unless they are taking antihistamines. As one hay fever sufferer observes: "The sore throat feels different from the kind of sore throat you get with an infection. It comes and goes, and it can be terrible in the morning but then be gone by supper. Mine always seems to be worse in the fall even though I have nasal allergies at other times of the year as well." How the mucus causes a sore throat is far from clear. Some doctors believe that the mucus simply irritates the throat.

Deeper down in the chest, the trachea branches into two tubes, the **bronchi,** which lead to the lungs. It is the bronchi that produce attacks of **asthma,** and asthma is sometimes a response to pollen, although there are many other potential causes.

In the walls of each bronchus there are layers of muscle that can contract suddenly, making the bronchus much narrower so that it lets through less air. When this happens, asthmatics find it difficult to exhale and their breath, whistling through the narrowed bronchi, produces a characteristic wheezing sound. Because they cannot exhale properly, they cannot inhale either, and they feel short of breath and uncomfortably tight in the chest. (During more severe attacks, asthmatics may feel as though they are suffocating, but such attacks are rare with pollen asthma.) In most cases, the asthma attack passes as the bronchi relax, but a severe asthma attack can be fatal and should always be taken seriously. Advice on dealing with asthma is given in chapter 5.

Pollen does not need to actually reach the bronchi in order to bring on pollen-induced asthma: this can simply be a **reflex reaction** to pollen in the nose. A reflex is an automatic reaction produced by the nerves linking two parts of the body. Presumably the reflex exists so that the nose can alert the bronchi to the arrival of unwanted substances in the air, which the bronchi can help to keep out of the lungs if they contract a little. In an asthmatic attack, however, the contraction of the bronchi has gone way beyond any useful function.

The automatic link between nose and bronchi reveals how important it can be to treat rhinitis. Doctors have found that by treating the symptoms in the nose (with a nasal spray, for example), they can make asthmatic attacks less severe or less frequent, or both. Given the serious nature of asthma, this is undoubtedly worthwhile.

Even those hay fever sufferers with no signs of asthma often show an interesting change in the bronchi during the pollen season. Their bronchi are

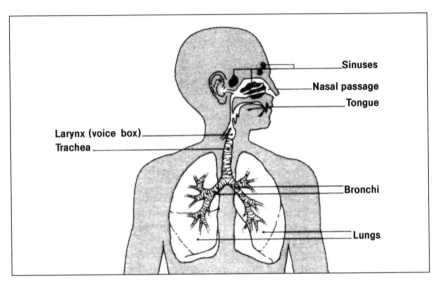

The airways

described as "hyperresponsive," which means that they will contract far more readily if submitted to a standard medical test with a substance known to cause bronchial contraction. Whether this hyperresponsive state can produce symptoms is unknown, but it might if the hay fever sufferer were exposed to an irritant such as sulfur dioxide, ozone, or cold air (see appendix 7).

Although a reflex reaction from the nose can produce asthma, for many pollen-sensitive asthmatics there is also a direct effect of pollen allergens on the bronchi. This raises an interesting question because most airborne pollen grains are too large for them to reach the bronchi, except in small numbers. Air has to travel through the nose or mouth and down the trachea before it reaches the bronchi, and most pollen grains never get that far. These relatively large particles are filtered out by the nose, and even if someone has a badly blocked nose and is breathing entirely through the mouth, most settle in the trachea.

So how can pollen allergens reach the bronchi? In 1972, researchers working on ragweed discovered that in releasing pollen, plants may also release much smaller particles that contain pollen allergens. The part of the flower that produces the pollen, known as the **anther,** may disintegrate as the pollen is shed. Since the anther contributed the proteins found in the pollen grain wall, it is not surprising to discover that it still contains some of those proteins. As it disintegrates, tiny particles containing these proteins—one of which is a powerful ragweed allergen—are scattered on the breeze. These particles are only a quarter the size of the ragweed pollen grain—five thousandths of a millimeter, compared to twenty thousandths of a millimeter. When inhaled, they reach the bronchi unhindered.

For a long time it was thought that these pollenlike fragments might be unique to ragweed, but researchers in Australia have now discovered equally allergenic particles coming from ryegrass plants. And in 1991 scientists found that Japanese red cedar also produces tiny fragments, far smaller than pollen itself, containing some of the pollen allergens. It now seems likely that many plants release allergenic pollen fragments as well as pollen itself.

Those who have both hay fever and pollen asthma find that the asthma attacks usually begin later in the pollen season than the hay fever symptoms, suggesting that repeated exposure is needed. However, the asthma may also continue long after the pollen season has ended because the sensitivity in the airways, once established, tends to perpetuate itself. Often, asthma that begins as a response to pollen continues throughout the year and eventually becomes a permanent part of life. An attack can then be brought on by all sorts of allergens and irritants, not just pollen. This tendency for asthma to self-perpetuate makes a powerful argument for using the available treatments during the pollen season, rather than letting hay fever and pollen asthma run their course.

Asthma is well known as a disorder that can be influenced by many different factors, some physical and some psychological. Often, the allergen alone merely makes an attack likely, while some other factor must come into play for the attack to start. In the case of pollen-induced asthma, for example, it sometimes takes a bout of vigorous exercise, as well as the presence of pollen in the air, to trigger an asthma attack. Psychological factors might also play a part (see page 72).

GENERAL SYMPTOMS

Some people feel feverish when they have hay fever, as already mentioned. In fact they usually do not have a fever—their temperature is normal. Other general symptoms during the hay fever season can include tiredness, irritability, and difficulty in concentrating.

RAY

Ray had suffered from hay fever since he was a boy and simply accepted the problem, rarely taking any medicines for it. In his mid-30's, he and his wife decided to move out of the city and bought a dilapidated cottage in the country. They moved in at the height of a beautiful summer and began clearing away the accumulated dirt of many years. Dust filled the air—and Ray's nose. He began to sneeze a little and within a few days he had a strange and unfamiliar feeling of tightness in his chest. During the following weeks, harvesting began in the surrounding fields, with several huge combine-harvesters working away all day and night. Ray noticed that, when outdoors, his eyes began to stream and the tightness in his chest became more noticeable. A few more days passed and Ray found it harder to breathe, so he reluctantly went to see the doctor. The diagnosis was asthma, and since that time, Ray has had to carry an inhaler containing a bronchodilator in his pocket wherever he goes.

Ray's case shows how someone who is already sensitized to pollen may be vulnerable to developing asthma. With Ray it was a massive dose of house dust, followed by the dust and mold spores generated during a cereal harvest. Since cereals are grasses, the dust that their dried leaves produce may well contain some of the same allergens as grass pollen—allergens to which Ray was already sensitive.

UNUSUAL REACTIONS TO POLLEN

There are some unusual reactions to pollen that do not involve the eyes, nose, or airways. Some are quite serious, but fortunately these are very rare.

Reactions in the digestive system include an upset stomach and, in a few instances, **colitis,** an inflammation of the large bowel. These conditions could be produced by pollen that settles on food and is eaten or by pollen that is inhaled and caught in the saliva, then swallowed.

Reactions in the skin include the allergic form of **eczema** and another allergic reaction known as **urticaria,** or hives, because it produces large, itchy bumps on the skin. In these reactions, bare areas of skin could be acquiring a dusting of pollen and reacting directly to this. Alternatively, pollen antigens that have entered the bloodstream (through tiny blood vessels in the nose) could reach the skin by this indirect route.

When urticaria occurs on the ankles after walking through grass, it is clear that direct contact is triggering the allergic response. While the pollen in the grass may be the prime culprit, its effects may be worsened by the juice that oozes from crushed grass leaves, because the leaves and stems of a plant often share allergens with its pollen. This is why some people with grass-pollen hay fever are so badly affected by mowing a lawn, even though the grass is not in flower. The action of the mower blades turns the grass juice into an **aerosol** of tiny airborne droplets that are inhaled by anyone near the mower. A few people experience allergic reactions when cutting privet hedges, and again the reaction may be to the juice of the crushed leaves, as well as to the pollen.

Among the very rare reactions to pollen are kidney disorders. As already mentioned, allergens from inhaled pollen pass into the bloodstream from the nose. The blood then carries them to all parts of the body, including the kidneys. Here the blood is purified in a process that involves it passing through very fine tubes. A strong immune reaction to pollen in the blood can affect the tiny blood vessels **(capillaries)** that lie around those tubes and stop the filtering process from functioning fully. The symptoms include puffiness, especially around the face and hands, and cloudy urine, which is also unusually plentiful.

Very occasionally, hay fever sufferers also report joint pains **(arthralgia)** during the pollen season. In these cases, the underlying mechanism is probably the same as that in kidney disease: the immune reaction to pollen in the blood produces an inflammatory reaction in the blood capillaries of the joints, which results in joint pain.

Migraine is another symptom that sometimes accompanies hay fever, but this too is rare. Usually people find that their migraines occur throughout the year but are more frequent in the pollen season. Some effect on the blood vessels, due to the immune response to pollen, is probably responsible for this reaction. A few women with hay fever experience irritation of the vagina during the pollen season.

ELIZABETH

Elizabeth had suffered hay fever in the spring since she was 9 years old, and hay fever in the late summer since she was 15. When she was 21, she developed an unpleasant itchy rash on her hands during August. This died down of its own accord at the end of September, and only a trace of the rash remained during the winter and spring. The following August it flared up again, and this was repeated in the third year. The doctor tried skin-prick tests (see chapter 6), but these gave many positive results; Elizabeth reacted to house dust, mold spores, feathers, wool, skin particles from cats and dogs, various foods, and many different pollens. It was impossible to tell which of these allergens might be causing the problem, and the doctor remained puzzled.

By chance, Elizabeth discovered the cause herself. The following summer she happened to take a holiday in late August in a mountainous area far from her home town. Here her rash cleared up at the same time as her hay fever vanished. The vegetation in the mountains was quite different from that at home, and one of the weeds whose pollen had produced a major reaction on skin-prick testing did not grow there. Clearly, this weed pollen was producing both hay fever and the rash on her hands.

RELATED CONDITIONS

Hay fever is just one form of **rhinitis,** the technical term for inflammation *(-itis)* in the nose *(rhin-)*. The more precise term **allergic rhinitis** is usually employed, to make it clear that this reaction is due to an allergy rather than to a cold or any other cause. Various forms of **nonallergic rhinitis** are also known, and some of these are discussed in chapter 13.

Not all allergic rhinitis is due to pollen. Several other airborne allergens can produce these irritating reactions in the nose, the most common ones being house dust (or, rather, the allergens it contains, mainly those produced by mites) and particles from cats or other pets. In all these cases the symptoms are generally less violent than in hay fever, but this is small compensation for the fact that they may well last all year long.

A few allergens other than pollen can produce seasonal symptoms, notably molds and outdoor insects (see pages 218–219) .

Chapter 12 looks in more detail at the various allergens, other than pollen, that can cause allergic rhinitis.

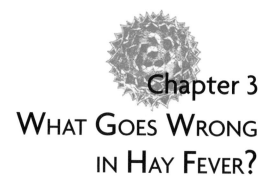

Chapter 3
WHAT GOES WRONG
IN HAY FEVER?

In the early 1980s, a boy in Houston, Texas, suddenly became famous throughout the world. He was photographed by newspapers and magazines and filmed by television crews as he played, ate, and slept inside a large plastic "bubble." The boy had spent his entire life, since early infancy, inside the bubble, sealed off from normal human contact. He could not even breathe the air that most people breathe because he had been born without a fully functioning **immune system** (the system that defends our bodies from disease). The air going into the bubble was treated to remove bacteria and viruses. Food was sterilized before being passed in through a special protected entry-port. The boy in the bubble was healthy, but only because his world had been made unnaturally safe.

When the boy was 12, surgeons attempted to transplant bone marrow from a relative. Bone marrow is the major source of immune cells in the body and such transplants can sometimes re-create a functional immune system. Unfortunately, the operation failed and the boy died.

The case of this little boy, and other children like him, suddenly makes us uncomfortably aware of how dangerous the natural world really is. The fact that we are normally oblivious to these dangers is a testament to the efficiency of our immune systems in dealing with the constant threats from disease-causing microbes.

The immune system comes into play even before we are born, although it is aided, at that stage, by immunity provided by the mother. At birth, a baby still carries some of this **passive immunity** acquired from its mother, and continues to be protected for many months. During this time, the baby's own immune system is maturing and taking stock of the world around it. An important part of that process is learning which items entering the body need to be attacked, because they cause disease, and which do not. Among those that do not need to be attacked are **pollen grains** (see chapter 1). There are also many other harmless items that the immune system must learn to ignore, including food molecules (the chemical constituents of food), dust particles, fragments of mites and insects, and other items in the air.

If the immune system *does* attack these harmless items, and if it does so vigorously enough to produce unpleasant symptoms in the person concerned, the reaction is known as an **allergy.** (The word simply means "altered reactivity.") The classical allergies include hay fever, asthma, and food allergy, and two skin disorders, eczema and urticaria (although these are not always allergic in origin). Allergy to pollen can play a part in *all* these reactions, although it is mainly associated with hay fever.

To understand allergy, it helps to know a little about how the immune system normally works. But first a word of warning: If the immune system were a movie, it would have a cast of thousands and a very, *very* complicated plot. Most filmgoers would leave before the end. What follows is a simplified account, with many of the key players omitted and the rest of the immune system explained as clearly as possible. Even so, it is not an easy read, and if you wish to pass on quickly to the next chapter, feel free to do so—the rest of the book can still be readily understood. We believe that it is worth trying to explain immunity and allergy because such knowledge can help people in understanding their illness and in making more informed decisions about their treatment. We hope, therefore, that you will read this chapter and find it interesting, but it is not essential.

THE FIGHT AGAINST DISEASE

The immune system consists of millions of free-ranging cells that permeate the whole body—guerrilla fighters in the war against disease. The bloodstream provides an important transport route for these **immune cells,** but once they reach the parts of the body where they are needed, they must leave the bloodstream by squeezing through gaps in the blood vessel walls. The immune cells pass through the tissues of the body and may become involved in any skirmishes with invaders that are going on there.

The fluid that bathes these tissues is constantly draining into special channels called **lymphatic vessels,** and as it does so it takes the immune cells, living or dead, along with it.

Lymphatic vessels permeate the body and are connected into larger lymph vessels—a collection and transport network known as the **lymphatic system,** which most people are quite unaware they possess. The colorless fluid that flows through it, with its precious load of immune cells, is called **lymph.**

Having been collected from the most distant parts of the body, the lymph is eventually channeled into a single large lymph vessel, called the **thoracic duct,** which pours lymph back into the bloodstream at a point near the heart. En route to this point, the immune cells pass through **lymph nodes.** These are

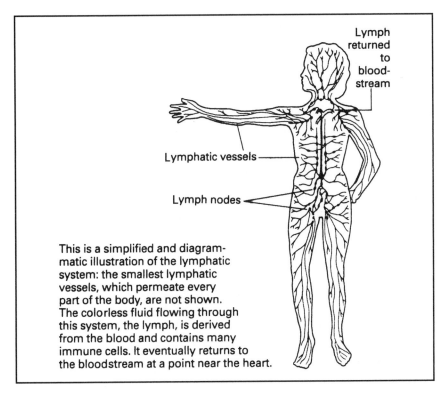

Lymph returned to blood-stream

Lymphatic vessels

Lymph nodes

This is a simplified and diagrammatic illustration of the lymphatic system: the smallest lymphatic vessels, which permeate every part of the body, are not shown. The colorless fluid flowing through this system, the lymph, is derived from the blood and contains many immune cells. It eventually returns to the bloodstream at a point near the heart.

The lymphatic system

concentrations of specialized immune cells that assess the guerrilla fighters to see what invaders they have encountered (they are carrying identifiable fragments of those invaders) and then react accordingly.

It is in the lymph nodes that many **antibodies** are produced, although they can be generated in other parts of the body as well. Of the many useful weapons deployed by the immune system, antibodies are probably the best known to people outside the medical profession. They are special molecules that bind to other molecules in a discriminating and highly selective way, rather like search dogs—one dog goes for the scent of cannabis, another for the scent of explosives, another for the scent of a particular criminal. In the same way, each antibody has a particular chemical target, called its **antigen.** These targets are used to pinpoint bacteria, viruses, or other microbes that can cause disease.

An antibody is like one of those toy arrows with a rubber sucker at their tip—all it can do is stick to its target, not penetrate or kill it. Nevertheless, antibodies can stop infections in a variety of ways. With viruses, which are very small and need to invade the body's cells before they can proliferate, antibodies may be able to stop them in their tracks just by sticking to them. With bacteria, however, antibodies alone would be largely ineffective because the bacteria are so much larger than the antibodies (see the illustration on pages 34–35).

Help is needed to defeat the bacteria, and the antibodies summon this help from other cells and molecules in the immune system, ones that have the power to kill. Frequently, hundreds of antibodies stick to the outer surface of a bacterial cell and this stimulates action by the immune system's assassination teams.

Antibodies would not work unless they were highly specific for their targets, the antigens. An antigen is an individual chemical, usually a protein (see the box "Understanding Proteins" in chapter 1), on the outer surface of the invading microbe. However, molecules on the outside of other items, including pollen grains, can also act as antigens. If they did not, hay fever and other allergies would simply not occur. (When an antigen provokes an allergic reaction it is known as an **allergen.**)

As noted in chapter 1, an antigen must have something distinctive and unusual about it—an unmistakable chemical feature known as an **epitope**— by which it can easily be recognized. By homing in on this epitope, an antibody should bind to one type of antigen only, and therefore to one type of microbe only. (In practice, things are not always quite that simple, and cross-reactions can occur. This is something we will come back to later, as it is an important factor in allergy.)

To combat all the many infectious microbes in the world, the body produces a vast range of different antibodies—millions of them. These antibodies are not "tailor-made" for the antigen as you might expect but are "off the rack." Very early in life, the millions of different types of antibody are generated randomly on a needed basis. (In this sense, they are quite unlike the tracker dogs mentioned earlier, which are *trained* to go for particular targets. The antibody comes into the world with the chemical nature of its target already fixed.) Most of the antibodies we generate are useless because they never meet an antigen that they can bind to. Others do encounter such an antigen, and if this turns out to be an antigen that requires an immune response, the body begins producing that antibody in large quantities. (During this production process, the antibody may change a little so that it becomes an even better match for the allergen. It is rather like buying an off-the-rack suit, but having the sleeves shortened and the waist taken in a bit to give a perfect fit.)

This system may seem rather wasteful and badly organized, with so many antibodies being generated and then not used. But it has the merit of being able to respond instantly to any new threat that comes along. Among the millions of different antibodies waiting around for something to happen, there is bound to be at least one that binds to antigens on the new invader.

THE TWO ENDS OF THE ANTIBODY MOLECULE

An antibody molecule is shaped like a slingshot. At the tips of the two arms (where the elastic should be tied on) are the sites that bind to antigen—two binding sites per antibody molecule, specific for the same sort of epitope. The other end of the molecule—the handle of the slingshot—interacts with various immune cells and molecules.

Not all antibodies are the same in the "handle" region. There are about eight different forms that the antibody handle can take, giving eight different **isotypes.** The characteristics of the handle region are of crucial importance because they determine which immune cells or molecules the antibody reacts with. This, in turn, determines what effect the antibody has on the rest of the immune system.

When the antibody has bound its antigen at one end, that fact is communicated to whatever is bound at the other end, which may be a potent killing cell, or a molecule with the power to cause inflammation, or some less violent immune agent that deals with things far more quietly. As a result of the differences in the handle region, some antibody isotypes raise hell when they encounter their antigen, while others contain the problem with a minimum of fuss.

The isotype that causes allergy is, unfortunately, one of the hell-raisers. It is known as immunoglobulin E, or **IgE** for short, and its handle end can bind to many different immune cells. However, it has a special affinity for some of the most disruptive and damaging cells in the body, the **mast cells** and **basophils.**

THE MIGHTY MAST CELL

Mast cells and basophils are basically very similar, but they patrol different territories in the body: basophils circulate in the blood, while mast cells are found fixed to the tissues of the body, including the membranes inside the nose and airways. Since mast cells play the major role in hay fever, we will deal only with them from this point onward, but basophils react in much the same way.

A single mast cell can carry as many as 100,000 IgE molecules on its surface. To trigger a reaction by the mast cell, several IgE molecules on its surface have to bind to the same antigen—they must be cross-linked by that antigen molecule. Although IgE molecules are the major trigger for mast cells, they are not the only ones. Different triggers probably produce different levels of reaction in the mast cell.

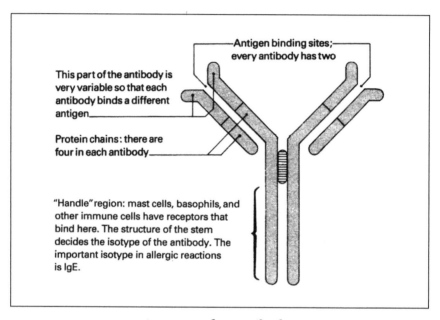

Anatomy of an antibody

Mast cells are packed full of large, round granules. Each granule contains a cocktail of powerful chemicals that can produce dramatic effects on the body when released. Among these chemicals are **histamine** and **leukotrienes.** The first of these will already be familiar to many hay fever sufferers because drugs that block the effects of histamine, called **antihistamines,** are widely used for hay fever. (Histamine is also found in the sting of a nettle plant, which injects it under the skin by means of sharp, hollow hairs. The hot, itchy bump that a nettle sting produces is an indication of what histamine can do to the tissues of the body.)

In the past few years, antileukotrienes have joined antihistamines in the fight against allergy as researchers have devised drugs that prevent leukotrienes from being produced or block their action in the body.

Histamine, leukotrienes, and other chemicals in the mast cells are collectively known as **mediators** because they mediate changes in the body. The main change they produce is an increase in the size of the tiniest blood vessels, the capillaries. The capillaries also become more leaky so that immune cells can pass in and out of them more easily. This produces **inflammation** in the area where the mast cells have discharged their contents—it may look red and swollen if it is in a visible part of the body.

The mast-cell mediators also act as distress signals, summoning more immune cells to the scene. Finally, they make surrounding membranes produce more mucus, hence the runny nose of hay fever (although this can be partially due to other causes as well; see the box "Nerves in the Nose" in chapter 13).

If there are enough of these mast-cell mediators on the loose, they will make certain types of muscle contract, including the muscles that surround the **bronchi,** the tubes leading to the lungs. Contraction of these muscles narrows the bronchi, and the hollow core can be made narrower still by a swelling of the membranes that line them. This swelling is due to inflammation. Extra mucus may also be produced inside the bronchi, making matters worse. These three reactions can all contribute to an asthma attack, when the bronchi become so narrow that breathing is difficult (see "The Lungs and Airways" in chapter 2).

A mast cell has dozens of granules stored inside it, and it can let off these chemical bombs gradually, a few at a time, or all at once in a massive "explosion." In general, far more is known about the spectacular explosions (which involve IgE as the trigger) than about the gradual piecemeal reactions (which probably involve other triggering mechanisms). Exactly what role these different reactions have is not yet known, especially in the case of the milder reactions, but we can make educated guesses.

Given the evidence now available, it seems likely that the two types of reaction are directed at different groups of invaders. The massive explosions seem to play a major part in combating large parasites such as tapeworms, roundworms, and liver flukes. Unlike bacteria, which are small enough to be engulfed by a suitable immune cell, these worms and flukes are veritable giants being attacked by an army of Lilliputian immune cells (see the illustration on page 34). Because of their great size, they need some special and rather drastic immune reactions to combat them. If mast cells lining the intestine release all their histamine and other chemicals simultaneously, the violent muscular spasms that follow, along with the inflammation and prolific mucus secretion, may be enough to dislodge many of the parasitic worms that have made their home there.

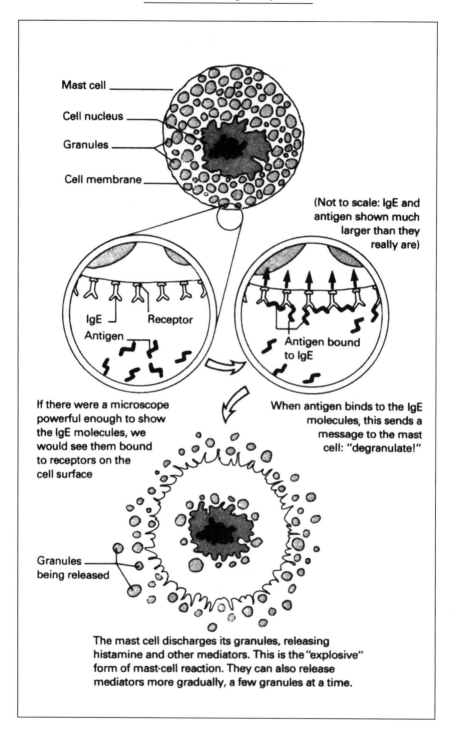

Mast cell

Cell nucleus

Granules

Cell membrane

(Not to scale: IgE and antigen shown much larger than they really are)

IgE — Receptor

Antigen

Antigen bound to IgE

If there were a microscope powerful enough to show the IgE molecules, we would see them bound to receptors on the cell surface

When antigen binds to the IgE molecules, this sends a message to the mast cell: "degranulate!"

Granules being released

The mast cell discharges its granules, releasing histamine and other mediators. This is the "explosive" form of mast-cell reaction. They can also release mediators more gradually, a few granules at a time.

How a mast cell is triggered into action

The gentler bit-by-bit release of granules probably plays a part in entirely different immune reactions, perhaps in those directed against bacteria or in the specialized defensive actions launched against viruses. A steady trickle of the mast cell's chemical contents may serve to summon other immune cells to the vicinity and keep them active there. This is largely speculative at present, but it seems plausible. For one thing, it would explain why there are so many mast cells in the eyes, nose, and airways. Their presence is definitely a puzzle if mast cells are involved only in combating worms and other large parasites. None of these parasites enters the body through the eyes or nose—most come in with food, or burrow through the skin, or are transmitted by biting insects. Mast cells in the eyes, nose, and airways must be there to combat some other type of invader, probably bacteria.

What seems to happen in hay fever is that the mast cells produce the violent, explosive reaction in the wrong place (the nose rather than the gut) and in reaction to the wrong item (pollen rather than parasites). This presumably happens because the normal control mechanisms, the restraints that keep the mast cells in check, have somehow broken down. To understand these control systems, we must first return to IgE, the antibody involved in allergy.

CHECKS AND BALANCES

All immune reactions have to be controlled, and while researchers have discovered a great deal about how this is done, many details remain unclear. This, then, is the story so far—an incomplete picture that we hope will be filled in by more medical research.

Antibodies are manufactured by special cells called **B cells.** Each B cell produces just one type of antibody, which, as already noted, may or may not turn out to be useful. B cells spend most of their lives waiting for their moment of glory to arrive, and if it does arrive—their particular brand of antibody is suddenly needed—they divide rapidly and produce hundreds of young B cells, all capable of mass-producing antibodies.

Each B cell, and all its offspring, produces antibodies that bind to a particular antigen because they all have the same sort of antigen-binding site. In general, they bind that antigen and that antigen only. (There are exceptions to this, where another antigen is similar and a **cross-reaction** occurs—see "Cross-Reactions" later in this chapter.) By controlling the activities of particular B cells, therefore, the production of particular antibodies can be regulated.

If an item (such as a pollen grain) has been classified as "safe" by the immune system, then various sorts of control are possible. One is to block the production of *any* antibodies to the antigens on that item. Another is to only

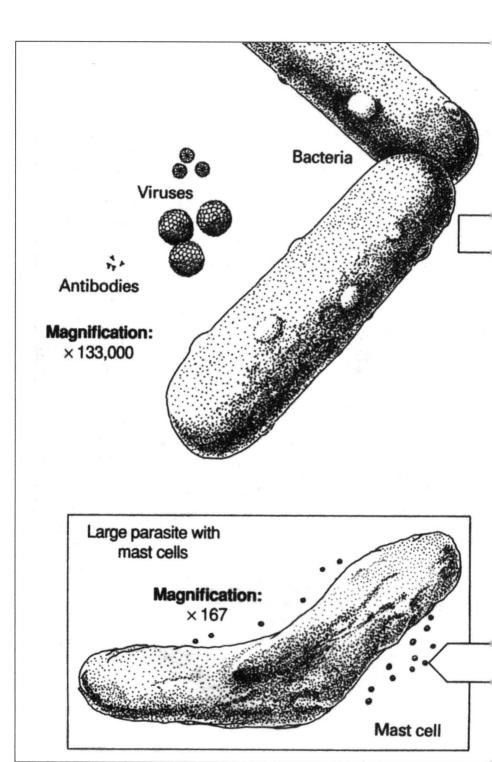

Pollen, microbes, and immune cells

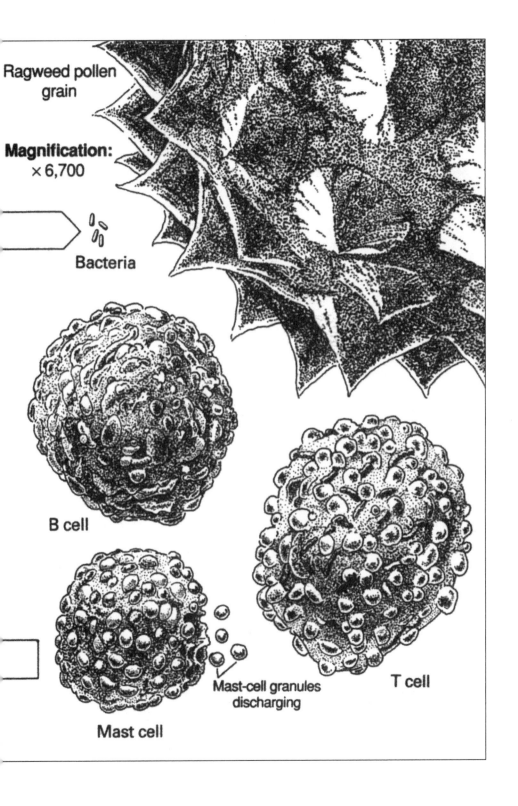

Ragweed pollen grain

Magnification: ×6,700

Bacteria

B cell

Mast cell

Mast-cell granules discharging

T cell

produce antibodies of particular isotypes. By opting for the "minimum fuss" isotypes, the immune system can clear the item out of the body (which may be necessary if it is plentiful) without instigating any violent, damaging reactions to it.

Both these forms of control work at the level of the B cell. The main way in which B cells are controlled is through another set of cells called **T cells.** To interact with a B cell, the T cell must be specific for the same antigen—it has receptors on its surface that are just as specific as antibodies. In effect, the T cell binds to the same antigen as the B cell (although it often goes for different epitopes on the antigen) and then issues chemical commands that tell the B cell whether or not to start up antibody production.

One set of T cells, called **T helper cells,** issues the "go" commands. Another set of T cells, called **T suppressor cells,** issues "stop" commands. The B cell can be frozen into inaction in two ways, by the lack of a "go" signal or the presence of a "stop" signal, so there are two separate possibilities for control here.

T helper cells and T suppressor cells can also control the isotype (the "handle" end) of the antibodies produced. This is possible because a B cell can change the type of handle it puts on to the antibodies (change the isotype) while keeping the antigen-binding sites exactly the same. Thus, it can produce hell-raising antibodies or minimum-fuss antibodies for its antigen, and does so under the direction of the T helper cells or T suppressor cells.

In the past few years, immunologists have discovered that there are two sets of T helper cells with different "policies" on antibody production, rather like opposing political parties. One set of T helpers, the **Th2** set, favors IgE, while the other set, called the **Th1** set, favors less violent antibodies. The two opposing sets of helper cells issue their messages in the form of chemicals. The main chemical issued by the Th2 set is called **interleukin 4,** while the main chemical message from the Th1 set is **interferon gamma.** If Th2 cells, rather than Th1 cells, are involved in an immune reaction, then IgE will be produced instead of a less damaging antibody.

But who or what decides to involve Th2 cells rather than Th1 cells? The answer requires us to introduce yet another set of cells, called **antigen-presenting cells,** or **APCs.** One of the appealing things about APCs is that their name tells you exactly what they do: chew up the antigen into fragments and present it to other immune cells in such a way that they can recognize it. APCs are plentiful in the nose, airways, skin and any other site where invaders are likely to arrive. They are the front line of the immune system, and they have the power to favor either Th1 or Th2 cells. The nature of the antigen they have picked up somehow influences which set they favor.

CONTROLLING IgE

Suppose these control mechanisms are not entirely successful, and some IgE is produced anyway—how does the body cope? Fortunately, there are fail-safe mechanisms that can neutralize the IgE. One is the production of a free-ranging chemical called **S-Fc epsilon RII,** which can bind to the "handle" end of IgE and so prevent it from binding to mast cells. Recent studies in Japan have shown that those prone to allergy have lower levels of S-Fc epsilon RII in their blood.

Another form of control is the production of **anti-idiotypic antibodies.** These are the immunological equivalent of highly specific antimissile missiles. They spike the guns of an antibody by binding to its antigen-binding sites. In other words, if an IgE antibody is being made that is specific for a pollen antigen, the immune system can form *another* antibody that takes the place of the pollen at its binding sites. This prevents the pollen itself from binding.

Some patients with ragweed allergy undergoing allergy shots begin producing anti-idiotypic antibodies to their ragweed IgE. This could be a factor in reducing their symptoms, although it is certainly not the only one (see below).

Whether this form of control operates normally in people who do not suffer from allergies, or in those who lose their hay fever symptoms as they get older, remains to be seen. Certainly, those who spontaneously recover from hay fever in later life may still have high levels of IgE to pollen antigens, so something is acting to prevent that IgE from causing trouble. Similarly, if you take 100 people off the street and test them for high levels of IgE in their blood (or IgE to specific allergens, such as pollen and house dust), you usually find that over 30 of them have enough IgE to produce allergic symptoms. They are said to be **atopic.** Yet fewer than half of those 30 atopic people would actually suffer from allergies. Something is preventing the potentially damaging IgE molecules from doing any harm. If researchers could find out exactly what, they might be closer to preventing allergic reactions.

There are many other mechanisms involved in the allergic response and the control of allergy: we have mentioned only the major ones here. One thing that is clear from modern research is that the question "What goes wrong in allergy?" is a pretty stupid one, because every patient is different. It is rather like asking, "What makes a person turn to crime?"—you may be able to identify certain factors that are likely to produce criminal behavior, but there is no single explanation that applies to everyone.

One person may get an allergy because a certain control mechanism has broken down and a backup mechanism isn't working all that well either. In a

ATOPY AND ALLERGY

People who are **atopic** are producing enough IgE to develop allergies. The majority get through their lives without any sign of allergy, but about a third develop an allergy, usually as children or teenagers.

The curious thing about these people is that they may develop one allergy as babies (atopic eczema, for example, or an allergy to cow's milk), lose it as they grow older, then develop a new allergy later (asthma or hay fever, per-haps). The allergic tendency is there, but the allergy itself "wanders about" from one site in the body to another. The offending aller-gen may change or may stay the same.

In the same way, allergies run in families, but while a mother might have asthma, her son has eczema and food allergy, while his son later gets hay fever. It is the allergic pre-disposition—atopy—that is inherited, not a particular form of allergy.

second allergic patient, both these mechanisms may be fine but something else is at fault, something so fundamental that other control mechanisms cannot cancel it out. These differences explain why some people do well on one treatment but not so well on another.

Allergy shots throw an interesting light on these control systems. Researchers have looked at the people who respond well in the hope of finding out how the treatment works. (This may or may not show how allergies are prevented naturally in healthy people.) To their surprise and consternation, they have found that all these "cured" hay fever sufferers are actually reacting in different ways under the surface. Some show a fall in IgE levels; others do not. Most show an increase in pollen-specific antibodies of the "minimum fuss" isotypes, but not all do. A proportion show anti-idiotypic antibodies to their pollen-specific IgE. Some have more pollen-specific T suppressor cells. Others have mast cells that are less hasty in releasing mediators after their treatment. A patient may show any mixture of these reactions.

Most intriguing of all are the patients who respond well to allergy shots but have *no changes in their immune system as far as researchers can tell*. Nothing that doctors can currently measure has changed in these patients. This is a clear sign of just how ignorant we still are about allergic responses. Something must have changed to make these patients better, but whatever it is remains a mystery. Much is now known, but much remains to be discovered.

PRIMING

One of the unfortunate things that happens in hay fever is the reaction known as **priming.** When an allergic reaction starts up in the nose, all sorts of chemicals are released, as already discussed. Many of those chemicals act as messengers to other cells, bringing them to the scene of the action. Among the cells that make for the nose are young cells that can develop into mast cells, and this increases the mast-cell numbers. Basophils (the cells that circulate in the blood and are very similar to mast cells) also flood in. They too can produce histamine and other mediators when they encounter the pollen allergens. The result is that there are even more highly damaging immune cells available to react to the next day's intake of pollen, so symptoms generally get worse as the pollen season progresses. Priming seems to occur in about 50 percent of hay fever patients.

Cells known as **eosinophils** also move into the nose, particularly during the late-phase reaction (see below). They too can contribute to keeping hay fever going, even when the pollen count is falling, and can help to make the symptoms more severe.

As well as having more histamine-producing cells (mast cells and basophils), the hay feverish nose also becomes more sensitive to histamine and reacts more strongly to it. This is probably just part of its generally increased sensitivity, since it will also take far more objection to cigarette smoke and other pollutants than it usually does (see "Vasomotor Rhinitis" in chapter 13). This increased sensitivity adds to the priming effect.

THE LATE-PHASE REACTION

Patients with hay fever make very good guinea pigs for immunologists because they are not exposed to their allergen all year round. If a researcher can find a set of willing hay fever patients and arrange to test them with their pollen in midwinter, he or she can see exactly what happens when they are given just one brief exposure to their allergen.

If the original diagnosis was correct, within minutes of inhaling a dose of pollen they will all be sneezing, blowing their noses, and wiping their eyes. The measurements are taken, a box of tissues provided, and in a while the symptoms pass . . . But something odd happens a few hours later: some of these people find themselves blowing their noses again, with an uncomfortable blocked-up feeling. This can begin 2 hours later or as much as 12 hours later, and it affects up to half the people tested. What these patients have experienced is a **late-phase reaction.** Like the initial reaction, it passes in time. Normally, during the pollen season, hay fever sufferers are unaware of the late-phase reaction because it simply merges with the initial reaction to a new dose of pollen being inhaled.

During the late-phase reaction, many immune cells are attracted to the nose, especially two groups known as **eosinophils** and **neutrophils.** The eosinophils, in particular, are thought to cause inflammation in the nose during the late-phase reaction.

A late-phase reaction also occurs in asthmatic patients, and it has been much more fully studied in asthma. The bronchi are generally slower to react to pollen than the nose, because fewer pollen antigens reach them (see "The Lungs and Airways" in chapter 2). But once asthmatic attacks have begun, the late-phase reaction that follows each attack helps to make the bronchi inflamed, sensitive, and overreactive, so that the smallest dose of allergen or irritant will set off a new attack. The late-phase reactions of the separate attacks eventually run together in an unbroken pattern of oversensitivity. For this reason, asthmatic symptoms often continue long after the pollen season has ended.

Occasionally, pollen-induced asthma turns into year-round asthma as a result of these self-perpetuating reactions. Treating the asthma at an early stage, before the pattern of repeated attacks and repeated late-phase reactions is established, has obvious benefits. It can prevent the bronchi from becoming habitually inflamed and oversensitive.

GENES AND AGE

An allergic response to a harmless substance such as pollen depends, first and foremost, on making IgE to that substance. As we have already seen, not everyone who is atopic (who makes enough IgE to suffer from allergy) actually develops allergies. Other control systems must also have failed for this to happen. In most studies, about a third of atopics are found to show allergic symptoms, but the number can be higher than this in certain circumstances.

It has been known for many years that allergies run in families. Modern research has been able to show that where some members of a family have allergies, several others are atopic but symptom-free. Clearly, the underlying tendency to allergy is inherited.

Not all members of a family will have high IgE levels, however. There are usually some "anti-allergy genes" in the family mix as well as the "pro-allergy genes" that produce high IgE, and some children are lucky enough to get only the good ones.

If *both* parents suffer from allergies, the outlook for their children is less promising. They are both putting in some pro-allergy genes, so there are more in the mix, and the chance of their children acquiring them is therefore quite high. But even people with allergies are probably carrying good versions of the relevant genes as well as the pro-allergy ones—the pro-allergy version may be masking the effects of the good one. With luck, one or more of their children will get the good versions only.

Given two children who are both atopic, why does one go on to develop allergies when the other does not? (This can happen even with identical twins who have exactly the same genes and are brought up in the same household.) The last chapter of this book looks at this question more fully and considers how vulnerable children can be protected from developing hay fever and asthma. Briefly, some aspects of the environment do seem to make a difference, especially in the first year of life.

Although the crucial environmental influences may operate in the first year of life, it is very unusual for hay fever actually to appear then. Usually it begins many years later. Why this should be is not fully understood, but it seems clear that, in immunological terms, the scene is set for hay fever in infancy, or early childhood, whereas the actual appearance of hay fever depends on certain changes in other departments of the immune system—changes that only come on several years later. The immune system certainly changes as we mature, and these changes affect the appearance (and disappearance) of hay fever. The positive aspect to this is that most people also grow out of hay fever as they get older.

As a broad generalization, most people with hay fever begin having symptoms in their teenage years or early 20s, but some start earlier, during childhood. Very few people first develop hay fever in their 30s or 40s, although this is not unknown. For those who develop hay fever as children or teenagers, there is a good chance that they will grow out of it in their twenties, or later. As already noted, they do not necessarily lose their high IgE levels, so clearly some other form of control is coming into play.

Exactly what this control might be is still unknown, but an interesting observation on AIDS patients may shed some light on this. Several cases are now known of patients who had suffered from hay fever or other allergies in childhood, but had then grown out of them many years before contracting the AIDS virus. Within a few months of the onset of AIDS symptoms, their allergies returned, although it was not always the same type of allergy that they had experienced in childhood. One man of 36, who had suffered asthma in his teens, developed eczema and hay fever as AIDS began. Others who have suffered hay fever as teenagers develop asthma or food allergy as they succumb to AIDS. This sort of pattern fits in well with the "wandering" nature of atopy (discussed earlier in this chapter).

The virus that causes AIDS is known to disable the T helper cells. We have already seen how the T helper subsets, Th1 and Th2, differ in their "policies" on IgE production. In the case of AIDS patients, it seems to be the lack of Th1 cells that is causing the allergy problem. Th1 cells, you will recall, influence B cells by producing interferon gamma, a chemical messenger that discourages the production of IgE. By treating AIDS patients with interferon gamma, which is available as a drug, their allergic problems can be brought under control. (Interferon gamma is of no use to most people with allergies, however.)

Perhaps hay fever sufferers who find themselves spontaneously cured as they grow older are experiencing a natural shift in their helper cells. If a shift occurred, away from Th2 cells and toward Th1 cells, this would reduce their production of IgE and thus their allergic tendencies.

CASTOR BEANS AND OTHER BADDIES

The immune system has to "decide" when producing IgE might be a good idea (in response to a liver fluke or tapeworm, for example) and when it is definitely a bad idea (in response to pollen). How this decision is made we do not know, but medical researchers have found that they can play a part in that

PAUL

Neither of Paul's parents had any signs of allergy, but it ran in both their families—several aunts, uncles, and cousins had asthma, hay fever, or urticaria (hives). The young couple assumed that because they were free of allergies, their children would be too, but they were wrong.

Both were carrying some genes for allergy, even though the effects were masked. Of their four children, only Paul was affected, and he developed eczema and asthma as a baby. The eczema did not last long and at the age of five the asthma disappeared, but hay fever then began. Every year Paul sneezed and blew his nose throughout the first eight weeks of summer. The doctor diagnosed hay fever to grass pollen. This continued until Paul was 12,

when the family moved from an unspoiled rural area into a large city with fairly high levels of air pollution. Within a few months his asthma had returned, and the following summer his hay fever was worse than ever before. Both continued until Paul was in his mid-20s.

Paul was unfortunate in suffering from so many different allergic disorders, and in starting asthma and hay fever at such an early age, but in many ways he is a good example of an atopic—someone with an allergic disposition.

As his case illustrates, that disposition can express itself in several different parts of the body, and may show up in different places (nose, bronchi, skin, and digestive system) at different phases of a person's life.

decision, at least in the laboratory. By adding certain substances to an injection containing an antigen, they can persuade the immune system to produce IgE to that antigen. The substances that have this effect are known as **IgE-specific adjuvants.** Presumably they mimic certain effects of large parasites in some way, thus promoting IgE production.

One of the most powerful IgE-specific adjuvants is found in castor beans, the raw material from which castor oil is made. During oil production, a dust comes out of the milling machinery and fills the air all around. It has unpleasant effects on many people working at the oil mills or living nearby. Dockers who handle castor beans may also be affected. Allergies to the dust are remarkably common, and it can also induce allergies to other substances, suggesting that the castor-bean dust contains both a powerful allergen and an IgE-specific adjuvant. Castor-bean dust often affects people with no previous signs of allergy.

Platinum salts are likewise known to favor IgE reactions to antigens *and* act as antigens themselves. However, this only affects workers in platinum-using factories.

Some IgE-specific adjuvants are simply particles that attract and hold proteins. These particles pick up protein antigens that originated elsewhere, resulting in a large antigen-coated particle that apparently stimulates the immune system to produce IgE. This effect can occur with a variety of particles including carbon particles, the soot produced by burning various fuels. The possible link between pollution and hay fever is one we will return to in the next chapter.

CROSS-REACTIONS

Most people have had the experience of seeing someone they know, saying hello, and then realizing, with great embarrassment, that they have made a mistake. The reason for the mistake is usually clear—the stranger's nose, mouth, or some other feature is similar to that of an acquaintance or friend. Exactly the same thing can happen to antibodies. Just as one nose can resemble another, so one epitope (see page 10) can resemble another, chemically speaking. If two epitopes are reasonably similar, then one antibody may bind to both of them. If those epitopes are on different chemical molecules (different antigens), then a **cross-reaction** has occurred. Usually the antibody has multiplied in the body as a response to one antigen, but then reacts to a second one as well.

In terms of fighting disease, cross-reactions often make sense. Many microbes occasionally undergo a **mutation**—a change in their hereditary material.

This can change the antigens in their outer coats, helping them to escape immune attack, so it pays if antibodies ignore minor alterations. Cross-reactions may also help the immune system if it has to tackle a related microbe, a type similar to one that has already been encountered and successfully defeated. It will already have a plentiful stockpile of B cells that make a suitable antibody for this new intruder.

Cross-reactions become a problem when they occur in allergic reactions because they can make a patient sensitive to a second item as well as to their original allergen. As one might expect, many cross-reactions in hay fever are between related plants. Because they are related, their pollen antigens can be chemically similar, and they may share key epitopes. This type of cross-reaction is very common in the grass family (Gramineae or Poaceae), where patients are often sensitive to pollen from several different species of grass. There are some other plant families where such cross-reactions are common (see chapter 11).

If a chemically similar antigen is found in food as well as in pollen, then this too may produce a cross-reaction because the relevant IgE molecule can be produced anywhere in the body, not just in the nose. The most common reaction is a tingling or itching sensation in the mouth, but sometimes a more violent and potentially dangerous immune reaction occurs (see the box on Jack's story on page 168). Many cross-reactions between pollen and foods have now been documented, and a list of all those currently known is given on page 165.

Finally, one very curious cross-reaction should be mentioned. To understand this particular medical tale, you must remember that all living things are descended from a single ancestor, a little nondescript blob of a thing that squidged about in the sea more than 1,000 million years ago. Although we may have come a long way since then, some of our most basic life processes are still the same, which means that some of the chemical "nuts and bolts" are also unchanged.

Among those nuts and bolts is a protein called **profilin,** a chemical heirloom so useful and precious that almost every living thing on Earth has hung on to it. Profilin is found inside human cells and in amoebas, yeasts, slime molds, mice, and cows. As you may have guessed by now, profilin is also found in pollen. In 1991, researchers in Austria discovered that it was one of the minor allergens in birch pollen, provoking an IgE response in 10 percent of those who are sensitive to birch pollen. When they took IgE from these patients, it bound equally well to human profilin as to birch-pollen profilin. Other tests showed that human profilin could probably trigger allergic responses in these patients.

The discoveries about profilin raise the intriguing possibility of patients being "allergic to themselves," or to some small part of themselves, at least. The idea of the immune system turning on the body itself—the biological equivalent of a military coup—is not unheard of. There are many diseases caused solely or partly by such **autoimmune reactions,** including one form of diabetes. Cross-reactions are thought to play a part in some of these. Whether an autoimmune reaction is actually occurring in the case of profilin is not known. Perhaps one of the body's control mechanisms intervenes and prevents a reaction to homegrown profilin. Certainly, if the body is reacting to its own profilin, there are no obvious symptoms in these patients as a result— only the symptoms of hay fever.

The Austrian researchers who discovered the profilin cross-reaction speculate that the body's own profilin may help to perpetuate hay fever: its presence all year long may maintain the level of IgE against pollen profilin. Profilin is also found in some other pollens, so this reaction may be important there too.

WHY US?

When people fall ill, they often ask indignantly, "Why me?" In the case of hay fever, it would be quite reasonable for *Homo sapiens* as a whole to demand "Why us?" Hay fever is very uncommon among other animals.

It is not that animals do not show allergic reactions at all—they do. Food allergies are known in dogs, pigs, and cows, mainly when they are fed an unnatural food such as soy, but sometimes in response to natural foodstuffs as well. Dogs sometimes develop itchy skin conditions in reaction to allergens they eat or inhale. Here pollen *may* play a part, one of the rare instances of a natural allergic reaction to pollen—but it does not generally produce symptoms in the nose. (Dogs may sneeze if they inhale a large dose of pollen when sniffing around in vegetation, but this is rarely a true allergic reaction; rather it is a simple response to the irritant effects of the pollen when inhaled in such quantities.)

According to Professor Brunello Wüthrich, who studies hay fever in Switzerland, the Swiss cow is sometimes afflicted by hay fever. However, this has not been observed in other countries. The only animals to show a condition resembling hay fever with any regularity are horses, notably thoroughbred horses. They sometimes also suffer from allergic reactions to the mold spores found in stored hay.

Efforts to induce hay fever in rats and mice, for the purposes of studying the disease and testing new treatments, have failed. There is no allergic reaction to pollen unless it is inhaled along with a powerful adjuvant (see the

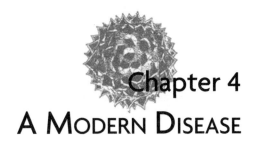

Chapter 4
A MODERN DISEASE

"At first I did not know what I had, and neither did any other doctor I encountered in the next two or three years. I gradually recognized that it was not an ordinary cold and that the symptoms were much worse on the golf course or even during a nice day rowing on Loch Lomond." These are the recollections of Dr. John Morrison Smith, who developed hay fever in the late 1930s while at medical school in Glasgow. "I do not remember seeing a case of hay fever as a student or being aware of any of my contemporaries suffering similarly . . . I do not believe any relative of mine for two or three generations in the past suffered from hay fever, but two of my own children have been affected by it."

That was just over 50 years ago. The idea of a succession of Scottish doctors being baffled by hay fever symptoms today is unthinkable.

Medical statistics tell much the same story as Dr. Morrison Smith's family history: hay fever has been steadily rising throughout the past 200 years. Before 1800, it seems to have been unknown. Today, in most developed countries, one teenager in six suffers from the disease.

From time to time, people cast doubt on the statistics showing that hay fever has increased dramatically: as we all know, there are "lies, damned lies, and statistics." The skeptics suggest that people simply did not bother about such minor ailments in the past, and did not visit the doctor with them, so hay fever never figured in the medical records. Another line of argument is that people just dismissed hay fever as a summer cold. Dr. Morrison Smith's account makes such theories seem extremely unlikely. Here was a young medical student on the lookout for an explanation of his unusual symptoms, which, unlike a cold, were worse on a fine day in the countryside and persisted for two months. If hay fever was as widespread then as it is now, how could he have missed it in his friends, relatives, and fellow students? Fortunately, one of the earliest hay fever sufferers was also a doctor who made a point of trying to find others with the same complaint. Dr. John Bostock (see chapter 2) had suffered from his summertime symptoms, which included itchy eyes, a constantly running nose, and paroxysms of sneezing, since the age of eight, but he first reported them to the medical world in 1819, when in his 40s. He continued to study the disease after 1819, and within nine years he had collected 28 fellow sufferers. (Today you could find that number of hay fever sufferers in a few hours if you simply stopped passersby on a busy street.) Bostock made extensive inquiries among other doctors and reported, "One of the most remarkable circumstances respecting this complaint is its not having been noticed as a specific affection, until within the last ten or twelve years."

Another oddity struck Bostock: all the patients he had collected were from "the middle or upper classes of society, some indeed of high rank." A tireless investigator by the standards of his time, Bostock decided to make sure this observation was correct: "I have made inquiry at the various dispensaries in London and elsewhere, and I have not heard of a single unequivocal case occurring among the poor." Medical historians today are able to confirm this particular report because dispensaries kept records and published them. At a dispensary in a very poor district of northwest England, the sale of medicines for "catarrh" (the general name used for a blocked or runny nose) was high in winter but low throughout the summer.

As the 19th century progressed, the disease became better known, but was still far from common. In 1837 a distinguished physician observed, "I have now seen several unequivocal instances of it—very few persons in comparison with the entire community are susceptible." The link with the upper classes was still there: "You may read almost every year in the newspapers that one of our English Dukes has gone to Brighton to escape the hay fever," he continued. (Brighton was the aristocracy's seaside resort—sea breezes, then as now, bring relief to hay fever sufferers.) The disease had became fashionable and newsworthy.

Soon afterward, a case of summer catarrh was recorded in Bordeaux, in the south of France, where it was attributed to sunlight. In 1852, Dr. J. Swett, unaware of any of the reports from Britain or France, described two forms of summer catarrh in the United States, one a reaction to grasses, the other to ragweed. Unlike Bostock, who blamed heat and sunlight, Swett shrewdly came to the correct conclusion about the cause of the disease at once. In Britain, it was the public who identified the origin of the illness.

By 1859, hay fever was known in Germany as well, and a Professor Phoebus of the University of Giessen, who collected information on the problem from both Britain and Germany, was able to report that there were fi-

HAY FEVER PIONEER: CHARLES BLACKLEY

Charles Harrison Blackley was a physician working in Manchester, England, and, like Bostock before him, was a sufferer from hay fever. Between 1859 and 1871, he carried out a series of experiments on the possible cause of hay fever. Among the causes that had already been suggested were benzoic acid, perfumes and odors, ozone, heat, and light. Each of these he tried in turn, but none produced the characteristic symptoms. Dust collected from a roadside did, however, and when he inspected it under the microscope he found that it contained grass pollen.

Blackley then collected grass pollen during the summer, stored it for several months, and inhaled some on a winter's day. The effect was immediate and dramatic, confirming the public hunch about the cause of hay fever (see chapter 2). Blackley collected other pollens—from garden flowers, weeds, and trees—and found that he reacted to them all (his hay fever must have been particularly bad).

Other experiments included flying a kite with a sticky glass microscope slide attached and then observing the slide under a microscope. This showed that pollen floated about high up in the atmosphere.

Blackley also invented a pollen trap and made the world's first pollen counts. For one man, working alone, he achieved a remarkable amount, and put the study of hay fever on a serious scientific footing.

nally some sufferers who were "not of the higher members of society." Hay fever, after 60 years or so, had reached the lower middle classes, but it took a few decades more to really conquer the proletariat. In the 1870s, English physician Charles Blackley found that hay fever was almost wholly confined to educated and professional people, and suspected that there was a "predisposition which mental culture generates." He thought that the rise in standards of education might be part of the reason for the spread of hay fever.

The numbers were growing all the time. The United States Hay Fever Association was founded in the 1870s and had almost 200 members. By 1903 there were thousands applying to join. A medical journal published in London in 1907 described hay fever as "a very common complaint."

In 1925 the disease was sufficiently well known for Noël Coward to discard *Oranges and Lemons* as the title of his new comedy about an eccentric English family entertaining guests during a summer weekend at their country house and call it instead *Hay Fever*. (The connotations of "midsummer madness" must still have been there in the 1920s, a distant memory of the time when English dukes galloped off to Brighton to escape their aristocratic malady.)

Attentive readers will have noticed what seems like a contradiction here. By 1925 hay fever is sufficiently well known to serve as the title of a play in London. Yet almost 15 years *later,* as a young medical student sneezes his way across Loch Lomond, no local doctor can identify his symptoms. This paradox cannot easily be explained, but it is certainly the case that hay fever affected some countries, and some districts, far earlier than others. Clearly the disease took longer to gain ground in Scotland, although today it is as common there as anywhere else in Britain.

TOWN AND COUNTRY

Reliable data are hard to find, but it does seem that, during its early days, hay fever was something of an urban disease. In the 1870s, Charles Blackley observed that hay fever was virtually unknown among the British farming community. Another author, writing in 1871, remarked that "in Ireland hay-fever is seldom heard of."

Fortunately, there is some solid evidence from Switzerland, where a doctor carried out a careful survey in 1926 and found that cases were ten times as common in the town as in the country. Roughly one urbanite in every hundred was affected, compared with only one per thousand in rural areas.

When a similar survey was carried out in Switzerland in 1985, 10 percent of the population suffered from hay fever, and there was no difference between the town and the countryside. Nor is there any difference between urban and rural populations in Britain today.

In some countries, hay fever is still a little more common in towns, but the tenfold difference recorded in the 1920s is never seen now. In southern Spain, for example, olive pollen sets many of the citizens of Cordoba sneezing, while those working in the olive groves on the hillsides beyond the city (where pollen counts reach far higher levels) are less likely to be affected. In Norway, Sweden, and Finland hay fever is still more common in the urbanized and industrialized areas. The same is also true of many east European countries, notably Czechoslovakia, where very high levels of hay fever and other allergies are found among children in industrialized areas. Italian city dwellers are twice as likely to have hay fever as those in the country. (There are some exceptions to this rule. Occasionally rural populations today have more hay fever than those in nearby towns, but this is generally in hot, arid countries such as Israel, where there is extensive irrigation to create farms. What happens is that the plants flourish and pollinate as vigorously as they would in a damp climate, but there is no rainfall to wash the pollen from the air. As a result, it builds up to massive levels.)

Today, in undeveloped regions of the world such as rural Africa, it does seem that hay fever is still unknown, or very rare, although no one has made a proper scientific study of this. In India, hay fever is quite common.

Just as the old link between hay fever and urban living lingers on in places, so there is still a ghost of the old link with social class. In some studies, but not all, hay fever is more common among the educated and upper classes. A recent study in the United States found it to be more common among those with higher incomes and among the better educated. In Switzerland, there is apparently a huge class difference—hay fever is three times as common among professional people as it is among manual laborers. This is not the case in Britain, but researchers *have* found that upper-class people with hay fever tend to get diagnosed more accurately than those in the lower classes, whose hay fever is more frequently mistaken for an infection. Could the differences between classes seen today in countries such as Switzerland therefore be illusory, or exaggerated? This is difficult to say, but the inquiries made by Bostock and others in the 19th century can make us confident that the class difference was there in the past.

Before we attempt to explain the strange and sudden rise of hay fever—a rise that still seems to be continuing—there are two other important pieces of evidence that must be included. One is the rarity of hay fever among animals, described in the previous chapter. The other comes from a mammoth medical survey that included 17,414 children.

During one week in March 1958, every child born in Britain became part of medical science. These children were studied at birth and again at the ages of 7, 11, and 23, when they or their parents were asked about a huge variety of symptoms. Many different aspects of their living conditions and social status were also recorded. This sort of information is a treasure trove for medical scientists, who can, with the aid of modern computers, scan the data for possible links and associations. One researcher has done just that for hay fever, but he found very few important links. Being born in the town or the country made no difference, nor did social class, nor did smoking by the parents (although this is known to affect asthma).

The one factor that did correlate remarkably well with hay fever was family size. An only child was much more likely to have hay fever than one with several brothers and sisters. Explaining away such a finding seems simple enough at first sight. Minor illnesses tend to attract less attention and concern among large families than they do in the cosseted only child, and parents with few children might have noticed hay fever more readily. Yet the difference was equally pronounced at the age of 23, when the young adults were reporting their own symptoms.

There is another possible explanation here. We know that susceptibility to hay fever and other allergic diseases is genetically inherited (see "Genes and Age" in the previous chapter). Perhaps atopic parents—those predisposed to allergy—simply have fewer children? Other evidence suggests that this is unlikely. What is more, if this explanation were true, allergies in general would show the same association with family size as hay fever. While eczema does show the same pattern as hay fever, asthma does not.

When the figures were looked at again, it became clear that family size was only part of the story anyway. Being the firstborn or the baby of the family also made a huge difference. Those least likely to develop hay fever were the youngest children from large families. Someone with four older brothers or sisters, for example, had only one quarter the chance of developing hay fever as someone with no older brothers or sisters. (To have four *younger* brothers and sisters also reduced the chance of hay fever, compared with the chance for an only child, but not nearly as much.) The differences persisted long after the children were grown up—in fact, they were more pronounced at age 23 than they had been at 11. Another large group of children, all born in 1970, has shown the same puzzling pattern.

PIECING TOGETHER THE PUZZLE

What could explain the quirky history of hay fever and the puzzling pattern still shown by the disease today? What, after all, could single out 19th-century aristocrats and the eldest children of 20th-century families, favor town dwellers at first but not later, and cause hay fever in human beings but not in most animals? Let's look at some of the suspects that have been arraigned over the years.

SUSPECT NUMBER ONE:
THE FINELY CHISELED NASAL ORGAN

In 1887, Dr. Edward Noakes of London concluded that hay fever was mainly due to a lack of space within the nose that compressed and irritated the membranes within. "Perhaps this latter fact," wrote Dr. Noakes, "may explain the observation that the disease is most prevalent among the aristocratic classes, who are generally accredited with possession of that refined contour and delicate chiseling of the nasal organ, which necessarily diminishes the space for the internal structures, and compels some of these to lie in contact with each other."

SUSPECT NUMBER TWO: CHANGES IN THE POLLEN

Some change in the pollen—either its quantity or its type—has been a popular culprit ever since the 19th century. In Britain people blamed the Corn Laws, the greater amount of hay being grown to feed the horses of urban populations, grasses grown on "rich soils," and anything else that looked like a possible scapegoat. However, these explanations were, and are, extremely implausible. The pollen count may change from time to time as agricultural practices change, but there has always been a fair amount of grass pollen in the air—enough, certainly, to spark hay fever if the human population was susceptible to it. Indeed, it was on the grassy plains of Africa that human beings evolved, and our ancestors' exposure to grass pollen then must have been massive. Breathing plenty of pollen, particularly grass pollen, is an age-old part of human life.

Looking at hay fever around the world, there are certainly specific instances of new pollens causing outbreaks of hay fever. In Florida and California, for example, various imported species grown in gardens have begun to cause severe hay fever symptoms. In India, epidemics of hay fever have been sparked by introduced weeds, such as Santa Maria feverfew. The spread of ragweed in various parts of the world also brings more hay fever in its wake (see page 130). But these are specific and isolated instances: in general, changes in pollen cannot be blamed for hay fever. As with grasses, many of the major allergens are from plants with which we have happily coexisted for thousands of years.

SUSPECT NUMBER THREE:
A GENETIC CHANGE IN HUMAN BEINGS

The tendency to allergy is inherited, and the genes producing that tendency must have been in the human population for thousands of years. Allergies are nothing new. We can state this confidently because the medical writers of ancient Greece gave clear descriptions of food allergy and asthma. They did not, however, mention anything remotely resembling hay fever, nor were there any convincing descriptions of it until Bostock's account. (There are sporadic reports of something called the "rose cold" in earlier times, which produced sneezing and was apparently brought on by roses. Its sufferers "held the smell of roses in deadly hatred." Some have suggested that this was actually hay fever, but it seems more likely to have been vasomotor rhinitis, which can be triggered by strong scents—see "Vasomotor Rhinitis" in chapter 13.)

The noses of our ancestors, even those ancestors who were atopic, apparently had the wisdom to tolerate pollen. They do not seem to have extended this tolerance to other airborne allergens, however. Reports from A.D. 41 tell of a violent allergy to horses seen in the son of a Roman emperor, and there are later reports from Germany of allergies to horses, dogs, and mice. Baker's asthma, a reaction to inhaled flour, was also known.

Could there be another genetic mutation that, when added to the genes for atopy, made the nose intolerant of pollen? If such a mutation had appeared in the late 18th century, this would perhaps explain the sudden appearance of hay fever. It is a nice idea, but it does not hold water. New genes spread very slowly. Calculations show that it would be impossible for a mutant gene to spread so rapidly as to affect 10 or 15 percent of the population in the space of 200 years.

WHAT SORT OF CULPRIT ARE WE LOOKING FOR?

With the three obvious suspects eliminated from the inquiry, we can be more precise about the sort of culprit we are seeking. It is something that acts on atopics (people who have a predisposition to allergy) and somehow makes them react allergically to pollen.

To put the matter another way, it somehow stops them learning to tolerate pollen. The immune system, as explained in chapter 3, has to sort out the difference between harmful invaders and harmless ones, so that it can react effectively and promptly against disease-causing microbes but not mount any damaging reactions against harmless items coming into the body, such as food molecules and pollen grains. The process of learning to shrug off harmless items is called **tolerance induction,** and it occurs when we first encounter a new allergen, usually as babies or young children.

It is difficult to investigate tolerance induction in human atopics directly, so we have to rely on studies with rats and mice. These show that an antigen that is inhaled *automatically* induces tolerance, in the sense of preventing production of the allergy antibody IgE. The action is specific: it applies only to the particular antigen that has been inhaled. It works by means of T suppressor cells, which can block the production of a particular type of antibody in response to a particular antigen. The T suppressor cells are like roving superintendents of the immune system, which patrol the body ensuring that other cells do not produce IgE to particular antigens, in this case pollen antigens.

That is what happens with antigens inhaled by adult mice and rats, and it is fair to assume that something similar happens in healthy humans encountering a new inhaled allergen as well (although there are other ways in which the allergic response is suppressed; see page 37). However, the system is not yet established in newborn mice and rats, which cannot produce the T suppressor cells. During the first weeks or so of life, they can be sensitized by inhaled allergens. They do not start producing high levels of IgE immediately because they cannot produce much IgE at this stage—but the scene is set. Once they become old enough to produce IgE abundantly, the lack of T suppressor cells to the inhaled antigen becomes evident, and they can produce IgE to that antigen (although they do not get any symptoms in the nose itself).

Even in adult rats and mice, and young ones past the vulnerable newborn state, certain things can interfere with the induction of tolerance, including nitrogen dioxide. If animals inhale fairly high concentrations of this gas, it irritates the nose and airways. If they then inhale an antigen that they have never been exposed to before, they do not become tolerant as they normally would. (Again, there are no symptoms in the nose of the rodent, but a blood test shows them producing IgE to the antigen.)

How far can we apply these discoveries to human beings? That is a difficult question to answer, but studies of children with allergies, and the conditions they were born into, show some interesting associations. For example, being born just before the pollen season may make hay fever as a child or teenager a little more likely. The general impression is that there is a period of particular vulnerability for the newborn child that lasts for three months or more. This could correspond, in some respects, to the brief period of vulnerability in the newborn mouse or rat, since human babies develop at a far slower pace.

However, looking back in time, it is clear that 300 years ago, babies (even atopic babies) did not react in the same way. They breathed pollen in their first few months, yet did not develop hay fever later. Something must have changed.

This could be something in our diet or way of life that influences the immune system and makes for a longer or more marked period of vulnerability in the young baby. Alternatively, it could be something in the air that irritates the airways, and thus directly interferes with tolerance induction by airborne substances when they are first encountered. This irritant could affect babies or children breathing in a potential allergen for the first time, but it might also affect adults in certain circumstances—immigrants from lands with different vegetation, for example. (It is known that immigrants sometimes develop hay fever; if they do so, it is within two or three years of arriving in their new country.)

Whether airborne irritants such as nitrogen dioxide really can prevent tolerance induction in humans, as they do in mice and rats, is unknown at present. Scientists generally assume that they can, but there is no proof, and extrapolating from animals to humans is always risky. (Whether irritants can *break down* tolerance that has already been induced is an even trickier issue, but one that is relevant to those who develop hay fever late in life; see "Genes and Age" in chapter 3.)

The information about tolerance induction is useful in compiling our list of suspects. It is clear that we are probably looking for something that is able to affect atopic babies very early in life, when they will first be exposed to certain airborne allergens.

SUSPECT NUMBER FOUR: AIR POLLUTION

As far as many journalists are concerned, this suspect has already been interrogated, charged, tried in a court of law, and found guilty. "Hay fever: the pollution sickness" was one memorable headline from 1992. To anyone who knows all the evidence in the case, however, it is obvious that this verdict is premature. There are too many facts that do not fit:

- Hay fever began not among the urban poor, living in the shadow of the Industrial Revolution and breathing the foul air of its foundries and factories, but among the upper classes. It then spread among the middle classes, and eventually reached the working class almost a century after it had begun.

- Hay fever does not naturally affect animals, with a few, rare exceptions. Our dogs, cats, cows, and sheep share the same polluted air that we do, so why has hay fever not affected them?

- Hay fever is *four times* more common among eldest children and only children than it is among the youngest in a family, a huge difference that the "pollution theory" cannot apparently explain.

That is the major evidence against. The historical evidence in favor lies in the link between hay fever and towns, a conspicuous link early on but one that has gradually disappeared during the 20th century. Some researchers believe that the spread of road traffic can explain this particular pattern: air pollution, originally a monopoly of urban areas, has now spread to the countryside with the growth in the number of cars and trucks.

Superficially, this is an attractive theory, but to accept it involves classing *all* forms of pollution as one, and assuming that smoke from factory chimneys has the same effect on the nose as car-exhaust fumes. Careful study of this subject makes it clear that "air pollution" is not just one suspect, but rather a group of individual suspects. To lump them together and call them "pollution" simply leads to muddled thinking. The different types of pollutant must be considered separately.

Motor Vehicle Exhausts

The best evidence on exhaust fumes comes from Japan. Researchers have studied the incidence of hay fever to Japanese red cedar, comparing people from different areas. Those with the highest incidence of hay fever were living along busy roads lined with these trees. They were three times more likely to be affected than people living near forests of red cedar but well away from traffic pollution. Those breathing plenty of traffic fumes and only a little pollen came somewhere in between.

Japanese scientists looking for the cause of this phenomenon have made detailed studies of diesel particulates, tiny sooty particles that come from the exhaust pipes of trucks and diesel cars. When a bus or truck spews out black exhaust fumes as it starts up, these particles are momentarily visible, but for the most part they are too small and too dispersed in the air for us to see. Nevertheless, they are there, and an urban commuter could inhale as much as 500 millionths of a gram of diesel particles every day. According to the Japanese researchers, just 1 millionth of a gram can boost IgE production to 100 times its normal level when placed in the nose of a mouse along with an antigen that has not been encountered before. The evidence suggests that diesel particles interfere with tolerance induction.

Could other constituents of modern exhaust fumes be playing a part, perhaps augmenting the effect of carbon particles from diesel engines? Nitrogen dioxide is known to interfere with tolerance induction in rats and mice and it is one of the gases found in car-exhaust fumes. However, the link is not that straightforward because the levels used in the experiments described above were about *a thousand times* higher than those on a polluted city street. Nevertheless, nitrogen dioxide may still be relevant here. Laboratory tests show that this gas, if it becomes concentrated in the air we breathe, acts as an irritant to the human nose and airways. Although the levels needed to produce symptoms are up to *a hundred times* higher than those found on city streets, a very different picture emerges from studies of nitrogen dioxide in the home. Here it is produced by gas stoves in poorly ventilated conditions and by old-fashioned paraffin or kerosene heaters.

A study of children in Great Britain showed that heating with propane gas or paraffin significantly increased the risk of their developing hay fever and year-round nasal allergies. In this study, and in one from Austria, gas central heating also emerged as a factor that increased the risk of hay fever. Electric heating was the option with the lowest allergy risk.

Another notorious gas produced by traffic should be mentioned here. Ozone is formed mainly in the summer months, and it too causes irritation of

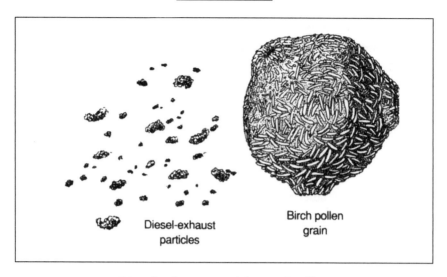

Diesel-exhaust
particles

Birch pollen
grain

Diesel-exhaust particles and pollen

the nose and airways. It can easily build up to levels that affect those with asthma, making attacks more likely. During a photochemical smog (see appendix 6), the levels reached will affect the breathing of healthy people too. Recent studies have shown that ozone also makes hay fever symptoms a little worse, producing more sneezing and itching of the nose. However, there is no evidence that ozone can interfere with tolerance induction in animals or humans. Making hay fever worse is one thing—starting it off in the first place is another.

Other Forms of Air Pollution

Unfortunately, evidence about other forms of pollution is much less satisfactory. Apart from soot particles, the only pollutants that have been studied in relation to allergy are sulfur dioxide and sulfuric acid.

Sulfur dioxide is a gas produced by coal fires, power stations burning coal, smelters, and some factories. It was a major ingredient of the smogs of former days, and a lethal ingredient for those with bronchitis, the elderly, and the very young. Sulfur dioxide is acidic and can severely irritate the airways, producing inflammation. In asthmatics, it can provoke an asthma attack (see "Coping with Pollen Asthma" in chapter 5). Thanks to antipollution measures, sulfur dioxide is far less of a problem in cities today.

Studies of the effect of sulfur dioxide on tolerance induction in animals show that it may prevent tolerance from developing, even at quite low concentrations, such as those that could still be encountered in a polluted industrial area today.

Tiny droplets of sulfuric acid in the air are another form of pollution that affects the airways. No one has looked at the effect of this on tolerance induction, but it could well be similar to the effect of sulfur dioxide.

There are many other types of modern pollutant, and few have been studied for their effect on allergy.

CAN WE REACH A VERDICT ON POLLUTION?

There are clearly some aspects of the hay fever epidemic that pollution totally fails to explain (see "Suspect Number Four: Air Pollution," earlier in this chapter), but if we accept that there are likely to be several causes rather than a *single* cause for this epidemic, pollution could be partially guilty. It seems probable that traffic pollution is playing some role in the present increase in numbers, and that smoke and sulfur dioxide may have been a small part of the problem in the recent past. But if smoke and sulfur dioxide had a major effect, it would not have taken so long for hay fever to touch the factory workers and poor city dwellers of the 19th century. This type of pollution was a widespread feature of industrial areas in the early 19th century, and even in the 18th century. In London, where nuggets of poor-quality coal from seams under the sea were regularly washed up on the shores of the Thames, people had been burning this fuel to warm their houses for centuries. One writer of the 17th century recorded a "hellish and dismall cloud of sea-coal" over London, while King James complained that St. Paul's Cathedral was being corroded by the smog. Sea coal, which can still be found today, produces an unpleasant acidic smoke full of sulfur dioxide. If such smoke could promote hay fever on a grand scale, why did it not do so in the 17th and 18th centuries?

Having dealt with pollution, there are two remaining suspects to consider.

SUSPECT NUMBER FIVE: "MODERN LIVING"

It is tempting to look for some aspect of modern living that was first enjoyed only by the very wealthy but then gradually spread to the middle classes and is now available to all sectors of our egalitarian society. If that luxury item was something that could irritate the nose, or subtly influence the immune system of a young child, it might qualify as a suspect.

A more varied and abundant diet is one possibility—perhaps it could affect the immune system in some way. No one has yet investigated this. Bottle-feeding has been suggested, but it does not seem to have much influence on hay fever, despite its effects in promoting food sensitivity (see page 249). Something in paper or printing ink—an obvious culprit given the long-standing link between hay fever and education—has never been looked into, as far as we know.

However, there is one aspect of modern living that has been investigated thoroughly in the past few years: hygiene.

SUSPECT NUMBER SIX: A DECLINE IN INFECTIONS

Certain infections have declined in the past 200 years, a decline that began long before vaccination was widespread, and which was due largely to better hygiene and sanitation. The suggestion that fewer infections could mean more allergy was seen only a decade ago as a rather wacky and implausible theory. Most doctors and medical scientists were preoccupied with the fact that virus infections (such as colds and flu) frequently trigger asthma attacks, and that one virus (called RSV) can make asthma more likely to develop in a child. The prevailing wisdom was that infections tended to pave the way for allergies, rather than protect against them.

A few scientists thought differently and began researching their hunch. They suggested that some infections—perhaps bacterial infections—might be capable of protecting children against allergy.

The evidence that this was indeed so came from a great many different sources in a surprisingly short space of time. During the late 1990s there was a sudden spate of research publications that broke down all the previous objections and firmly established the "hygiene hypothesis" as the new orthodoxy. These are some of those research findings:

- Doctors in Austria, Finland, and Germany all discovered the same thing, in separate studies: there was a lower rate of allergies, especially hay fever, among children raised on a farm with animals, compared with children living in the same villages without farm animals. The Austrian study established that regular contact with livestock and poultry was the most important factor: children not living on farms but having close contact with farm animals were also at lower risk. The Finnish study identified the period from birth to 6 years as the crucial time period.

- A large group of Italian military cadets were assessed for allergies, including nasal allergies. At the same time, blood samples were taken and tested for antibodies to common infections: this allowed doctors to see what diseases the men had been exposed to early in life. Among men with antibodies against three common infections that are dispersed via food and feces—hepatitis A, *Toxoplasma gondii,* and *Helicobacter pylori*— allergies were least frequent. Only 8 percent of the cadets in this group had allergies. Among the men with no antibodies against any of these infections, 20 percent had allergies. The doctors carrying out this experiment believe that these three infections are not necessarily important in themselves, but that they identify individuals who were "reared in an environment that provides a higher exposure to many other orofecal or foodborne microbes." In other words, they grew up in the kind of household where you didn't bother washing your hands before meals. Incidentally, the military cadets were also checked out for antibodies to measles, mumps, rubella, chicken pox, and herpes. None of these infections gave protection against allergies—only infections carried in food and feces did.

- Studies from the former East Germany (carried out in 1992 to 1993, when a lot of children still went to a nursery at 6 months old, as in the communist era) showed that if children from small families went to a nursery when they were between 6 and 11 months old, they were substantially less allergy-prone than if they went later. The allergy risk was highest for only-children who did not go to a nursery until they were over 2 years old. This throws light on the previous finding that having older brothers and sisters reduces the risk of allergy. The East German data showed that mixing with lots of other children in a nursery produced more infections and also gave protection against allergy— suggesting that the protective effect of siblings is indeed due to infection.

- U.S. scientists looked at babies under 2 years with history of wheezing and gave them skin tests for common allergens. They also tested the dust in the children's homes for bacterial endotoxins. All the babies who were sensitized to one or more allergens lived in homes with relatively low levels of endotoxin in the house dust. Children from homes with high levels of bacterial toxins in the household dust did not seem to have developed allergic responses.

- A huge survey of children in 16 countries—including the United States, Australia, and New Zealand, as well as various European nations— showed that having a dog in childhood, sharing a bedroom, and having a large family could all protect against allergies. Brothers were more protected than sisters—perhaps because boys are stereotypically dirtier than girls.

- In several studies, children with pets at home during early childhood have lower rates of allergy (although if they do develop allergies, these may well include allergies to the pet). Most interesting, the benefits of pet ownership are much more pronounced for children without brothers and sisters, suggesting again that minor infections are the key—a dog can take over the role of a grubby older sibling in protecting a child from allergy.

- A British study showed that children who wash their hands more than five times and have two baths a day are almost twice as likely to get asthma as children who wash their hands less than three times a day and have a bath every other day. (Asthma is not necessarily fueled by allergies, but in children it generally is.) This could be an effect from harmless bacteria found in garden dirt, which are known to influence the immune system away from allergy-type responses (see below).

- Several studies have now produced evidence of a link between antibiotic use before the age of 1 or 2 and the later development of allergies or asthma or both. One study, by doctors in England, followed 1,900 children up to the age of 16. Among children at risk of allergy (because their mothers had allergies), taking antibiotics before the age of two was linked with an increase in the rate of allergy from 32 percent to 54 percent. The more courses of antibiotics a child received, the greater the risk. The type of infection for which the drugs were prescribed was not important, but broad-spectrum antibiotics, which kill a wide range of bacteria, were more closely linked with allergies—suggesting that the depletion of friendly bacteria in the gut (the gut flora) could be responsible for increasing the allergy risk. Penicillins seemed less likely to promote allergies than erythromycin or cephalosporins.

Looking back into history, the hygiene hypothesis can explain so much—why, for the first century of its existence, hay fever was a disease of the urban upper classes, only gradually working its way down to the poor and to rural communities. This fits in well with the gradual spread of more hygienic ways of life, especially the habit of keeping children clean and encouraging them to play indoors rather than outdoors. The hygiene hypothesis can also explain why hay fever is still virtually unknown in most poor developing countries but starts to boom when living conditions improve. And it can explain why animals don't get hay fever.

THE LAST PIECES OF THE PUZZLE

Research has now begun to reveal exactly how bacteria might affect the development of allergy. A newborn baby, as it turns out, is an allergic reaction just waiting to happen—its immune system is geared up to respond to the environment with the production of IgE (the allergy antibody) rather than less troublesome antibodies. This is because the pro-allergy Th2 cells are far more numerous and active than the Th1 cells (see page 36) at this stage of life. Why?

The answer lies with the pregnant mother-to-be, whose immune system has to be prevented from following its usual course—attacking anything that is alien in the body. Unless held in check, a woman's immune system could reject a fetus (or at least retard its growth) in just the same way that heart transplants are rejected. To prevent attacks on the fetus, the immune system is retuned during pregnancy, with that aspect of immunity—the part that rejects transplants and could reject a fetus—being reduced.

It happens that this particular aspect of immunity is coordinated by the Th1 cells, so they are told to be less active, which inevitably means that the Th2 cells become dominant.

This change of emphasis occurs in the mother's immune system, but it carries over into the immune system of the fetus because they are sharing the same blood supply. The blood contains the messenger substances that choreograph the immune system's day-to-day performance.

Immediately after birth, the baby's immune system is still following the same pattern, continuing to "up-regulate" Th2 cells and "down-regulate" Th1 cells. This is what sets the stage for allergic sensitization.

What should happen, just after birth (and what would have happened in the past), is that the outside world gives the baby's immune system a sharp nudge in the opposite direction and gets it operating in a healthy, non-allergic way. That nudge comes from a dose of bacterial products—something that we would inevitably have encountered when we lived closer to nature. For example, ordinary garden dirt contains harmless bacteria that do not cause any symptoms but do tweak the immune system toward Th1 cells and away from Th2 cells. Indoor bacteria can do the same—in the study of babies and bacterial endotoxin in dust, described above, high levels of endotoxin in a house were associated with high levels of Th1 cells in the resident baby's blood.

Living in the far-from-natural modern world, lacking close contact with soil, animals, and unwashed human beings, the baby's immune system flounders in limbo without clear guidance. Worse, the baby may be born by cesarean section and not even pick up the normal and healthy gut flora from its mother's vagina during birth. Or the gut bacteria may be obliterated by a course of broad-spectrum antibiotics. Robbed of all the natural cues that should teach it how to operate correctly, the immune system wanders off down the allergic path, setting a course for eczema, hay fever, and asthma later in life.

Of course, many modern children are brought up in ultrahygienic conditions and emerge allergy-free. You may be asking why all children don't get allergies, if the way we live is so important. The fact is that the unfortunate overemphasis on Th2 cells probably occurs in all newborn babies, but in some children—those who are atopic or allergy-prone—there are genetic factors that make it more marked. At the same time, some of the internal checks and balances that could still prevent allergy, even in our sterile modern world, are lacking in these children (see "Controlling IgE" in chapter 3). This is a genetic vulnerability that became apparent only with the emergence of modern living conditions.

Chapter 5

TREATING HAY FEVER AND POLLEN ASTHMA: SELF-HELP AND MEDICAL HELP

Far too many people with hay fever choose to suffer in silence—if you can describe volleys of explosive sneezes and regular snorting into handkerchiefs as "silence." According to one survey, for every hundred people with hay fever, fewer than 25 are getting treatment that relieves their symptoms fully. No doctor, however optimistic, would suggest that all the hundred could be entirely freed from their symptoms, but it is certainly true that many more people could be helped, and that many could experience far greater relief by reassessing their current forms of treatment.

Reassessment requires knowledge of the disease, knowledge of all the treatments now available, a consideration of the individual's lifestyle and preferences, and some intelligent experimentation. Unless family doctors were to devote themselves full time to hay fever, abandoning interest in all other diseases, they would be hard-pressed to do this for everyone who needed such help. Consequently, there is a real role for patients to play here—in reassessing their own treatment and in calling on their doctor for professional help when it is needed.

Do not expect a panacea—a single treatment that clears up your hay fever unaided. For the lucky few there will be a treatment that produces such magical effects, but for most the battle against allergy is one that has to be fought on several fronts at once.

The two primary forms of treatment—medicinal drugs and pollen avoidance—are dealt with in detail in chapters 7 and 8, respectively. In brief, as far as drugs are concerned, there have been several major innovations in the past few years, including drugs with far fewer side effects. One of the newer drugs may help you, even if you have, in the past, experienced unpleasant reactions to drug treatments.

Pollen avoidance can range from a few simple measures (such as wearing sunglasses or protective glasses and keeping windows closed at certain times of day) to high-tech "pollen-proofing" of your home and car, combined with protection of your nose and eyes when out-of-doors. These measures are particularly useful to people with severe hay fever who are not helped very much by drugs or who have strong objections to taking them.

Allergy shots are another option for such patients, and this is fully described in chapter 9. The orthodox method, hyposensitization, is explained, along with two relatively new alternative treatments.

Finally, chapter 10 deals with other treatments, mostly unconventional ones, such as dietary supplements, inhalations, homeopathy, hypnosis, herbal remedies, and acupuncture. Some of these may work; others are probably a waste of money.

By reading each of these chapters in turn, you will have a clear idea of what you could do to tackle your hay fever symptoms. You can then choose from the various options available, selecting those that suit your home and lifestyle, your financial situation, your preferences for drug or nondrug treatments, and the severity of your symptoms. Be prepared to try different approaches and different combinations until you find one that suits you. Everyone is different.

As a very first step, however, you do need to be sure that you are actually suffering from hay fever. Chapter 6 looks at how hay fever should be diagnosed. It suggests how you can diagnose yourself and when a doctor should be called on to confirm the diagnosis.

If you are allergic to other airborne allergens, not just pollen, you may have a more complex task in dealing with your allergens. Chapter 12 describes these airborne allergens, and the avoidance measures needed for each of them, in detail. The clearest sign of multiple allergies is if your symptoms continue at times of the year when no plants are in flower. Even though the symptoms may be very mild at these times, and seem scarcely worth noticing compared with what you go through in the pollen season, the other allergens are definitely worth investigating. It may be that the year-round effects of other allergens are making the nose unduly sensitive to pollen when it arrives. By dealing with the other allergens, therefore, you could make your hay fever much less severe. The most common allergens involved are those produced by dust mites, molds, and pets—and the good news is that control or avoidance of these allergens is much easier than pollen avoidance.

Allergens encountered at work that can produce rhinitis are also dealt with in chapter 12, and this section looks in some detail at **sick building syndrome.** Finally, chapter 13 discusses nonallergic forms of rhinitis, such as **vasomotor rhinitis,** and deals with sensitivity to food, which can produce a variety of symptoms including rhinitis. The last part of the chapter explains how to carry out an elimination diet to diagnose such food problems.

Occasionally, people with hay fever are allergic to another airborne substance but never suspect that they are because they have symptoms only during the pollen season. What happens is that the response to the secondary allergen (such as the dust-mite or cat allergen) remains under control when the nose is in good health. But when spring or summer arrives, and the nose becomes inflamed by the reaction to pollen, it also becomes "primed" to react to the other allergen. The basic mechanism underlying "priming" is described in chapter 3. To put it simply, once the nose becomes disrupted by its annual quarrel with pollen, it is oversensitive and easily upset by other allergens. You should suspect this if any of the following apply to you:

- Your hay fever is just as severe indoors with the windows closed (either at home or at work) as it is outdoors

- You seem to sneeze or blow your nose a lot when close to a cat, dog, or other pet (but bear in mind that pets coming in from outside can carry pollen in their fur)

- You sneeze a lot first thing in the morning (most often a sign of dust-mite allergy or, less frequently, feather allergy)

- You are affected far more in some houses or buildings than in others, even though windows are closed in both

- You sneeze or blow your nose a lot when close to sources of mold spores such as compost heaps, dead leaves, and rotten wood (see "Mold Spores" in chapter 12 for a full discussion)

If you are reacting to other allergens during the pollen season, it is highly likely that they are aggravating your hay fever symptoms. Chapter 12 will help you to identify the culprit, and gives specific advice for avoiding that allergen.

IS IT ESSENTIAL TO SEE A DOCTOR?

It is traditional, in self-help books such as this, to play it safe and advise people to visit their doctor before trying to treat themselves or changing their current treatment. However, a great many people with hay fever already treat themselves, and many have never consulted a doctor about the problem. In most cases, this is probably quite satisfactory. Given the large numbers of people who now have hay fever, it would surely be an unnecessary burden on family doctors to have to see yet more hay fever patients, unless those patients have a specific need for professional help.

Self-treatment, based on pollen avoidance and medicinal drugs, should work well for all straightforward cases of hay fever. There are now several drugs that can be bought without a doctor's prescription. Only if these fail, or cause side effects, should you need to consult your doctor about trying other drugs. Pollen avoidance is thoroughly covered in chapter 8, and it is unlikely that a general practitioner will be able to offer any additional advice.

The situations in which you should definitely go to see an allergist are as follows:

- If you have symptoms in the eye that include inflammation and/or swelling of the eyelids. This can progress to blistering and ulceration, and may cause blindness if left untreated.

- If you suffer from asthma, either during the pollen season or at other times of year. Check the next section for asthma symptoms; these can be quite mild, and you could suffer from asthma without having recognized the fact.

- If your rhinitis persists for most of the year, or well beyond the flowering season for plants, and you cannot identify a year-round allergen that might be causing the problem

- If your "hay fever" has come on suddenly and is very severe

- If your "hay fever" has come on following an accident that involved injury to the head, particularly to the face or nose

- If your mucus or saliva tastes salty; make a point of mentioning this to the doctor

- If you are suffering pain in the nose or face or have earache; make a point of mentioning this to the doctor

- If you are suffering from nosebleeds

- If nonprescription drugs have failed to help you much and you are still suffering hay fever symptoms, despite pollen avoidance measures

- If you are not sure which pollen causes your hay fever and feel that you need to know; your doctor can give you a skin-prick test (see chapter 6)

- If your nose becomes completely blocked

- If your rhinitis is so severe that you have lost your sense of smell, cannot sleep properly, cannot work or study, or feel generally unwell

- If you would like allergy shots

On *very* rare occasions, cancerous growths in the nose have been mistaken for an allergic condition because they have produced symptoms that were almost exactly the same. If you have visited your doctor repeatedly and none of the medicines prescribed has had any effect, do go back again. The most likely explanation is that your allergy is highly resistant to treatment, but there is a remote chance of something more serious being wrong, and this should be investigated.

Another condition that can resemble allergic rhinitis is a leakage of the fluid that surrounds the brain (the **cerebrospinal fluid**) following injury to the face. The leakage may be intermittent, and it may not be apparent until some time after the accident. The tell-tale sign in this case is that the fluid is more salty than normal mucus from the nose and that your taste buds detect this. Again, this is a rare condition.

COPING WITH POLLEN ASTHMA

Only a minority of patients with hay fever develop pollen asthma as well, but this can happen. The asthma tends to begin later in the pollen season than hay fever, and to continue for longer afterward (see page 21).

Some hay fever sufferers may experience asthma in response to other allergens, such as dust mites, mold spores, and skin particles from animals (see chapter 12). This could simply be making the pollen asthma worse during the summer or causing asthma attacks to continue into the winter months. Skin-prick tests (see page 77) are valuable to pinpoint other allergies of this kind.

Most people think of asthmatics as suffering from severe attacks of wheezing and shortness of breath. This is indeed the case for many, but asthma can produce much milder symptoms instead. Feeling tight in the chest, having a persistent dry cough, and feeling short of breath when out in cold air are all possible signs of asthma. For some people, asthma comes on only when they exercise vigorously. If you have any of these symptoms, you should see your doctor for advice.

As well as taking the drugs prescribed for your asthma, it is important to treat the symptoms in your nose. Recent research shows that there is a nerve reflex between the nose and the airways of the lungs (see pages 19–20), and that inflammation in the nose will make the airways more sensitive and prone to asthma attacks. So keep on top of your hay fever or perennial allergic rhinitis if you want to be free of asthma symptoms. Detailed advice about coping with asthma can be found in *Asthma,* by Jonathan Brostoff, M.D., and Linda Gamlin (Healing Arts Press, 2000).

If someone suffers from pollen asthma, heavy exposure to the allergenic pollen should be avoided in case it triggers a severe asthma attack. For example, a child with hay fever and pollen asthma who is sensitive to grass should be kept away from a lawn that is being mowed or a hay meadow being harvested.

It is a good idea to avoid heavily polluted areas if you suffer from asthma because several pollutants can make attacks more likely. The three most heavily implicated are ozone, sulfur dioxide, and acidic droplets (sulfuric acid) in the air. Ozone is most commonly found during the summer. Sulfur dioxide and sulfuric acid droplets are associated with domestic coal fires, industrial areas, and fuel-burning power stations. Further details can be found in appendix 6.

Sulfur dioxide is also used as a preservative in certain foods, and significant amounts may be given off when eating these. Sometimes this is sufficient to bring on an asthmatic attack. If you know that sulfur dioxide affects you badly, you should avoid all foods containing it, or approach individual foods cautiously to see if they affect you. The foods concerned are listed in appendix 7. If you have never reacted badly to any of these foods, there is no need to avoid them.

For anyone with severe asthma, cross-reactions are a potential hazard. Sometimes allergens in pollen cross-react with those in a food, and while most of these reactions to food are mild, they can be vigorous and produce anaphylactic shock (see the box on page 135). This is especially dangerous for an asthmatic. Cross-reactions are described more fully in chapter 11.

Another hazard, but one that is easily avoided, is aspirin. Some asthmatics know that they are sensitive to aspirin (see "Aspirin Sensitivity, Asthma, Rhinitis, and Nasal Polyps" in chapter 13), but others can take aspirin with no apparent ill effects for many years, then suddenly develop a sensitivity to it. A bad reaction to aspirin can be life-threatening, so it is probably best avoided by all asthmatics. These are the aspirin and aspirin-like drugs:

aloxiprin
aspirin
benorylate
choline magnesium trisalicylate
diflunisal
salsalate

Note that these are the generic names of the drugs, not the brand names (which are impractical to list, being so numerous and with new brands introduced all the time). You'll have to read the small print on the packet to find the generic name, and it may be easier just to ask the pharmacist before you buy any drugs. Always buy painkillers, headache remedies, and the like from a pharmacy where you can get expert advice.

Another group of drugs are chemically similar to aspirin and carry the same risk. They are collectively known as nonsteroidal anti-inflammatory drugs, or NSAIDS. The most commonly used drugs are:

felbinac
fenbufen
fenoprofen
flurbiprofen
ibuprofen
ketoprofen
naproxen
tiaprofenic acid

Again, these are generic names, not the more familiar brand names. Most of these are prescribed drugs, used for conditions such as rheumatoid arthritis, but some are available without prescription, as headache remedies and general painkillers. These should not be taken by asthmatics. In the case of prescribed drugs, discuss with your doctor whether these are safe for you to take.

There are many ways in which asthmatics can help themselves. Knowing how to use inhalers properly and understanding when to use the drugs are two essential steps toward coping with asthma. If you feel unsure about these points, do go to see your doctor again—you will not be wasting his or her time. Self-help groups (see appendix 5) can also be very useful.

Using a **peak-flow meter** can also be very valuable. Your doctor should be able to provide you with this piece of equipment and show you how to use it. The meter measures how fast you can expel air from your lungs when breathing out as hard as possible. This gives a good idea of how much narrowing

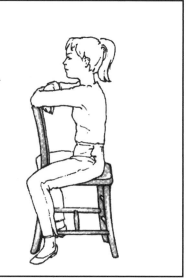

The most important thing to remember during an asthma attack is to stay calm. Sitting upright with your elbows resting on the back of a chair can be helpful. If the back of the chair is not high enough, add a pillow or two. Sitting in this position lifts your rib cage and reduces the amount of muscular effort needed to breathe. A large group of anxious onlookers tends to increase the asthmatic's anxiety and thus make matters worse.

Coping with an asthma attack

there is in your bronchi. Doctors use peak-flow meters in the office to diagnose asthma, especially where the only symptom is a cough or tightness in the chest. At home the peak-flow meter should be used daily and the meter reading recorded. This regular reading helps to show whether or not your asthma is improving in response to drug treatments. It can also identify deterioration in your condition before the effects become noticeable.

Asthma attacks can be frightening, but if one does occur, it is important to stay calm. The emotions play a crucial role in asthma, and anxiety will make the tightening of the airways far worse. (Sometimes attacks are actually triggered by tension and anxiety alone, although there is almost always an underlying cause for the asthmatic condition, usually an allergic one.) For a child, in particular, panicky adults are likely to make matters a great deal worse, whereas a soothing and reassuring person can actually alleviate the attack. For this reason, it is vital not to be overprotective with asthmatic children, and not to make them unduly fearful of their disease. They need to have as much freedom as possible, combined with a realistic understanding of the risks and their own limitations. This rhyme, written by an asthmatic boy with an asthmatic brother, sums up the ideal outlook for a child:

> *Brothers are we,*
> *Both strong as sailors,*
> *But we never go nowhere,*
> *Without our inhalers.*

Make sure that asthmatic children get enough exercise by taking them to an indoor swimming pool, for example, where the amount of pollen in the air will be very low. Vacations by breezy coasts or high in the mountains are also beneficial, since pollen counts are usually low in these places (mountains are also inhospitable to dust mites, if these are an additional allergen).

Chapter 6
DIAGNOSING HAY FEVER AND IDENTIFYING THE POLLEN CONCERNED

Hay fever follows the seasons of the year more closely than any other disease, and for this reason the timing of the symptoms plays a major part in arriving at a diagnosis.

In many parts of the world the hay fever season is so clearly defined that patients can be diagnosed on this alone; if they have the right symptoms, and have them at the right time of year, then hay fever will be considered overwhelmingly likely and no further tests will be carried out.

This approach works when there are just two or three major pollen allergens whose times of release do not overlap too much. The cooler regions of the world are more likely to fall into this category because their vegetation is less varied and the growing season for plants is strictly limited. With only a few warm months available for growing, plants confine flowering to a brief interlude only, although pollen production may be prolific during that time to compensate.

In northeastern Canada, for example, birch pollen and grass pollens are the two major allergens. The birch season runs from May to June, then stops fairly sharply. (Although research shows that people with birch pollen hay fever often react to other plants as well, it is mainly birch pollen that is causing their symptoms.) The grass season occurs in July. Most people with seasonal rhinitis suffer in one or both of these seasons. With only two principal allergens, each having a clear-cut season, skin-prick tests (explained in detail later in this chapter) are not used for the majority of patients. The sharply seasonal nature of the symptoms answers two questions at once: it shows that patients have hay fever rather than some other form of rhinitis *and* it pinpoints the pollen primarily responsible. These are the two major aspects of diagnosis.

This diagnosis-by-season approach tends to be far less useful in warm, moist areas such as Florida, California, and northeastern Australia. Here there is highly varied vegetation, including both native and introduced plants, and some very long pollination seasons. In southern Florida, for example, growing conditions are good all year round, and there is grass pollen in the air during every month. Someone with year-round symptoms might be sensitive to grass pollen, or to mold spores or dust mites, or to some combination of these items. Other pollens might also play a part. The patient could, alternatively, have a nonallergic form of rhinitis (see chapter 13). In such a situation, skin-prick tests or other forms of medical diagnosis are vitally important.

In most regions of Canada and the northern United States the major allergen is ragweed, which pollinates from August to October. However, there are other allergenic weeds pollinating at this time, and skin-prick tests are helpful in pinpointing the culprit pollen. There is also a fairly well-defined grass season, usually from May to July. Those with hay fever symptoms in early spring may be reacting to one of a range of different tree pollens. In these regions, a rough diagnosis can be made on the basis of the season when symptoms occur, but skin-prick tests are useful in reaching an accurate diagnosis.

Appendix 1 lists the major allergenic pollens in different regions of the world, together with their pollination seasons. By noting when your symptoms occur and studying the list for the region where you live, you may well be able to identify your problem pollen. Check the illustration on pages 110 and 111 (or with a local plant or tree field guide) to see if the likely culprit actually grows in the area where you live. If it grows densely in the surrounding area, then you can fairly assume that it is the problem. However, its apparent absence is not proof of its innocence. Pollen can travel for many miles on the warm airstreams of spring and summer, so even if the plant is not growing around your home area, it could still be affecting you. Check what plants grow in the surrounding countryside and in the areas from which the prevailing winds blow.

IS IT ESSENTIAL TO IDENTIFY THE POLLEN CAUSING HAY FEVER?

If it is not obvious which pollen causes your hay fever, you may be wondering whether it is crucial to identify your problem pollen and whether you should therefore pay a visit to your doctor.

For those people who can control their hay fever symptoms well enough using antihistamines or other medicinal drugs, the answer to this is probably no. For those who do well with general avoidance measures, such as keeping windows closed when they have hay fever, the answer may also be no.

Identifying the pollen becomes important only if your symptoms are really troublesome and you want to try taking more specific avoidance measures—then you do need to know which plant causes your symptoms. Occasionally, the plant is growing in a very limited area indeed and can actually be eliminated. For example, one patient with hay fever and pollen asthma discovered, through skin-prick tests, that the cause of the trouble was cypress pollen. Since she lived in a rural area of Australia, and the row of trees lining the driveway to her house were the only cypresses for miles around, eliminating cypress pollen from her life was a simple task.

The other situation in which it may be vital to identify your problem pollen is if you intend to travel abroad. The culprit pollen may be far more common at your destination than in the area where you currently live, resulting in a severe hay fever reaction that could spoil your trip. For example, someone with hay fever to "tree pollen" might travel to Sweden during May (when birch pollen counts can reach 3,000 grains per cubic meter of air) and discover, to his or her cost, that the previously unidentified "tree" causing the problem was birch.

DIAGNOSTIC TESTS FROM THE DOCTOR

The tests a doctor can offer you show whether your body *could* mount an allergic reaction to a particular pollen, not whether it actually does so. They are rather like the test used for the brakes of an elderly car: if this shows that the brakes are not all that good any more, it suggests that the car might become involved in an accident. The brake test does not predict absolutely that the car will have an accident tomorrow, because other factors are involved besides the condition of the brakes.

The medical test most commonly used for hay fever involves introducing a small amount of a specific pollen allergen—grass pollen, for example—into the skin and then seeing what reaction this provokes. If there is a reaction, this shows that the allergy antibody IgE (see "The Two Ends of the Antibody Molecule" in chapter 3) is present in the skin, and that it is an IgE specific for grass pollen allergens. That is as far as the test goes. It does not show that the person tested has hay fever to grass.

The interpretation of the test is based on previous medical research and runs as follows: If there is IgE to grass pollen allergens in the skin, then there are probably identical IgE antibodies in the nose, and if these are present in the nose, they could produce grass pollen hay fever. However, this is by no means certain. As explained in chapter 3, the body has a great many different ways of regulating allergy, and even though it has produced IgE against grass pollen, it could well have seen the error of its ways and instigated a control mechanism to keep that IgE in check.

Skin tests, then, are only a clue to the nature of your rhinitis. They should always be looked at in the light of other evidence, such as the time of year when you suffer symptoms and the local types of vegetation. In this way, they can be used to confirm a suspicion about particular pollen allergens.

Alternatively, if someone has rhinitis all year round, a skin test can be used to suggest likely allergens, such as dust-mite and cat allergens. These suspects must then be investigated in other ways—usually by trying to eliminate or avoid them and seeing if there is any improvement in the symptoms.

The Skin-Prick Test

This is the most commonly used skin test for classical allergies. A slightly different technique, the puncture test, is preferred by some doctors. The term "prick-punture test" covers both these techniques, which are very similar. A third variant, the scratch test, is also used by a few doctors, but is losing popularity because the results are less consistent.

The skin-prick test is usually carried out on the lower part of the arm, using the soft, hairless skin on the inner surface. Sometimes the skin on the back is tested instead. An extract of the allergen is used, with a single drop being placed on the skin. A pointed instrument known as a lancet is then used to lift the skin under the drop, puncturing it slightly so that some of the allergen extract enters the skin. This process is repeated for each of the allergens to be tested, usually 10 or more, and sometimes up to 30. Surplus extract is dabbed off, and the skin is left to react for between 10 and 20 minutes. At the end of this time, the area of skin around each prick test is examined for signs of inflammation—this reveals whether the skin contains IgE antibody specific for that allergen. If there is any reaction, the size of the bump around the test site gives a rough idea of how strong that reaction is.

Antihistamine drugs, which can be bought without prescription, will interfere with skin-prick tests by inhibiting the reactions to allergen. If you are taking antihistamines and require a skin-prick test, you must stop taking the drugs at least two days before the test. Since the test is quick and easy, it will probably be carried out at a first appointment, so it is worth stopping antihistamines before you see the allergist for the first time—assuming that you can manage without them. Always inform the doctor that you have been, or are taking, antihistamines.

After the skin-prick test, you may suffer a delayed reaction at one or more of the test sites. This can come on many hours later and can produce a large bump that is painful or itchy. It is just one example of the late-phase reaction (see "The Late-phase Reaction" in chapter 3). Should you experience such a reaction, it is nothing to worry about, and it will clear spontaneously within a day or so.

Intradermal Testing

In many countries, including the United States and Canada, skin-prick testing (described above) is used almost exclusively, and intradermal testing is rarely practiced. In some other parts of the world, however, intradermal testing is still the norm.

This test involves using a larger amount of allergen (but a weaker concentration) than the skin-prick test and injecting it a little more deeply into the skin. As more allergen is used, there is a very small risk of **anaphylactic shock,** a major allergic reaction involving the whole body, which can be fatal if not treated promptly (see the box "Anaphylactic Shock" in chapter 9). If you suffer from asthma (whether to pollen or to some other allergen), make sure the doctor knows this before intradermal testing is carried out—the dangers of anaphylaxis are higher for anyone with asthma.

Blood Tests

These are tests for the amount of IgE (the allergy antibody) in the blood. Usually the test is for a particular type of IgE, such as IgE to grass pollen antigens. There are two versions of this test, whose technical names are the radioallergosorbent test (RAST, for short) and the enzyme-linked immunosorbent assay (ELISA, for short).

Such a test is far more expensive and troublesome than a skin-prick test, yet it does not tell the doctor very much more. One occasion when it might be used is for a patient with a severe skin disorder that prevents a skin-prick test being carried out. It can also be valuable for patients taking antihistamines who are unable to stop taking them even for a few days for skin testing. Finally, there are patients who might be given a RAST rather than a skin test because they have suffered anaphylactic shock in the past and are regarded as a high-risk case by the doctor. This is probably overcautious, as anaphylactic reactions to skin-prick tests are virtually unknown, but given the severity and danger of anaphylactic shock, caution is probably wise.

The total amount of IgE in the blood (rather than particular types of IgE) can also be measured. This is rarely done for adults, as it does not generally tell the doctor anything useful. However, it may be a valuable test for new-borns who are considered at risk of allergy (see page 245).

Intranasal Provocation Tests

In chapter 4, the pioneering studies of Charles Harrison Blackley were de-scribed. This 19th-century doctor, as you may remember, was a hay fever suf-ferer himself and the first to identify the true cause of hay fever. He did so by saving pollen during the summer, then inhaling it in midwinter to see what

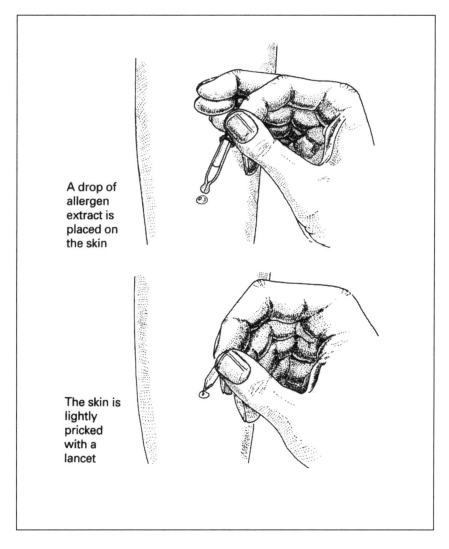

A drop of allergen extract is placed on the skin

The skin is lightly pricked with a lancet

The skin-prick test

happened. He sneezed, and the rest is history. This seems to be the best, simplest, and most direct test for hay fever, so why is it not used by doctors today? The answer is that a test of this type *has* sometimes been used in the past; it is known as a **nasal provocation test.** But it has fallen from favor because it is difficult to "standardize"—that is, to ensure that all patients are given the same dose of pollen allergen and to measure their reaction in an accurate and scientific way. There is also some risk of provoking a severe reaction in the nose or, worse, an asthma attack.

However, if you are sufficiently curious about the cause of your hay fever and have not managed to identify the pollen responsible by the usual routes, then you could follow in Blackley's footsteps. Collect a few different pollens for comparison. Be very cautious about how much pollen you inhale—begin with the tiniest of pinches, spread it out on your hand, and sniff very gently. *(Do not try this method at all if you have ever had an asthma attack.)* If there is no reaction, try a larger sniff. You may need to repeat this daily for a few days to get a reaction.

For a truly scientific approach, you should label the containers on the base and not look at the label until you have carried out all the tests. In other words, test each pollen without knowing what it is at the time. This avoids the result being biased by your expectations. Test one pollen each day, without looking at the label either before or afterward. Slip the container into an envelope that you have labeled with the day and any symptoms you experienced. Repeat this until you have tested all the pollens, then open the envelopes to see which plants provoked your symptoms.

LIMITATIONS OF SKIN TESTING

Standard forms of testing available from the doctor have certain limitations. One that has already been mentioned is the chance of a **false positive**—a positive skin test (or blood test) to a pollen or other allergen that does not actually cause symptoms. It occurs fairly frequently, especially with dust-mite allergen.

The opposite can also occur—the skin test can be negative even though the person *does* have symptoms in response to that allergen. This **false negative** reaction is most unusual, however. It occurs only when there is IgE for a particular pollen in the lining of the nose but none in the skin. An allergist will usually look into such discrepancies using a nasal provocation test, although this too has its problems, described earlier.

Compared to the skin-prick test, the intradermal test has a greater chance of a false positive reaction and a lesser chance of a false negative.

One major shortcoming of all tests is that they can find only what they

BARBARA

Barbara's day always began with a bout of exhausting sneezes. Wherever she lived it was the same. She had moved from New York to Israel to Britain, but the sneezing always followed her. During the rest of the day she suffered from a constant runny nose.

Several doctors had wondered if she might be allergic to dust mites, and had given her skin-prick tests, but none was positive. Some had gone further and tested her blood for IgE antibodies to dust mites, but again there was nothing. Finally, an allergist decided to test her nose directly. She carried out the test several times, sometimes puffing dust into Barbara's nose, sometimes an inert powder. Barbara was never told which it was, so her reaction was not prejudiced. The house dust produced severe sneezing and watery mucus, while the inert powder did not. Clearly, Barbara was allergic to something in house dust, probably dust mites. Although she was quite severely allergic, the skin tests and blood tests did not show this. Such **false negative** tests can happen with medical tests because the allergy antibodies (IgE) may be present in the nose but not in the skin or bloodstream. Although this is relatively unusual, doctors should always bear in mind that it can happen. Reducing the mite population in her house (see "House Dust" in chapter 12) produced a remarkable improvement in Barbara's health.

look for—and they mostly look for reactions to common allergens. If you are allergic to anything out of the ordinary, it is unlikely that the allergen concerned will be included in the set of extracts that the doctor has available. Some allergists will make up their own extracts to test likely suspects.

Occasionally, patients have strong suspicions about a particular pollen, only to be told that it cannot possibly be a cause of hay fever. This may happen with garden flowers (which are pollinated by insects) and with pine trees, both of which have gone down in medical lore as *never* causing hay fever. It is true that these two groups are not often implicated in hay fever, but there are plenty of exceptions among both insect-pollinated plants and conifers (see "Bees or Breeze?" in chapter 1).

UNSUSPECTED ALLERGENS?

Until the late 1970s, tests for cockroach allergy were rarely carried out in the United States. Then allergists began testing for this particular sensitivity and found that it was remarkably common. Up to 30 percent of people with allergies are sensitive to the feces and skin particles of cockroaches. In some inner-city areas in the southern states, where the warm climate suits cockroaches perfectly, they are the most common cause of allergy.

Looking at a range of houses and using sensitive techniques to detect cockroach allergens, researchers found evidence of them in most samples of house dust. Even houses with no sign of cockroach infestation could show cockroach allergens in their dust, suggesting that if cockroaches are common in an area, they may pay flying visits to every house on the street.

When the researchers looked at commercial extracts of house dust used for skin testing, they found that some contained cockroach allergens while others did not. Thus, a person with cockroach allergy might seem to be sensitive to house dust on the basis of one test, but if tested with house-dust extract produced by a different company, the test would be negative.

One intriguing aspect of cockroach allergy is that in cool climates cockroach numbers fall in winter and rise in the warm summer months. The amount of cockroach allergen in the air follows suit. Thus, someone with a runny nose or asthma due to cockroach particles might suffer symptoms only during summer or might get much worse then. At present, such people would undoubtedly be diagnosed as having hay fever. If a skin-prick test were carried out, it could show no reactions to any of the allergens included, or it could show positive reactions to some allergens, including pollens. This might indicate that the patient is allergic to pollens as well as to cockroach allergen, or the pollen reaction could be a false positive. Either way, the patient would probably be diagnosed as having hay fever when, in fact, this has little or nothing to do with the symptoms. The error should be obvious to the patient, because there will be far more symptoms indoors than outdoors. (This is unlikely to happen with hay fever unless you have a source of pollen indoors—see pages 112–118—or you live in a tower block; see page 112.) It is up to the patient to impress this fact on the doctor and to ask for a further set of tests.

Other insect allergies may also be more widespread than is commonly thought. Researchers in Japan decided to test this idea using skin-prick tests, and found a remarkable number of people who were allergic to insects such as silkworms and caddis flies. These are insects that generate a lot of airborne particles at certain times of year, and again they could produce seasonal symptoms that resemble hay fever (see the box "Cross-Reactions Involving Airborne Allergens" in chapter 12).

Could there be pollens that are a widespread cause of hay fever but are not usually included in skin tests? Probably not, but there may be some exceptions. Scientists trapping pollen at the University of Cordoba in southern Spain found very large amounts of cypress pollen in the air during the winter months. They asked local doctors about cypress allergy and were told that it was unknown—but since no one tested for it, this was hardly surprising. Eventually, the doctors were persuaded to include cypress pollen extract in their skin tests, and it turned out that cypress hay fever was quite common in the Cordoba region. Because the trees pollinate in winter, patients with this problem had always been diagnosed as having a prolonged cold, and therefore had been treated with entirely inappropriate medicines.

Ferns are another unexpected source of allergies. They produce large numbers of tiny spores that can generate new fern plants. The documented cases of fern allergy that have reached the scientific journals so far concern ferns kept as houseplants. One woman had suffered from persistent sneezing and a constant runny nose for two years before her doctor pointed the finger of suspicion at the large fern in her living room. Although her symptoms were present most of the time, they were much worse at home. Could spores from outdoor ferns—plants that are common in some areas, usually in cooler climates—have kept the reaction going? Possibly, but the fact that removing the fern from her home put a stop to the symptoms suggests that they were not a major factor. How widespread fern allergy is nobody knows. Again, it is something that is rarely tested for.

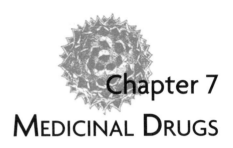

Chapter 7
MEDICINAL DRUGS

Attitudes toward drugs present one of the most curious paradoxes of the modern age. On the one hand, there are a surprising number of people in our society who celebrate Saturday evening by sniffing an anonymous white powder or swallowing an unlabeled white tablet, the powder or tablet being of unknown composition and bought from a dubious character with absolutely no qualifications in pharmacy. Many more people regularly inhale another drug, supplied in a package that is clearly labeled CAUSES LUNG CANCER. At the other extreme, large numbers of people are terrified of taking any tablets, even those whose ingredients are known and carefully standardized, produced by reputable pharmaceutical companies, tested extensively for safety, and approved by the government.

In between these two extreme groups, the rest of the population hovers uncertainly, not sure whether medicinal drugs are a blessing or an insidious threat to its health. One of the problems lies in the word "drug" itself, which includes everything from cough medicine to crack cocaine in one great tar-spreading brush stroke. The well-publicized scandals involving medicinal drugs, notably those about *thalidomide* and Opren, have kept the fears going, and for many people the sense of mistrust is extended indiscriminately to all medicines.

In the case of allergy, particularly hay fever, we believe that this is unfortunate and deprives many people of the most useful help they can obtain. Drugs are not the only form of help, as the next two chapters will make clear, but they are not an option to be dismissed lightly, especially if your symptoms interfere with your life to any degree. Spring and summer are the best times of year—times to be enjoyed rather than endured.

Compared to the risk of driving down a highway for an hour, the risk of taking an antihistamine is, for most people, very low indeed. Driving a car is dangerous, however good a driver you may be, but few of us give up driving because of the risks. Occasionally spending an evening in a room full of cigarette smoke is slightly dangerous, but who would give up socializing to avoid this remote risk of lung cancer? In other words, we take some risks all the time, unconsciously weighing them against our pleasure or convenience and deciding that the pleasure is worth the risk. Enjoying the sunny summer months is a pleasure one should not forgo unnecessarily.

This chapter is intended to inform you fully about the drawbacks, side effects, and risks of the drugs available for hay fever, other forms of rhinitis, and asthma. It does not minimize them but instead presents them in full. It explains, as far as possible, how the drugs work and why they may cause side effects. With this information you know what the "cons" are. Discovering the "pros" is up to you—you would have to try the drugs and see how much they help you. Once you know both the pros and the cons, you can make a balanced and rational decision about taking drugs.

For anyone who is already taking medicines, this chapter can be of use in two ways. First, it can help to identify alternative drugs that may control the symptoms of hay fever or pollen more effectively, or simply cause fewer side effects. Second, the chapter explains how to get more out of the drugs by using them more effectively. Many people with hay fever do not get the full benefits of the medicines they take because they start them too late in the season.

If you are already taking a medicine and do not know exactly what type of drug it is, you can use appendix 4 to find out. There, and in the text that follows, the generic names of drugs (names that are used worldwide) are shown in italic (e.g., *chlorpheniramine*), while the trade names or brand names used in the United States are shown with a capital letter (e.g., Aller-chlor, Chlor-Pro, Phenetron, or Teldrin. With nonprescription drugs, the generic name of the drug used is always given on the packet, although you may have to look hard for it. There are sometimes two drugs in a medicine, so be sure to check both drugs in appendix 4 and to read the information on each.

The information given here is intended as a guide only. If you buy nonprescription medicines and feel you need further information, ask to speak to the pharmacist at the store where you buy them. The pharmacist can advise you on the safety of the medicine and whether you should consult your doctor before taking it. With prescription drugs, be sure to tell the doctor about anything that may be relevant to the choice of drug, such as other nonprescription drugs you are taking or high alcohol consumption, or if you are pregnant or trying to conceive.

MAST-CELL STABILIZERS

There are only two well-established drugs in this category at present, *cromolyn* and *nedocromil*. They are very safe drugs, with fewer risks or side effects than any of the other anti-allergy medicines.

How They Work

These drugs are thought to tackle the allergic reaction at an early point by making mast cells more stable—that is, less likely to discharge their granules (see "The Mighty Mast Cell" in chapter 3). However, there is some question about exactly how they work. Whatever their effect, they need to reach the mast cell before the allergen does.

Minor Side Effects

Sneezing, stinging, and smarting are fairly common reactions, but they are not a cause for concern as long as they pass quickly—which they usually do. With inhalers and nebulizers containing these drugs, there can be a transient cough as a result of throat irritation. Rinsing out the mouth with water after inhaling the drug will reduce these side effects.

On rare occasions, when used as a nose spray or as an asthma treatment, these drugs have actually brought on an attack of asthmatic wheezing. If this happens, consult your doctor.

Even more rarely, there can be a true allergic reaction to the drug, in which case it must be discontinued immediately. You should see your doctor if you have these side effects or if you suffer a rash.

Precautions and Interactions

Cromolyn is considered safe for use by anyone, even pregnant women and breastfeeding mothers. *Nedocromil* should not be taken during pregnancy.

Usefulness

Suitable for symptoms in the eye or nose, and for asthma. These drugs do not work for everyone, but when they do work they are very effective. Since they are so safe and free of side effects, they are worth trying.

Mast-cell stabilizers are particularly useful for young children if the doctor is reluctant to prescribe corticosteroid nose drops.

In the case of eye drops, those containing mast-cell stabilizers are considered much safer than corticosteroid drops.

How Taken

Eye drops for conjunctivitis. These contain *cromolyn* (Opticrom).
Nasal spray or drops for hay fever. These contain *cromolyn* (Rynacrom, Nasalcrom).
Aerosols, nebulizers, or spinhalers for asthma. These contain *cromolyn* (Intal), or *nedocromil* (Tilade).

Maximizing the Benefits

With mast-cell stabilizers, it is important to take them before encountering your problem pollen. If they get to the mast cell before the allergen, they are far more effective in stalling the allergic reaction. An asthma attack that has already begun cannot be relieved with this drug. However, some patients with hay fever do find that they are helped by these drugs, even after the symptoms have appeared.

The benefits gradually build up, particularly with asthma and perennial (year-round) rhinitis. It can take up to six weeks of regular dosage for the antiasthma effect to be established. With eye and nose symptoms due to pollen, the good effects are seen much more quickly, usually within a few days. But it is important that you use the drug regularly, and at the correct intervals, to gain the full benefit. Some doctors recommend starting the drug two or three weeks before the pollen season to ensure maximum effectiveness. The nose drops need to be used at least four times a day, so if you lead a hectic life and are not much good at remembering such things, this may not be the best drug for you.

With nose drops, a nose that is already profoundly blocked may be impermeable to the drops. In such cases, drops or spray containing an unblocking agent called a **sympathomimetic** (see page 94–96) can be useful, in the short term, for opening up the nose to the mast-cell stabilizer, but they should not be taken for too long.

Some good effects will persist for several days after the treatment is stopped, but if you have asthma, or if the pollen season is still in progress, you should not discontinue the drug suddenly without consulting your doctor.

ANTIHISTAMINES

These are the drugs most widely used for hay fever. There are several kinds that can be bought without a prescription because they are considered very safe.

How They Work

Antihistamines work by interfering with the activities of histamine. This is a mediator (chemical messenger) released by mast cells (see "The Mighty Mast Cell" in chapter 3), the cells that cause the allergic reaction. Although mast cells release several different mediators, histamine is probably the most powerful of them all.

When histamine is released into the bloodstream by mast cells, it affects the blood vessels themselves and certain muscles, known as smooth muscles. These smooth muscles are the ones over which we have no voluntary control, such as those in the bronchi, the digestive system, and the bladder. Histamine makes these muscles contract, and the effect is particularly noticeable in the bronchi, where muscle contraction causes narrowing of the airways—an asthma attack. The effect of histamine on the blood vessels is to make them more leaky, so that immune cells can escape into the surrounding tissue—part of the process of inflammation. Histamine also has several other actions that promote inflammation.

Histamine exerts its effects by binding to **receptors** on its target cells—cells lining the blood vessels, for example. When histamine binds, the receptor molecule passes on a message to the cell itself—it is rather like a doorbell that can be rung only by one specific messenger, histamine. Antihistamines work by being a little bit like histamine—similar enough to bind to the receptor, but not similar enough to make the receptor "ring the bell" of the cell. They block the path of histamine so that it cannot bind to the receptor.

Like many of the chemical messengers in the body, histamine has a number of different jobs. It is released by various other cells in the body, not just mast cells, but in these cases histamine simply acts as a local messenger substance, carrying instructions to cells in the immediate vicinity only.

To allow messenger substances to have multiple jobs in the body, there is usually more than one type of receptor for each messenger. Cells in the brain, for example, may have a different kind of receptor from cells in the heart, so that the messenger can have different effects on each. In the case of histamine, three types of receptor are known, called Hl, H2, and H3. It is the Hl receptors that are involved in the inflammation response and which antihistamines block. The proper pharmaceutical name for antihistamines is "histamine Hl-receptor antagonists." They do not bind to the second type of receptor for histamine, the H2 receptor, which is found in the lining of the stomach.

Minor Side Effects

There is a range of antihistamines on the market, some of which have been in use for decades while others are relatively new. A full list of those taken in tablet or liquid form is given below. Antihistamines in drops and sprays are listed under "How Taken" on page 92.

Older Antihistamines:

(Several of these older antihistamines are also available combined with a sympathomimetic—see page 96)

azatadine (Optimine)

brompheniramine (Dimetane, Veltane)

chlorpheniramine (Aller-chlor, Chlor-Pro, Phenetron, Teldrin)

clemastine (Contac Allergy 12 Hour, Tavist)

cyproheptadine (Periactin)

diphenhydramine (Allerdryl, Allermax)

hydroxyzine (Atarax, Apo-Hydroxyzine, Multipax, Vistaryl, Vistazine)

phenindamine (Nolahist)

pheniramine (available only in combination with a sympathomimetic drug)

promethazine (Anergan, Phenazine, Phenergan, Prothazine)

trimeprazine (Temaril)

triprolidine (Myidyl)

Nonsedating antihistamines:

acrivastine (Semprex)

cetirizine (Zyrtek)

fexofenadine (Allegra)

loratadine (Claritin, Claritin RediTabs)

mizolastine (Mizollen)

The older types have quite a few side effects, notably drowsiness. There can also be dizziness, nervousness, tremors, stomach upsets, dry mouth, blurred vision, and, occasionally, impotence. In children, they sometimes have the opposite effect to drowsiness, making the child hyperactive. They have these effects because part of the histamine molecule is quite similar, chemically speaking, to some other messenger substances, including **adrenaline, serotonin,** and

acetylcholine. All these substances are involved in passing messages between nerve cells. Because of the chemical similarities, antihistamines can bind to some of the receptors for these nerve-cell messengers, partially blocking their action. Drowsiness results from antihistamines blocking the action of adrenaline; the dry mouth and stomach upsets are a result of their blocking acetylcholine.

Anything affecting the nervous system has very noticeable effects, even if the degree of interference is actually quite small and causes no serious damage. This is generally the case with antihistamines, and the side effects are usually nothing to worry about—they should certainly not discourage you from trying a different antihistamine. Having said this, a minority of people do need to be careful about taking antihistamines because of preexisting medical problems; these are listed under "Precautions and interactions" on page 91.

As everyone's body chemistry is different, these symptoms will be experienced to different degrees. Some people can even take the old-type antihistamines with no side effects at all. Others find that the side effects vanish if they persist in taking the antihistamines. The disappearance of the side effects is due to an adjustment of the receptor-messenger interactions that were involved, and it is most unlikely that any damaging long-term effects are occurring. At the end of the pollen season, when antihistamines are no longer being taken, the system will shift back to its original equilibrium.

Although the side effects of antihistamines can be distressing, they are not indicative of any major damage being done to the body. The only two side effects to be a major cause for concern with most antihistamines are a skin rash and hyperactivity in children. If either of these occurs, stop taking the drug and consult your doctor.

Indirect harm is the greatest danger with antihistamines, because drowsiness is risky if you are driving a car or working close to machinery. It is important to check the effects of antihistamines before getting behind the wheel. This is less of a problem with the newer, nonsedating antihistamines (see below), but even with these you should proceed cautiously at first. Note that alcohol and other sedatives will make any such side effects far worse.

The newer, nonsedating antihistamines have more difficulty in crossing the barrier that exists between the bloodstream and the brain, so fewer antihistamine molecules reach the brain. They should not cause any drowsiness, although a few people do still find that they have this effect.

If you have tried one of these newer antihistamines and still suffered side effects, it is well worth trying another one. They are different chemically, and there may be one that is just right for you. If you have found that they make you sleepy when combined with alcohol, try *cetirizine* or *loratadine,* neither of which has this effect.

Precautions and Interactions

There are a few situations in which antihistamines *might* be genuinely harmful. You should discuss the matter with a pharmacist or doctor if any of the following apply:

- You are pregnant or breast-feeding (see "Coping with Hay Fever or Asthma When Pregnant" later in this chapter)

- You have epilepsy, even *petit mal,* in which case the side effects on the nervous system may be problematic

- You have liver or kidney problems, or urinary retention

- You have glaucoma

- You have prostate enlargement

- You are taking antidepressants, anti-anxiety drugs, or sedatives

- You have a thyroid disorder

- You have a heart condition or high blood pressure

- You have porphyria

- You have a stomach or duodenal ulcer

- You have Parkinson's disease

One of the newer antihistamines, *mizolastine* (Mizollen), has occasionally had side effects on the heart, causing abnormal heart rhythms. The same precautions apply as with other antihistamines (see above), but in addition you should:

- Take care never to exceed the stated dose

- Avoid drinking grapefruit juice, except in small amounts

- Tell your doctor if you have ever suffered from abnormal heart rhythm, or any other heart disease that he or she may not know about

- If you have liver disease, make sure your doctor remembers this when prescribing *mizolastine*

- Remind your doctor about other prescription medicines you are taking, and mention any nonprescription medicines. You should not take *erythromycin* or *ketoconazole* while taking *mizolastine*. Certain other drugs may also interact with this antihistamine.

Usefulness

Antihistamines are very effective in reducing most of the symptoms of hay fever, but they do not relieve a blocked nose. For this reason, they are often combined with a sympathomimetic (see the following section). Corticosteroids, given as drops or spray, are useful for reducing nasal congestion, but not if the nose is absolutely blocked. In such cases, sympathomimetic drops or spray may be used first to open up the nose for the corticosteroid; alternatively, corticosteroid tablets may sometimes be used (see page 103).

In the case of asthma, antihistamines are not particularly helpful. This is because asthma is a complex reaction in which other mediators besides histamine play a major role. The medicines used for asthma are described in the last two sections of this chapter.

Certain antihistamines have other actions as well and therefore deserve a special mention. *Ketotifen* (Zaditen) acts as both an antihistamine and a mast-cell stabilizer. It has proved useful in preventing asthma attacks, but may have side effects similar to those of the older antihistamines. This drug is available in Canada but not in the United States.

If antihistamines are taken regularly for many years, they may eventually become less effective. Switching to another form of treatment, such as corticosteroid nose drops or a mast-cell stabilizer, may be the best course of action in such circumstances.

How Taken

Antihistamines are mainly taken by mouth in tablet, capsule, or liquid form. They are carried around the body in the bloodstream and reach the nose and eyes in this way. Many can be bought without a prescription, but if none of these works for you, it might be worth asking your doctor about those available on prescription.

Eye drops containing antihistamines are also available for anyone with conjunctivitis. The new antihistamine *levocabastine* is especially good for eye symptoms, and is found in drops under the brand name Livostin. There are also older types of eye drops that contain the antihistamine *antazoline* combined with a sympathomimetic (in Otrivine-Antistin, for example). The presence of the sympathomimetic means that such drops should not be used for too long, but a few weeks is probably safe.

Levocabastine, which is highly specific in its effects and a very powerful blocker of histamine, is also available as a nasal spray which, like the eye drops, is also sold under the brand name Livostin. Alternatively, there is *azelastine* (Astelin), which is also very effective. Current trends in drug use favor drops and sprays, which put the drug exactly where it is most needed. This more precise targeting of drugs means that the dosage can be much smaller, minimizing possible effects on other parts of the body.

Maximizing the Benefits

A knowledge of how antihistamines work can help in using them to best effect. To do their job, the antihistamine molecules must bind to the Hl receptors for histamine before histamine arrives. If histamine is already there and securely bound, the antihistamine cannot dislodge it. In time, the histamine will become detached from the receptor naturally, and an antihistamine can then take its place, but by then the allergic reaction will already have begun, and the most the antihistamine can do is to prevent the next influx of histamine from making matters worse.

Once some histamine has been let loose and has bound its receptors, various changes take place that make the nose and eyes far more sensitive to pollen—the effect known as "priming" (see "Priming" in chapter 3). Among other changes, more mast cells and basophils will gather in the nose, so more histamine can be released next time. This makes the task of the antihistamine far more difficult.

For these reasons, starting antihistamines a little *before* the hay fever season, and continuing them without a break, makes excellent sense. They can give far better results for the same dosage, and may even allow the dosage to be lower. If you do not have a personal record of when your hay fever symptoms began in the past, you can use appendix 1 to work out when your problem pollen is likely to become airborne. Start taking the antihistamines a few days beforehand, or a week to be on the safe side. For summertime pollens, such as those of grasses, the season will begin up to three weeks earlier if the spring weather has been unusually warm, so adjust the time accordingly. Some pollen information services, such as those available on special hotlines or the Internet, include a prediction of when the grass pollen season will begin.

Acrivastine (Semprex) is faster acting than other antihistamines and is useful as a "rescue" treatment. It is not available in Canada, but in the United States it can be purchased over the counter.

SYMPATHOMIMETICS IN NOSE DROPS, NOSE SPRAYS, OR EYE DROPS

These drugs are for short-term use only. As long as this point is understood, they are very safe. They are widely available without prescription and, unfortunately, are often misused.

How They Work

Sympathomimetics are drugs that mimic the effects of naturally produced adrenaline, the messenger molecule that produces the "flight or fight" reaction. Adrenaline has various effects, but one is to make the small blood vessels (capillaries) contract. Thus, it has an opposing effect to histamine.

By applying a drug that mimics adrenaline, the blood vessels in the nose can be persuaded to contract. This immediately reduces nasal congestion and makes it easier to breathe. If there is blockage of the sinuses or the Eustachian tube (see "No Nose Is an Island unto Itself" in chapter 2), this will be relieved. When the drug is applied directly to the nose, only a very small dose is needed, and there should be little effect on the rest of the body.

Sympathomimetics are also included in some eye drops to reduce redness, swelling, and pain.

Minor Side Effects

As with most nose sprays, there may be some irritation at first. Stinging can also occur with eye drops, and there may be some blurring of vision. Check that you are not affected by this before driving a car.

If significant amounts are absorbed from the nose into the bloodstream, effects will be noted similar to those of adrenaline: a faster or more noticeable heartbeat, irritability, insomnia, and headache. Reduce the dose and these effects should disappear. These side effects are harmless to most people, but may pose a risk to some because of other medical conditions (see below).

Precautions and Interactions

For certain people, even a small amount of sympathomimetic reaching the bloodstream can pose some risk. Older people should use a lower dose, and young children should not be given these drugs at all. Discuss the use of these drugs with a pharmacist or doctor if any of the following apply:

- You have a heart condition

- You have high blood pressure

- You have epilepsy

- You have a thyroid disorder

- You are taking antidepressants (monoamine oxidase inhibitor–type) or have taken them within the past two weeks

- You have glaucoma

- You are pregnant

The major risk with nose drops and sprays containing sympathomimetics, and one that affects everybody using them, is that the nose itself can become dependent on them. This usually occurs when the drops are used for more than two weeks, but it can happen more quickly, after just five days of continuous treatment. If you then stop using the drops, the nose goes "cold turkey" and becomes completely blocked. The medical term for this is **rebound congestion.** Continuing with the drops will not solve the problem because the nose will gradually become more blocked, and increasing the dosage will produce side effects on the heart.

Once the drops are discontinued, the rebound congestion will slowly sort itself out and the nose will return to normal, but the intervening period may be most uncomfortable.

It is vital with sympathomimetics to use the drops or spray as recommended on the package, and never to increase the amount or take an extra dose. If you find that your nose is becoming more congested, or the effects of each treatment do not last as long, then begin to phase them out. Even if the drops are working well, you should stop using them as soon as you can, preferably within a few days. Never continue for more than 14 days.

If you experience any pain in the eye, palpitations, or chest pain, stop using the drops immediately.

In the case of eye drops containing sympathomimetics, these can generally be continued safely for a few weeks, but ask your pharmacist's advice.

Usefulness

For instantaneous relief of a blocked nose, sympathomimetics applied directly to the problem are unrivaled, but it must be remembered that they are not treating the underlying condition. You could find them useful at the very height of the hay fever season or at a time when a blocked nose is a serious problem—when taking an exam or giving a speech, for example. They can also be useful occasionally if your blocked nose is preventing you from sleeping well.

The nose can also be unblocked in other ways, such as inhalations and with nasal drops containing salt water (see "Treatments to Unblock the Nose" in chapter 10). Neither of these will give such dramatic relief as sympathomimetics.

One major use of sympathomimetic nose drops and sprays is in opening up a blocked nose for the delivery of other drugs, such as corticosteroids and mast-cell stabilizers. Use them only for three to five days.

How Taken

Nose drops and sprays. The main ones available are *oxymetazoline* (Afrin, Genasal, Nostrilla, Sinarest), *naphazoline* (Privine), *phenylephrine* (Alconefrin, Neosynephrine, Sinex), *tetrahydrozoline* (Tyzine), and *xylometazoline* (Otrivin). **Eye drops or nose drops, combined with another drug,** principally antihistamines (as in Dristan Nasal Spray and Otrivine-Antistin).

Maximizing the Benefits

Since you cannot use them for long, save sympathomimetic nose drops for when they can be most helpful—at the height of the pollen season, for example.

ANTIHISTAMINES AND SYMPATHOMIMETICS COMBINED IN TABLETS OR LIQUID

Another use for sympathomimetics is in a mixture with antihistamines, to be taken by mouth. All the mixtures contain the older type of antihistamines.

How They Work

Antihistamines tackle the allergic reaction (see "Antihistamines" earlier in this chapter), while sympathomimetics help to unblock the nose and overcome the sedative effect of the antihistamines.

Ideally, the side effects of the two drugs should cancel each other out: the "speed-you-up" effect of the sympathomimetic should counteract the "slow-you-down" of the antihistamine. At the same time, the sympathomimetic relieves the one symptom that antihistamines have little effect on: nasal blockage.

Minor Side Effects

The sort of side effects occurring with sympathomimetic nose drops (see previous section) can also occur when taking a mixture of antihistamine and sympathomimetic by mouth, but they are unusual. The drowsiness and other side effects typical of antihistamines (see "Antihistamines" earlier in this chapter) are more likely.

Precautions and Interactions

Those listed under "Antihistamines" also apply here.

Some of the risks associated with sympathomimetic nose drops also apply here, and anyone with a heart condition, thyroid disorder, or glaucoma should not take these tablets (see "Precautions and Interactions" in previous section). It would be a good idea to talk to the pharmacist before taking one of these mixtures, as there are several other medical conditions that make them unsuitable.

The problem of rebound congestion (see page 95) rarely occurs with these preparations, since the amount of sympathomimetic included is small, and they are not applied directly to the nose.

Usefulness

These mixtures were developed before the new antihistamines came on the market, at a time when all antihistamines had a sedative effect on a high proportion of patients. To a large extent, these mixtures have been superseded by the new non-sedating antihistamines, but they may still be useful, particularly if your nose is badly blocked when you have hay fever.

How Taken

The antihistamines used are mostly the same as the older antihistamines that can be taken alone (see "Antihistamines"). The sympathomimetics used are often different from those found in nose drops and sprays but have much the same effect. Although usually taken as tablets, liquid forms are also available.

Antihistamine/Sympathomimetic Mixtures

Brand name	Antihistamine	Sympathomimetic
Actifed	*diphenhydramine*	*pseudoephedrine*
Dimotane Plus	*brompheniramine*	*phenylpropanolamine*
Dristan Allergy	*brompheniramine*	*pseudoephedrine*
Hayfebrol	*chlorpheniramine*	*pseudoephedrine*
Sudafed Plus	*chlorpheniramine*	*pseudoephedrine*

Maximizing the Benefits

Follow the instructions under "Antihistamines."

CORTICOSTEROIDS

These are valuable drugs that need to be used with care, since too much can damage the body. However, when applied directly to the nose, in a nasal spray, there is very little risk involved, and the effect is superior to any other drug available for hay fever.

How They Work

These drugs mimic the action of one of the body's own hormones, **hydrocortisone** (also called **cortisol**). Hydrocortisone has a variety of effects. It controls the amount of sodium and potassium that the kidney allows to pass into the urine and releases glucose into the blood. It also moves protein out of the muscles and bones and influences the way fat is deposited. Finally, it suppresses inflammation, but only at doses far higher than those normally found in the body. This last effect makes corticosteroids useful in treating allergies.

In using corticosteroids to treat allergic reactions, the trick is to persuade the drug to reduce inflammation without carrying out any of its other actions. This has been achieved, to a large extent, by modifying hydrocortisone slightly. This chemical tinkering has produced *prednisolone, beclomethasone,* and *budesonide,* which suppress inflammation but have very little effect on the excretion of salt by the kidneys or on other bodily functions.

When corticosteroid drugs are taken by mouth or injected, they simply act on the outcome of allergic reactions, reducing the inflammation. But when corticosteroids are applied directly to the nose, they also stabilize mast cells and thus reduce histamine release. This double action makes corticosteroid nose drops a very useful form of treatment.

JOHN

For John, hay fever came on suddenly and without warning when he was 33 years old. Initially he thought he had caught a cold, but when the violent sneezing and runny nose persisted for eight weeks, this seemed unlikely. There was also an intense itching in his eyes and a congested feeling in the nose "that made ordinary existence almost impossible." His doctor suggested buying over-the-counter remedies, but John found that all antihistamines gave him a dried-out sensation in the nose and a "spacey" feeling. He decided he was more willing to endure the symptoms of hay fever than the side effects of the antihistamines. The next year, however, his symptoms were worse, and the doctor prescribed a nasal spray containing a corticosteroid. At the very first try he found that the spray gave him an immediate and intense headache.

When John reappeared at the doctor's office, it was clear to the doctor that this was a patient who was unusually sensitive to drugs. But he wondered if corticosteroid drops, which do not penetrate the sinuses as readily as a nasal spray, might be the answer. He therefore prescribed nasal drops, which turned out to solve the problem. They control John's hay fever very thoroughly and cause no side effects.

As John's case shows, it is always worth persisting with drugs until a suitable one is found. Sometimes the same drug will affect a patient differently depending on the way in which it is delivered—spray or drops, in this instance. The gas used in aerosol sprays can be an irritant for some people.

Minor Side Effects

There can be some stinging, burning, irritation, or sneezing when given as nose drops or sprays, and some forms affect the senses of smell and taste. Overuse of nose drops and sprays can dry out the nose, as well as cause crusting and nosebleeds. Some people suffer other side effects with the sprays (such as headaches) but do well on nose drops. There are also differences between the various corticosteroids, and one may irritate your nose while another does not, so be prepared to try different types. Using salt-water drops in the nose (see "Treatments to Unblock the Nose" in chapter 10), in between the doses of corticosteroid, may reduce the irritant effect of the drug.

The drug itself is only part of the story here—the way in which it is delivered can also affect the nose. Some preparations are water-based (aqueous) sprays, which are generally less irritating than aerosol forms. Other side effects include infections, which are a more serious matter and are therefore considered in the next section.

In general, corticosteroids have few obvious side effects, but can be dangerous if misused—the exact opposite of antihistamines, which tend to produce minor side effects quite often but are actually very safe.

PRECAUTIONS AND INTERACTIONS

The first thing that needs to be said here is that corticosteroids are quite different from the anabolic steroids that are misused the sporting world. Nor have they anything to do with steroid hormones involved in sex and reproduction, such as testosterone, estrogen, and progesterone. Rest assured, then, that taking corticosteroids will not turn you into the Incredible Hulk, allow you to win the Olympics, put hair on your chest, or stop you from getting pregnant. Great confusion has been spread on this topic because people use the word "steroid" indiscriminately for a variety of quite distinct substances.

What corticosteroids *can* do is to make infections more likely, particularly fungal infections such as thrush *(Candida)*. In suppressing inflammation, they hamper a valuable part of the body's fight against disease.

However, the use of corticosteroids for hay fever or perennial rhinitis does not seem to be associated with a great increase in the risk of disease, as the dosage used is generally low. *Candida* infections in the nose are very rare. Consequently, the drops are safe as long as there is no infection in the nose to begin with: *corticosteroids should never be used when an infection is already present.* (There are medicines that combine corticosteroids with an antibiotic, and these can be prescribed in such circumstances.)

If you are using corticosteroid nose drops or spray for year-round rhinitis, your doctor should see you every six months and examine the membranes inside the nose to ensure that no damage is occurring. Thinning of the nasal membranes is the most likely problem with continuous use of corticosteroid sprays and drops. This could be irreversible, so do take care. You can protect yourself in the following ways:

- When you insert the drops or spray, keep it away from the nasal septum, that is, the thin central part of the nose that divides one nostril from the other.

- After inserting the drops or spray, apply a little ointment, such as pure petroleum jelly (Vaseline). Don't use anything with lots of different ingredients, especially fragrances—you just want the plainest ointment possible, to keep moisture in the nasal membranes. (This will also help keep pollen out of your nose, incidentally—see "Protecting Your Nose from Pollen" in chapter 8.)

- Try using the drops or spray only once a day to see if you still get adequate control of your symptoms. Discuss this with your doctor first if the spray was prescribed for you.

Note that if you have nasal polyps, there is a particular way to insert corticosteroid drops that makes them far more effective—see pages 227–228.

Some people who experience stinging and burning after use of nasal drops and sprays are reacting to nondrug ingredients such as preservatives or to the pH (acidity/alkalinity) of the liquid. Ask your pharmacist about the possibility of trying different preparations—there may be a product containing the same drug but with different preservatives and a more suitable pH. Using one of these might resolve the problem.

With corticosteroid eye drops, there is a small risk of infections in the eye and care should be taken not to expose the eye to bacteria. Avoid, for example, rubbing the eyes with unwashed fingers, using grubby towels on your face, or applying makeup that has been open for some time. The herpes simplex virus, which causes cold sores and genital sores, is particularly dangerous to the eyes, and great care should be taken not to expose them to this infection.

Those with glaucoma should not use corticosteroid eye drops. If anyone in your family has ever suffered from glaucoma, you should mention this to the doctor.

A more insidious problem arises if corticosteroids are taken over a long period of time or at a high dosage, because the glands that produce hydrocortisone for the body feel somewhat redundant and tend to reduce their own production levels. Stopping the drug leaves the body with insufficient corticosteroids, which can lead in the worst cases to collapse. This means that corticosteroids taken as tablets should *never* be stopped abruptly if they have been taken for more than a few weeks. The glands must be given time to recover their natural level of activity by gradually reducing the dosage. Even after as little as two weeks, corticosteroids should be withdrawn gradually, by halving the dose each day, to avoid a flare-up of the original symptoms.

Someone taking corticosteroids by mouth should carry some kind of identification as a warning to hospital staff in the event of an accident; they need to know that the natural production of hydrocortisone may be suppressed. Your doctor can advise you on the most suitable form of ID for this purpose. Be sure to carry it at all times.

Corticosteroids are sometimes given as a "depot injection" for severe hay fever (see below). This slowly releases the drug into the bloodstream over the following weeks. The dose declines naturally, so the problem of suddenly stopping the drug does not occur. However, it is still important for medical staff to know about the treatment in the event of an accident. One problem with the injection method is that there can be some wasting of the muscle or slight discoloration of the skin at the site of the injection. This, however, is usually a temporary effect.

If you have been receiving a corticosteroid injection for hay fever every year for some time (it is the only form of therapy given as a single injection), then you may want to discuss the continuation of this treatment with your doctor. Perhaps, given the hazards involved, this approach should be reconsidered, especially if there are newer forms of treatment that you have never tried, such as nonsedating antihistamines and corticosteroid nose drops. In any event, you could be growing out of your hay fever now, making the injection unnecessary.

The problem of suppressing the body's own hydrocortisone production arises only when corticosteroids are taken by mouth or injected. There is generally no cause for concern with eye drops or nasal drops and sprays because the amount reaching the bloodstream is so small. The exceptions to this rule are young children under the age of 9, for whom any sort of corticosteroid preparation, even nose and eye drops, should be used cautiously. Significant amounts can be absorbed into the bloodstream and might affect the child's growth. Make sure that your doctor sees the child regularly.

Those inhaling *high-dose* steroids for asthma may have a certain amount of the drug reaching the bloodstream and should be checked regularly by a doctor. Note that most asthmatics are on low- or medium-dose steroid inhalers and there is little or no risk. For more information, consult *Asthma,* by Jonathan Brostoff, M.D., and Linda Gamlin (Healing Arts Press, 2000).

Usefulness

Corticosteroids are very useful for suppressing inflammation in the eyes, nose, and bronchi. They often work for hay fever when all other drugs have proved ineffective. A study by medical scientists at the University of Chicago, published in 2001, compared hay fever sufferers using corticosteroid nasal spray continuously during the hay fever season with others taking antihistamine tablets continuously. The former group had fewer symptoms. Most doctors agree, however, that this continuous treatment with corticosteroid spray is a good idea only for people with a relatively short case of hay fever during a few months of the year. People with prolonged hay fever symptoms (six months or more) or year-round nasal allergies should not be relying on corticosteroid spray or drops unless there is no other effective treatment: the risk of local side effects in the nose is too great. There are various alternatives: try drops containing a mast-cell stabilizer (see "Mast-cell Stabilizers" earlier in this chapter) or an antihistamine (see "Antihistamines" earlier in this chapter) first, and consider allergy shots (see chapter 9) for your year-round allergies.

Recent research shows that corticosteroid nose drops, used for hay fever, can also help to reduce asthmatic symptoms occurring in the pollen season, probably by interfering with the reflex reaction between the nose and the bronchi (see "The Lungs and Airways" in chapter 2).

With eye drops for conjunctivitis, it is a good idea to try out mast-cell stabilizers (see "Mast-cell Stabilizers" earlier in this chapter) before corticosteroids are prescribed. They may do the job just as well and are safer than corticosteroids. New eye drops containing antihistamine (see page 93) are also safe.

How Taken

Nose drops and sprays for hay fever and year-round rhinitis. Only a very small dose of corticosteroid is used. Although some enters the bloodstream, it is broken down promptly by the liver before it can have any effect on the rest of the body. However, you should not exceed the stated dose or use the drops continuously for more than six months without being examined by your doctor. The drugs used include *beclomethasone* (Beconase, Beconase AQ Nasal, Vancenase Nasal), *budesonide* (Rhinocort, Rhinocort Aqua), *dexamethasone* (Decadron Phosphate Turbinaire), *flunisolide* (AeroBid, Nasalide), *fluticasone* (Flonase), *mometasone* (Nasonex), and *triamcinolone acetonide* (Nasacort, Nasacort AQ).

Eye drops for conjunctivitis caused by pollen. The drugs used include *dexamethasone* (AK Dex, Decadron Phosphate, Decadron Ophthalmic Suspension), *fluorometholone* (Flarex, Fluor-Operation, FML, FML Forte, FML Liquifilm), *medrysone* (HMS), *prednisolone* (Econopred, AK-Pred, Inflamase Forte, Inflamase Mild Ophthalmic, Metreton, Pred-Forte, Pred-Mild), and *rimexolone* (Vexol).

Where there is a possibility of infection, nose and eye drops are available that contain an antibiotic as well as a corticosteroid; ask your doctor about these.

Tablets for dealing with a severe attack of asthma or controlling troublesome hay fever symptoms during examinations. Sometimes this is the only effective treatment, but it has certain risks (see page 101). Most doctors are cautious about prescribing such treatments. The tablets should be continued for a minimum of three weeks and then slowly withdrawn.

"Slow-release" injection into the buttock for controlling severe hay fever. A single injection at the beginning of the hay fever season leaves a reserve of corticosteroid in the muscle. This slowly leaks out into the bloodstream and continues combating inflammation for several weeks or months. As with corticosteroid tablets, this is a treatment with some risks attached, so it should not be used unless other methods have failed. (A similar form of treatment, in which corticosteroid is injected into the nose, is no longer being used because it carries a danger of blindness.)

Maximizing the Benefits

Corticosteroid injections are given before the hay fever season begins. With nose and eye drops, it is also useful to start the treatment before the pollen becomes airborne, preferably about a week before. However, starting early is not as vital with corticosteroids as it is with mast-cell stabilizers or antihistamines. If symptoms do appear, begin using the drops or spray as soon as possible to avoid "priming" (see "Priming" in chapter 3).

With nose drops and sprays, it is important to learn how to use them correctly; ask your doctor's advice. If your nose is very blocked, the drops may be unable to reach their target. A sympathomimetic can be useful, in the short term, for opening up the nose to the corticosteroid drops, but it should not be taken for too long (see page 95). The maximum benefits from nose drops may not be felt until you have been using them for a week or two.

ANTILEUKOTRIENE DRUGS

These are relatively new drugs that might be useful for some people with severe year-round rhinitis. They are also used for asthma.

How They Work

Among the messenger chemicals produced by mast cells (see chapter 3) during an allergic reaction are certain ones called **leukotrienes.** These help to perpetuate the inflammatory process begun by histamine, and they amplify the reaction by attracting more immune cells into the area.

Antileukotriene drugs fall into two distinct groups. First there are those that bind to the receptors for leukotrienes, called leukotriene-receptor-antagonists. Currently, there are three drugs in this group, *montelukast* (Singulair), *zafirlukast* (Accolate), and a newer drug called *pranlukast.* Second, there are those that block the production of the leukotrienes altogether, called 5-lipoxygenase inhibitors. There is only one drug in this group at present, *zileuton* (Zyflo). It is available in the United States but not in Canada.

In tackling inflammation, the antileukotriene drugs work in a completely different way from either steroids or *cromoglycate.* This makes them useful as an add-on treatment, supplementing the effects of existing anti-allergy drugs. They can also be used alone.

Minor Side Effects

Symptoms such as headache, infection, nausea, upset stomach, diarrhea, pain, cough, and flulike discomfort have been noted in preliminary trials. None indicates any serious underlying problem or damage.

Precautions and Interactions

According to the data gathered so far, serious side effects are rare. However, as with all new drugs, you should report any unusual symptoms to your doctor, just in case these represent a rare or long-term side effect of the drug that has not been picked up in preliminary trials.

Very occasionally *montelukast* causes anaphylaxis or other allergic reactions, such as itchiness, hives (urticaria), and swelling (angioedema). Stop taking the drug immediately if any of these occur.

Zileuton (Zyflo) and *zafirlukast* (Accolate) can cause liver damage, but again such reactions are very rare. Your liver function should be closely monitored by the doctor with regular blood tests, and the drug withdrawn at the first sign of trouble. You should not be given *zileuton* if you have liver disease.

The most alarming development noticed to date is the appearance, in a very few people taking *zafirlukast* or *montelukast,* of a disorder called Churg-Strauss syndrome. This syndrome is probably not due to the antileukotriene drugs themselves, but rather to a reduction in the dose of steroid tablets that was permitted by the use of these drugs. Doctors believe that all these patients were already suffering from an underlying eosinophilic disease, which was masked by long-term steroid tablet treatment. When the steroids were stopped, the disease became evident.

Usefulness

Antileukotriene drugs were originally designed to treat asthma. Their potential for treating other allergic diseases is currently being explored. Several studies show that they work well for perennial allergic rhinitis. In one trial involving people allergic to cats, taking an antileukotriene drug for a week reduced the symptoms brought on by cat allergen. They are especially useful for patients with aspirin sensitivity who suffer from rhinitis or asthma, or both.

How Taken

All the antileukotriene drugs are taken in tablet form. If you are trying an antileukotriene drug for the first time, there won't be any noticeable effects for about three days. Once you are taking the drug regularly, each dose requires

2 to 4 hours to have its full effect, but goes on working for 12 to 24 hours in total.

NEW DRUGS FOR HAY FEVER

There are various experimental drugs that may soon be available for hay fever sufferers. One is the genetically engineered drug *omalizumab* (brand name: Xolair). This novel drug works by inactivating IgE (the allergy antibody). It is an antibody itself, and it binds specifically to the "handle" end of the IgE antibody (see the illustration on page 32). This stops the IgE from interacting with mast cells or basophils.

In a recent study, 536 patients with ragweed allergy were given a shot of *omalizumab* just underneath the skin, before the ragweed season, and at 3 to 4 week intervals during the season. Compared to patients getting placebo injections, those who got the highest doses of *omalizumab* reported fewer hay fever symptoms, despite taking only half as many antihistamine tablets. The drug seemed to cause few side effects.

Unlike allergy shots, this is not a lasting reeducation of the immune system. To get continuous relief for year-round allergens such as dust mites, patients would probably have to receive the injections indefinitely.

German researchers have experimented with a combination of *omalizumab* and allergy shots (immunotherapy), and found that *omalizumab* can boost the benefits of the allergy shots. They studied patients aged between 6 and 17, with severe allergies to both grass and birch pollen. Their hay fever symptoms were reduced by 48 percent when *omalizumab* was given along with immunotherapy, compared with immunotherapy alone. The researchers believe this combined therapy would be good for "complicated allergy patients with multiple sensitivities."

Omalizumab is not yet approved by the U.S. Food and Drug Administration. Initially, the manufacturer of the drug is seeking approval for its use in the treatment of severe asthma.

COPING WITH HAY FEVER OR ASTHMA WHEN PREGNANT

This is obviously something that you should discuss with your doctor. The management of asthma during pregnancy is particularly important because the lack of oxygen during an asthma attack can increase the risk of the baby dying soon after birth, being born prematurely, or having a low weight at birth. These risks disappear if the asthma is managed well. Ask your doctor to refer you to a specialist if you are concerned that your asthma is not under good control.

Some of the drugs used for asthma are not considered safe during pregnancy, so your medication may have to be changed. But overall, the dangers to the baby from uncontrolled asthma are *far greater* than the dangers from asthma drugs.

If you suffer from hay fever and normally take nonprescription medicines, ask a pharmacist or doctor about their safety during pregnancy. Be sure that your doctor knows what you are taking, whether a prescription or a nonprescription drug.

With antihistamines, you should be aware of a danger that can arise in the very early stages of pregnancy, when you may not even know that you are pregnant. A few antihistamines carry a risk of deforming the baby, so you should not conceive while taking them, *nor for several weeks afterward.* Reliable contraceptive measures should be taken throughout this time. It is wise to treat all antihistamines with caution, unless your doctor advises you that a specific antihistamine is safe.

The safest drug to use during pregnancy and breast-feeding is *sodium cromglycate* (see "Mast-cell Stabilizers" earlier in this chapter), which can help with both hay fever and asthma. Sprays or drops containing nasal corticosteroids are also considered safe.

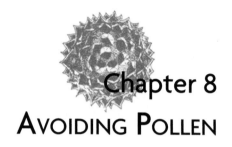

Chapter 8
AVOIDING POLLEN

Although you cannot evade pollen completely, you can certainly reduce the number of pollen grains you inhale every day. Indeed, some substantial reductions are possible if you are prepared to make certain changes. This could make your hay fever symptoms much less troublesome.

This approach may be sufficient on its own for some people, but for many more it will need to be backed up by use of medicinal drugs (see chapter 7) or allergy shots (see chapter 9). It can be particularly useful for those whose hay fever is only partially controlled by drugs.

THE INVISIBLE ENEMY

Most wind-pollinated plants scatter their pollen in the morning, but this is not true of all. The majority of grass species, for example, release their pollen in the morning, but a few species wait until the afternoon, so there is some pollen entering the air all day.

Knowing when pollen release is likely to begin in the morning is quite helpful. Grass pollen release occurs from about 7:30 A.M. onward on a warm summer morning when the ground and the grasses are dry, but if there is dew, the timing will change. Pollen has to be thoroughly dried out before the plant disperses it, so pollen release will be delayed on a dewy morning until most of the dew has evaporated. Rainfall the previous evening will have the same effect. Ragweed generally gets going much earlier than grasses, releasing its pollen between sunrise and 9 A.M., although certain weather conditions can delay release until as late as 2 P.M. No precise figures are available for other types of plant but one study found birch pollen to peak between noon and 6 P.M.

Plants respond to the weather and are more likely to release their pollen during a dry, sunny spell. Days that are dry and windy are the worst for ragweed. During cool, damp periods, pollen builds up in the flowers, so the next warm day is likely to see a bumper pollen count as all this stored pollen is liberated.

As the sun's rays warm the earth's surface, the air above it also warms up and then begins to rise, carrying the pollen with it. On a still day the rising pollen accumulates high up in the atmosphere. Ragweed pollen has been found two miles up in the air. When the sun sets and the earth begins to cool, the pollen is no longer buoyed up by currents of rising air, and gradually it falls to earth again.

How long this takes will depend on a variety of factors. It is much slower in built-up areas than in the country, because city pavements and buildings take longer to cool. In the countryside, most of the pollen descends between 8 P.M. and 10 P.M., but in the heart of the city the peak can be at midnight, and some pollen may not finally touch down until 2 A.M. This is why hay fever sufferers may wake in the night with an attack of sneezing.

The picture presented so far is a very simple one, which can be altered greatly by different weather conditions. Strong winds during the day will tend to blow away pollen and the heavy evening pollen-fall does not then take place. Should there be rainfall during the day, this washes most of the pollen out of the air, bringing relief to hay fever sufferers.

Inversions can make a big difference to the way pollen accumulates in the air. An inversion occurs when the air at ground level is slightly cooler than the upper layers of the atmosphere. The ground air cannot rise in the normal way, and the layer of warmer air above acts like a lid on a saucepan. This "lid" keeps in the ground air along with its pollen and any pollutants it may contain (see appendix 6). Cool temperate climates most often experience inversions in winter, but they can occur in summer too. In warmer climates inversions frequently occur in summer, and they are notorious in cities such as Los Angeles and Mexico City, where they contribute to smogs (see appendix 6). In mountainous regions, temperature inversions can occur in valleys, because cold air sinks down the mountainsides at night and can accumulate in the bottom of an enclosed valley. The layer of warmer air that sits like a lid over the valley can make pollen counts higher or lower. If the main source of pollen production is in that valley, then the pollen count will build up under the inversion. On the other hand, if the main pollen source is outside the valley, the inversion will keep that pollen out. When inversions are not present, the strong winds in mountainous regions tend to blow away pollen, and it is often blown straight across mountain ranges, missing the valleys.

Knowing the timing of pollen movements makes it possible to reduce your exposure. Stay indoors and keep windows closed when pollen is falling in the evening. For city dwellers, windows should remain closed at bedtime. To air the house, open the windows very early in the morning (to avoid grass

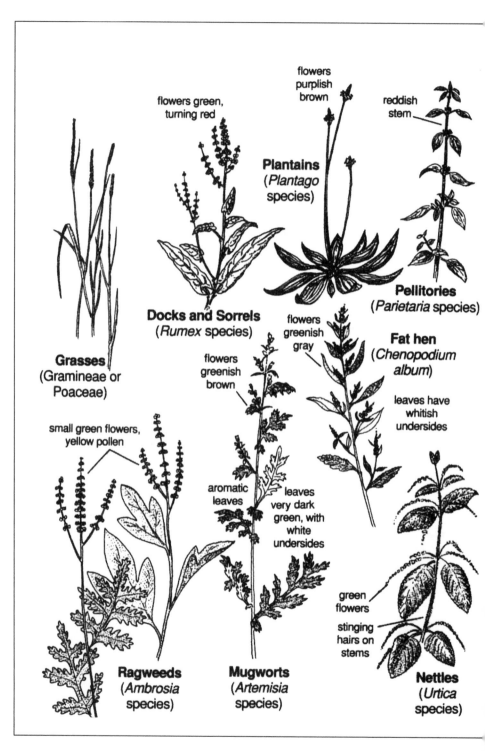

flowers green,
turning red

flowers
purplish
brown

reddish
stem

Plantains
(*Plantago*
species)

Docks and Sorrels
(*Rumex* species)

flowers
greenish
gray

Pellitories
(*Parietaria* species)

flowers
greenish
brown

Fat hen
(*Chenopodium
album*)

Grasses
(Gramineae or
Poaceae)

leaves have
whitish
undersides

small green flowers,
yellow pollen

aromatic
leaves

leaves
very dark
green, with
white
undersides

green
flowers

stinging
hairs on
stems

Ragweeds
(*Ambrosia*
species)

Mugworts
(*Artemisia*
species)

Nettles
(*Urtica*
species)

The major culprits in hay fever

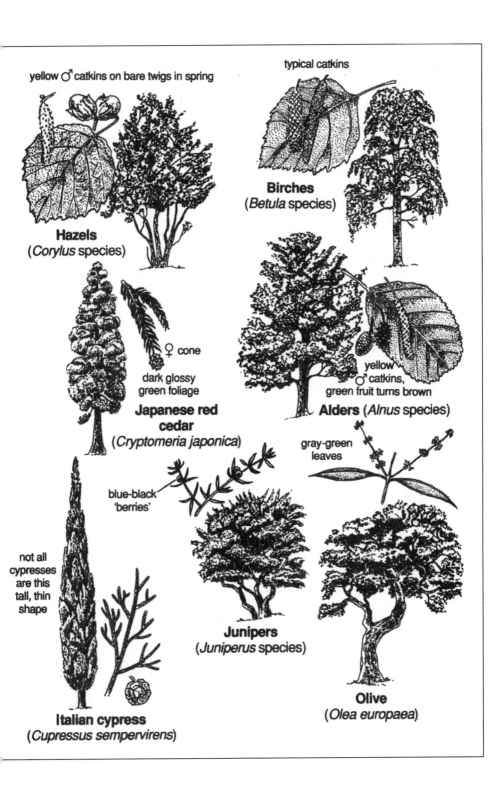

yellow ♂ catkins on bare twigs in spring

typical catkins

Birches
(*Betula* species)

Hazels
(*Corylus* species)

♀ cone

dark glossy
green foliage

**Japanese red
cedar**
(*Cryptomeria japonica*)

yellow
♂ catkins,
green fruit turns brown

Alders (*Alnus* species)

gray-green
leaves

blue-black
'berries'

not all
cypresses
are this
tall, thin
shape

Junipers
(*Juniperus* species)

Italian cypress
(*Cupressus sempervirens*)

Olive
(*Olea europaea*)

pollen) or in mid-afternoon (to avoid pollens such as ragweed that are re-leased at sunrise).

If you live or work in a tower block, you should be aware that the warm air rising during the day constantly lifts pollen upward, so the amount of pollen in the air at ground level may be quite low, whereas there are relatively high levels in the air ten stories up. Keeping the windows closed while at these levels is the only real solution, but if you can get down to street level, you may be more comfortable.

Pollen comes into cities from the surrounding countryside, but it is also generated locally, on railroad banks and waste ground, by trees growing in parks and gardens, and by those lining the streets. Lawns in parks are not usually a problem because they are mowed regularly, which prevents the grasses from flowering. The grass in garden lawns may be mowed less often, so may produce some pollen. If grass is your problem pollen, you should avoid areas with unmown grass in the morning, when the pollen is being released. In the evening, it will fall indiscriminately over everyone and everything, so any outdoor excursion will expose you to pollen.

Try to get out and exercise at times when the pollen count is lower—after rainfall, for example, or in the late afternoon and early evening, or very early in the morning if you are grass-sensitive. Exercise improves your general state of health and should not be abandoned during the pollen season. Indoor swimming pools are a good place for pollen-free exercise, or you could use a mask and/or protective eyewear (see "Protecting Your Eyes from Pollen" and "Protecting Your Nose from Pollen" later in this chapter), which would enable you to run or cycle.

AVOIDING POLLEN AT HOME

Pollen grains are fairly large particles, compared with some of the other items that can cause allergy, and this is one of their key advantages. The larger the particle, the faster it settles from the air. In an average room, with completely still air, all the pollen grains will have settled in about four minutes (see the box "Particle Sizes" in chapter 12). The time taken depends on the ceiling height as well as the particle size: if you live in a grand old mansion with ceilings 20 feet (6 meters) high, it will take eight minutes. Add another four minutes for every 10 feet (3 meters) of ceiling height.

This means that if you go into a room, shut the windows and doors, and sit fairly still, you should be breathing air that is virtually pollen-free within five minutes. It may take a little longer for your symptoms to subside but they should ease off within an hour. During a long spell of sunny weather, when you are exposed to pollen for many days in succession, you may well be experiencing **late-phase reactions** (see "The Late-phase Reaction" in chapter 3) to the pollen of the previous day. In this case, your symptoms will not disappear entirely when you sit quietly indoors, but they should lessen because the nose and eyes are not being challenged by any new intake of pollen.

Even with doors and windows closed, there will, of course, still be some pollen coming in from outside, with the air that sneaks in around the edges of window frames and under doors. This may be so little that it does not bother you, but if it is a problem, you can deal with it in other ways (see below).

You may not want to spend very long sitting still, but once the pollen has settled, you can move around fairly normally without disturbing the settled pollen too much. Obviously, more vigorous and rapid movements will cause more disturbance than simply walking about. It may help to change your clothing on arriving home, putting on something you do not wear outdoors —that way you are not carrying a layer of pollen around with you on your clothes, to be disturbed whenever you move. Rinsing your hair may also be worthwhile, especially if it is thick or long. This will wash out the pollen grains, again reducing the amount you are breathing while indoors.

When in bed, we probably inhale quite a lot of pollen from our hair, and a nightly hair-rinse can reduce this. Another measure that is worth trying is to cover the bed and pillow with a bedspread or spare sheet during the day, then carefully roll it up at bedtime. This will prevent pollen from settling on the pillow and bed during the day and evening, and thus reduce the amount inhaled while asleep.

If you live with others, especially children, still air is probably a rare commodity, and pollen will be continually disturbed in the home. In this case, you may want to use an air cleaner to reduce the airborne levels (see page 114–116). This is not the only solution, however; you can also take steps to reduce the amount of pollen waiting to be disturbed. Regular vacuum cleaning will help. Regular dusting using a wet cloth is also worthwhile; polished wood can be rubbed dry with another cloth to prevent marking. This will reduce the amount of pollen collected in the carpeting and on furniture, windowsills, and other surfaces. Air currents created by movement in the room, doors opening and closing, and other disturbances will then churn up less pollen into the air you breathe.

Pets coming in from outside carry quite a lot of pollen on their fur, so people with hay fever may be better off keeping their distance from the family dog or cat for a while. Alternatively, the pet could be excluded from the house during the pollen season. It should certainly be kept out of the patient's bedroom—this is a basic year-round precaution for anyone with allergies.

One rather obvious hazard for anyone with hay fever is bringing items into the house that produce the problem pollen. Hazel catkins and pussy willows, for example, might produce symptoms in some hay fever patients, particularly hazel, as there is often a cross-reaction from birch (see the discussion of the birch family under "Cross-Reactions between Tree Pollens" in chapter 11). In general, flower arrangements that contain only colorful flowers are unlikely to be a problem because these rarely cause hay fever (see "Fear of Flowers" in chapter 1). However, they may carry the pollens of other plants, such as grasses, on their leaves and petals. It is also possible that the scents of these flowers will be an irritant to the hay feverish nose.

Ferns grown as pot plants can sometimes cause hay fever–like symptoms (see page 83).

In the case of someone with ragweed sensitivity, there might be a cross-reaction with other flowers in the daisy family (Compositae or Asteraceae), many of which are pretty garden flowers. Goldenrod is the worst offender, but any daisy, aster, dahlia, marigold, chrysanthemum, thistle, or sunflower might cause problems. For more information on cross-reactions, see chapter 11.

If, despite these basic measures, you still suffer from hay fever symptoms when at home with the windows closed, there are further steps you can take. It may be that a large amount of air is still coming into the house from outside—under doors, around windows, through cat flaps or ventilation bricks. One obvious solution is to block off these entry holes, perhaps by installing better-fitting windows and doors, or by simpler measures, such as plastic taped over the openings. However, this has some drawbacks for people with other allergies besides hay fever. Someone who is allergic to cats or other pets, and still has those pets in the house, could be made much worse by a reduction in ventilation, which can lead to a massive buildup of small allergenic particles in the air (see page 206).

Blocking off drafts could well increase the moisture level in your house, and this will be a problem if you are allergic to either mold spores or dust mites (see chapter 12 for more information on both of these allergens). As a short-term measure, reducing drafts is acceptable, but the ventilation must be increased again at the end of the pollen season. (The only other option is to use a dehumidifier, which takes moisture out of the air; see appendix 3.)

Removing pollen grains from the indoor air, using an air filter or ionizer, is another option. With these devices, it is important to make sure that what you are buying is up to the job—that is, powerful enough for the size of the room. Appendix 3 gives guidelines for choosing an air cleaner or ionizer.

WHOLE GRAINS OR POLLEN PARTICLES?

A crucial question, in relation to any airborne allergen, is "How big is it?" The size of the particle carrying the allergen makes an enormous difference to its becoming airborne and staying aloft long enough to be inhaled. Combating a very small allergen is an entirely different process from combating a large one. "Very small" in this case means less than 4 microns (thousandths of a millimeter), while "large" means 20 microns or more. An illustration in chapter 12, "The Size of Airborne Particles," compares the sizes of major airborne allergens.

The size of the particle also influences the way in which it affects the human body. The size of pollen grains makes them highly likely to land in the eyes, which is why hay fever so often produces eye symptoms. Size also determines how deeply particles penetrate into the airways, an important factor in pollen asthma (see the box "Particle Sizes" in chapter 12).

Most allergenic pollens fall in the range from 15 to 40 microns (thousandths of a millimeter). A full list of the different sizes is given in appendix 2.

Life would be simpler if there were only intact pollen grains to cause hay fever.

Unfortunately, some plants also generate much smaller particles that contain pollen allergens. These are known for ryegrass, ragweed, Japanese red cedar, and Australian white cypress pine (Callitris). Whether they exist for other plants is uncertain, but it seems likely. The smallest of these particles may be a mere half-micron across. Whether they are an important factor in hay fever will depend on how abundant they are in the air. At present this is not known, and more research is needed on this topic.

If these smaller particles are causing your symptoms, your efforts to avoid pollen allergens will be affected, but not to any major extent. There are four possible effects:

1. The particles take longer to settle than whole pollen grains. Particles of 2 microns take six hours to settle from an average room, compared with four minutes for most pollen grains. Thus, simply sitting still indoors, with the doors and windows closed, will not give you any prompt relief from hay fever. This makes air-conditioning or an air cleaner a more attractive option.

2. A dust mask that could remove whole pollen grains might not be effective against these smaller particles; pollen fragments will probably require a higher grade of mask. As masks are fairly cheap, you can test one to see if it works for you and buy a better model if it does not.

3. Most good-quality vacuum cleaners that use paper (rather than fabric) collecting bags will retain the intact pollen grains that they pick up, but many smaller particles may escape and be given off as a fine spray into the air. If this is happening, you will be aware of hay fever symptoms when vacuuming or soon afterward (although this could also indicate an allergy to dust-mite droppings or something else in dust; see chapter 12). In such cases, there are specialized vacuum cleaners marketed for dust-mite allergy that can help considerably. For full information on these, see appendix 3.

4. Fine particles become airborne more easily, and research with cat allergens shows that an air filter with a powerful fan can churn up settled particles, offsetting its cleaning action to some extent (see "Cats" in chapter 12) If very small pollen particles are a problem and you opt for an air cleaner, you may also need to reduce the quantity of settled particles in the home by careful vacuuming and wet dusting.

One manufacturer produces a high-quality air cleaner that is also a powerful dehumidifier, capable of actually killing the dust mites in a room by making the air desert-dry for a few hours of the day when the room is not in use (see appendix 3). This machine could be very useful if you are sensitive to mold spores or dust mites as well as pollen, allowing you to keep the windows tightly closed without making the house damp and actually killing many mites as well.

Air-conditioning is also of benefit to hay fever sufferers, particularly ducted systems that cover the entire house. Because these take in only a small amount of air from the outside, less pollen enters the house, and much of that is removed during the cooling process anyway: cooling makes water condense from the air, and the tiny water droplets take pollen with them. The amount of pollen inside the house is small, and the coolness makes it far less of an ordeal to keep the windows closed. The moisture content of the air is controlled by the air conditioner, so there should be few problems with dampness and mold.

Scientists in Wisconsin have studied the effects of air-conditioning systems on ragweed pollen and found that they remove about 95 percent of the pollen. Adding a high-quality air-filtration unit to the intake on air conditioners reduced the pollen a little more—to about 2 percent of outdoor levels. This further reduction in the pollen level was found to lessen nighttime symptoms in ragweed-sensitive people a little, compared with air-conditioning alone, but the researchers concluded that the extra benefits were small.

Unfortunately, there has been no comparable scientific research on air cleaners. However, it seems likely that air cleaners and ionizers will remove significant amounts of pollen from the air, and hay fever sufferers who have tried them frequently report good results. Some suppliers may allow you to try out an air cleaner or ionizer in advance of buying it, by either renting it or selling it with a money-back guarantee. This enables purchasers to see whether a device is of any assistance to them, and to choose from the different types available (see appendix 3). If you do invest in an air cleaner or ionizer, remember that it will be effective only when the windows are kept closed.

Freestanding air-conditioning devices that treat a single room only are also available. No one has checked to see how much pollen they remove from the air, but they probably take out some, and they make closed windows more bearable. Again, there are suppliers who rent these machines, so that you can see how much they help.

A new product that has recently appeared on the market is a filter unit that fits into a partially open window. This is intended to allow fresh air to

SMALLER THAN SMALL?

While most hay fever involves pollen grains or pollen particles, some people are probably reacting to **volatile compounds** given off by plants. A volatile compound is any substance, solid or liquid, that readily turns into a vapor at normal temperatures. Any scent depends on volatile compounds—it is because the molecules become airborne that they enter the nose and trigger the sense of smell.

Obviously, scented flowers give off volatile compounds, but so do the leaves and stems of many plants. Not all of these compounds have smells that the human nose can detect.

Why are these substances produced by plants? In some cases, they are compounds that insects dislike, and are released to deter them from eating the plants.

The question of whether volatile substances can affect hay fever sufferers is a difficult one, but there is some evidence that they can.

One plant that is known to produce volatile compounds in abundance is oil-seed rape, the yellow-flowered crop plant that has lately been accused of causing minor hay fever epidemics in some areas where it is grown. The volatiles from rape may have an irritant effect on the nose that affects many people, not just those of an allergic disposition. It may be these that are responsible for the "hay fever" outbreak, especially when it affects those with no previous history of allergy. Since the volatiles are acting as irritants, not allergens, this is not genuine hay fever. However, some people are genuinely allergic to oil-seed rape pollen.

Some people with allergies to tree pollen begin reacting very early in spring, before pollen is released. It has been suggested that tree buds release volatiles as they swell and open in the spring, and that this may be provoking symptoms.

In Sweden, volatiles coming from birch twigs in the spring are known to affect some people with birch hay fever. They also affect just as many people with no sign of hay fever or other allergies.

Only a minority of people with hay fever are likely to be affected by volatiles. One possible sign of this problem is experiencing nasal irritation from the scent of flowers; your nose is clearly sensitive to the volatile substances making up the scent, and perhaps to other volatiles as well.

If you are sensitive to volatile compounds, how will this affect your efforts at pollen avoidance? Volatile compounds will not settle out of the air, although they will disperse very readily. They are unlikely to affect you at low concentrations, so you will probably find that, when outdoors, you are affected by them only if close to the source. Whether they penetrate indoors, and what happens to them there, is unknown at present. Your nose will simply have to be the judge of that.

Since volatile substances are not particles, they will not be removed by air cleaners of the electrostatic or HEPA types or by dust masks. The only type of filter that can take out these substances is one containing activated carbon (see appendix 3).

come in while keeping pollen out. Whether it actually achieves much is an interesting question—the air resistance created by the filter probably means that very little ventilation occurs. For more information on this and other products sold for allergy relief, go to the Allergy-Intolerance Web site at www.allergy-intolerance.com.

Teenagers represent a high proportion of hay fever sufferers, and it is often fairly easy to reduce the airborne pollen in a teenager's bedroom, by the methods already described, without affecting the activities of the rest of the household. This is worth the effort if the pollen season coincides with exams, because it gives the hay fever patient somewhere to study with a minimum of symptoms. One small additional measure that may help is to cover the desk and books with a sheet when not in use, and then roll it up carefully when studying begins. This will prevent a layer of pollen from accumulating on books and notepads, to be disturbed when the pages are turned.

REDUCING POLLEN EXPOSURE IN THE GARDEN

There is not a great deal that can be done here, and your neighbors' gardens will probably frustrate your efforts anyway, but you can avoid making your pollen exposure any worse.

Mowing a lawn can affect someone with allergy to grass pollen quite badly, even though the grass is not in flower. Tiny liquid droplets, containing similar allergens to those in the pollen, are thought to be at fault. The hay fever sufferer should not, therefore, cut the grass.

Cutting the lawn at frequent intervals will help to prevent it from flowering, although grasses will adapt to regular mowing and may flower when very short. Take a close look to see if flower heads are developing. Make sure that the edges of the lawn are trimmed and that grasses are cut down in the weedy corners of the garden.

Avoiding grass in the garden altogether is possible and may be valuable for those who develop a rash when sitting on grass. Chamomile lawns or herb lawns are an alternative (but chamomile is not recommended for anyone who also has ragweed allergy because the two plants are related and can cross-react). A good gardening book should tell you how to create such a lawn.

Certain plants should be avoided, such as ornamental grasses (e.g., pampas grass) and sedges if you are grass-allergic, and various members of the daisy family (see page 159) if you are sensitive to ragweed. If you are planning to plant trees, a skin-prick test may be advisable first, to find out whether any particular species could cause you problems. Birches are probably best avoided anyway. In warmer climates, hedges and windbreaks consisting of cypresses are quite often a source of hay fever problems. (Several plants seem to cause more problems in hot climates than cool ones, probably because the pollen becomes drier while on the plant and is therefore dispersed more widely by the wind.)

If you have a large yard with large patches of ineradicable ragweed, nettles, docks, or other weeds, at least cut them down before they flower. Remember that a single ragweed plant can generate a million grains of pollen in a day. Should you experience any symptoms while slashing or trimming the plants, these may be caused by droplets of plant juices in the air; get someone else to do the job for you next time.

PROTECTING YOUR EYES FROM POLLEN

Protecting the eyes from pollen is fairly easy. In fact, this is an area with considerable scope for self-help, and one that is often neglected by hay fever sufferers.

Many people with eye symptoms from pollen already wear sunglasses in spring and summer, but this is providing only rather limited protection. Researchers in New Zealand and the United States have found that the protective effect of glasses can be much improved by adding shields at the top, bottom, and sides of the frames. Simply adding shields to the top and sides of the frames can also be very helpful.

The cheapest way to achieve this is to make your own shields for an existing pair of glasses or sunglasses. Apart from low cost, the advantage of this is that you can extend the coverage right around the lens, giving thorough protection. Furthermore, the shape is personalized for your head, giving a very good fit.

The illustration on the next page shows how to make these shields. Clear plastic sheeting can be bought in model and hobby shops or in some shops supplying art materials. A thickness of 7.5 thou (thousandths of an inch) is the best because it wraps around the frame easily.

Use glue or double-sided sticky tape to stick the plastic to the glasses frame. If using glue, check first that it does not dissolve the plastic of the frame by testing a small inconspicuous area. Avoid "superglues" because you want to be able to remove all traces of the glue at the end of the pollen season. Check that the glue you plan to use can be rubbed off or removed with a solvent without damaging the frame. Should your glasses have plastic lenses, keep the glue away from these.

Cut a strip of plastic sheeting about 3 inches (8 centimeters) wide and 8 inches (20 centimeters) long. First, stick the plastic strip across the top of the frame (see illustration, page 120, step 1). Once the plastic is stuck firmly to the top of the frame, wrap the strip around, mold it to the side of the frame with

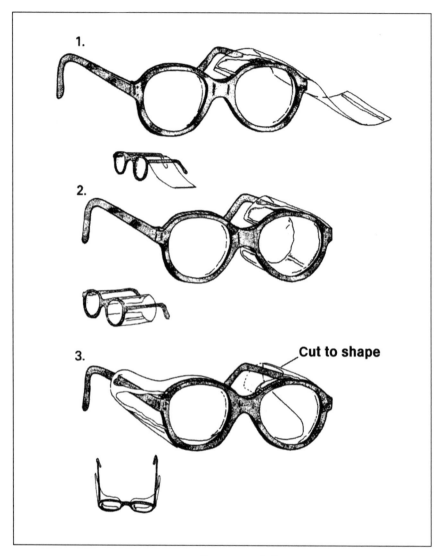

1.

2.

3.   **Cut to shape**

Keeping pollen out of the eye

your hand, and then stick it down. Leave to set firmly, then wrap the plastic around and stick it to the bottom of the frame (step 2). Repeat this process for the other lens.

Once you have a cylinder of plastic around each lens, you can cautiously cut away the plastic to fit your face (step 3). Do this a little at a time, using sharp scissors. Try on the glasses after each cut, feel where the plastic rubs your face, and trim off a little more at that point. When you have achieved a good fit, smooth the cut edge with an emery board or fine sandpaper.

Cliff

Cliff had one of the most severe cases of hay fever that his specialist had ever seen. He was still in his teens, and the fact that the grass pollen season coincided with his final school exams was a major problem. Allergy shots had been tried without success. Neutralization therapy did not work either, and antihistamines were of little help. The specialist then tried *cromoglycate* and corticosteroids, but these produced only a minor improvement. Cases such as this are rare, but when they do occur the only solution is to avoid pollen as far as possible. Cliff took to wearing sunglasses while walking outside, with a special filter mask over his nose too, at the height of the pollen season. His family kept the windows closed at home in the evenings and bought an air cleaner to reduce the pollen level in his bedroom. Although Cliff still suffered with hay fever, he found the symptoms were bearable and no longer interfered with his work.

When the weather is warm, there should be very little problem with condensation (misting up) inside your customized spectacles. If you do find them fogging over occasionally, there are special cleaning fluids available from opticians that are antistatic and make condensation less likely.

If you are prepared to spend a little more money, there is now a really good range of safety glasses that are designed to look like ordinary glasses. There are several excellent and fashionable designs that look nothing at all like the plastic safety goggles sold in do-it-yourself shops and could be worn with no embarrassment whatsoever. Choose ones that give good protection at the sides of the lens and a certain amount of protection over the top as well. The extent to which they shield the eye varies, but some models give very good top-and-sides coverage and a few extend below the lens.

These frames can be fitted with prescription lenses for those who wear glasses (see appendix 3). Alternatively, they can be fitted with tinted sunglass-type lenses, or plain glass lenses, for those with good sight or contact lenses. Many people with eye symptoms find that they dislike strong light, and dark glasses give them welcome relief from the sun. There are occasions, however, when sunglasses make things difficult socially; you may want to keep them on indoors if the windows are open, for example, but not taking sunglasses off when meeting people can seem impolite, especially in a work situation. Having both options available—a pair of protective glasses with tinted lenses and a pair with plain glass—is therefore useful.

Of course, plastic goggles sold for sports use or do-it-yourself protection can also be used against pollen. For a child who does not wear glasses, plastic sports goggles may be the simplest and cheapest option.

PROTECTING YOUR NOSE FROM POLLEN

The first person to use an umbrella was stoned by the outraged citizens of 19th-century London. Thirty years ago, someone running along the street in shorts and a T-shirt would have been regarded as an oddball, whereas joggers are now commonplace. Twenty years ago, cyclists wearing helmets were stared at and ridiculed. With so many people now suffering from hay fever, it will only take a few brave souls to start the ball rolling and make summertime dust masks seem entirely unremarkable. Already there are antipollution masks, aimed at city cyclists, which have been designed with looks as well as practicality in mind (see appendix 3), and increasing numbers of cyclists are wearing them.

Of course, there are other drawbacks to masks besides loss of street credibility. They inevitably make it a little harder to breathe and can become hot and uncomfortable in summer. However, if your hay fever is bad and drugs have not helped much, the discomfort of a mask worn only when outdoors may be much less than that of hay fever endured all day and night. Bear in mind that reducing your exposure substantially when outdoors can avoid the priming reaction that will make you ultrasensitive to pollen at other times, so the benefits could be substantial.

For some people, masks can prove useful as temporary protection from a particularly heavy load of their allergen—if they have to drive on a hot day, for example, or mow the lawn themselves. Some other instances in which masks can be valuable as a temporary protection are listed in appendix 3, where details of the different types of masks are also given.

A far less conspicuous way of protecting the nose is to insert a plug of foam rubber into each nostril. We know of only one hay fever sufferer who has tried this, but he reported excellent results, even when exposed to massive amounts of pollen, and says that the nose plugs cannot easily be seen when in place. The foam he uses is not the sort generally found in cushions or foam mattresses, where there are many small air bubbles within a solid mass of rubber. This type does not let the air through because the bubbles do not interconnect. The type of foam used is known as "windowless" or "reticulated" foam and looks like a tangled net of fibers. The holes in the foam should be about 1 millimeter across. The nose plugs do not filter out all pollen entering the nose, but much of it gets stuck to the strands of the foam, so that the amount inhaled is reduced considerably.

Obviously, the foam needs to admit enough air to make breathing through the nose easy. If there is too much air resistance from the foam, you may begin breathing through the mouth, and this will mean that more pollen and pollen fragments penetrate the airways, perhaps triggering pollen asthma. However, reticulated foam generally admits plenty of air.

Some hay fever sufferers report good effects from simply smearing petroleum jelly (Vaseline) on the skin just inside the nostrils. By making this surface sticky, it can detain some of the pollen that flows past on the incoming air, reducing the amount that reaches the delicate membranes beyond.

Farmworkers with hay fever who suffer serious symptoms when in contact with crops can use respirators designed for industrial workers. The high level of protection they offer may be valuable to anyone who cannot avoid contact with large amounts of their problem pollen or other allergen. Plant breeders, nurserymen, and laboratory technicians working with small animals are among those who could benefit from such devices. Suppliers are listed in appendix 3.

One of the best devices for all-day use is a powered respirator helmet. The helmet itself is fairly light and comfortable to wear. The air filter, powered by a battery, is carried in the small of the back, attached to a belt that buckles around the waist. Air is taken in by this unit, filtered, then pumped up a flexible tube into the back of the helmet. Channels within the helmet carry it over the head and pump it out over the forehead. A plastic face shield extends down from the helmet, and the filtered air being pumped downward keeps outside air from entering at the bottom of the face shield.

RICHARD

Richard first began to get hay fever when he was 13 years old, and at 40 he is still enduring the same symptoms, which last from early spring to midsummer, as he is sensitive to both tree pollens and grass pollens. His main problem is a very dry sore throat, a blocked nose, and sore, itchy eyes. As a young man he tried antihistamines, but the forms then available made him extremely sleepy and he had to give them up since his work as a traveling salesman required full concentration, especially when driving. Newer types of antihistamines have proved very effective for Richard and do not cause any drowsiness. He also uses eye drops that contain an antihis-

tamine and a sympathomimetic. The medicines keep his symptoms under control and allow him to lead a relatively normal life, but Richard still finds his hay fever a nuisance and sometimes a social embarrassment.

Five years ago, he began driving a car with air-conditioning and found to his surprise that he was substantially better. "I actually enjoy being on the road during the summer now," he says, "as it is the only time when I am relatively comfortable." For many people with hay fever, there is no single solution to their problems—they need to use several methods of coping with their illness, as Richard has done.

AVOIDING POLLEN WHEN DRIVING

There can be heavy concentrations of pollen in the air around country roads and particularly on highways. The movement of the traffic constantly stirs up pollen grains from the ground. In a long dry spell, when there has been no rain to wash away the pollen, a thick layer remains on the road and shoulders. Elsewhere, this does not easily become airborne again, but the considerable turbulence of air beside a highway produces high airborne concentrations. Hay fever when driving is often a major problem, especially if you have eye symptoms and it affects your vision.

The simplest avoidance technique is to drive with the windows closed, and this is the standard advice given to hay fever sufferers. Needless to say, it can be sheer hell to be stuck in a hot little metal box on a sweltering summer's day, and most people yearn for another solution. Even with the windows closed, there will still be some pollen intake, plus the pollen that was in the car to begin with.

The most sophisticated solution, if you can afford it, is a car with air-conditioning, which will cool you off and cut down the pollen load considerably, since the air conditioner takes a great deal of pollen out, along with moisture droplets. There are also cars that have special antipollen filters.

If a new car is beyond your means, there are various other solutions to pollen in the car. For example, filters can be fitted over the air intake or you could install a car ionizer or air cleaner (see appendix 3). These devices will reduce the quantity of pollutants inhaled, as well as protect you from pollen. But you will still have the problem of heat to contend with, because the windows must be kept shut for them to be effective.

If you are a passenger in someone else's car, or simply hate the thought of closing the car windows, a pair of protective glasses may help. You could also consider wearing a dust mask to protect your nose.

MAKING USE OF POLLEN COUNTS

Not so long ago, pollen counts were for one or two types of pollen only and simply told you what yesterday's pollen count had been. The situation now is much better and improving all the time. Several telephone lines and Internet sites currently offer pollen forecasts for the day ahead and general outlooks for the next three days. They also give pollen counts for a variety of allergenic species.

Not all services are the same. If the one you have been using does not offer pollen forecasts and outlooks, try another. Some early-morning television programs also give a pollen forecast for the day.

Pollen counts are always given in number of grains per cubic meter of air.

The figures are usually averages for a 24-hour period, which includes peak periods and low-pollen periods. The actual pollen count at peak times will therefore be much higher. Sometimes pollen counts that relate to levels during the peak period are given, but this will usually be stated. Bear this in mind when comparing figures from different sources. Some plant types provoke symptoms at quite low pollen counts; others reach high counts before they set people sneezing.

There is only a limited value in pollen counts that relate to the previous day (retrospective counts). These cannot help you to avoid pollen, but they may help to explain a change in your symptoms. If you are uncertain whether you are allergic to pollen or to some other allergen, then knowing how the pollen count changes and seeing if this fits in with your symptoms may be useful. However, if you are not entirely in step with the official pollen counts, this does not rule out sensitivity to the pollen in question. The changes in pollen levels in your immediate locality may be somewhat different from those elsewhere.

The pollen forecast is far more helpful in pollen avoidance, but it too has its limitations. The forecasts depend on computer models that predict pollen release based on the time of year, temperature of preceding days and weeks, predicted temperature, predicted rainfall, and other variables. Some of the crucial facts and figures that lead to the pollen count prediction are obtained from weather forecasting, so if the weather forecasters are wrong, the pollen forecast will also be inaccurate. Similarly, the pollen outlook is as dependable as the weather outlook for the next three days.

If you are planning to take your medicinal drugs before the pollen season starts—a good idea with antihistamines, mast-cell stabilizers, and corticosteroids—the pollen count may be helpful in deciding when to begin. The information source you use should include a prediction of when grass pollen will first appear.

Another use for the pollen forecast is in planning activities that involve high exposure to pollen, such as a trip to the countryside or to a park. The pollen forecast can help you avoid high-pollen days, but it will, of course, also help you avoid the best summer weather! If you are taking a long journey by car and do not have antipollen devices or air-conditioning in the vehicle, the pollen forecast can be very useful.

HAY FEVER AND THUNDERSTORMS

On the night of June 24, 1994, doctors in London emergency rooms were seeing an extraordinary number of people with asthma attacks. Almost half of them had never suffered from asthma before—and most of these people were hay fever sufferers.

"We had about seventy patients in the space of 15 or 16 hours, when normally we'd see about six asthmatics a day," recalls Dr. Julian Webb, then a doctor at St. Thomas's Hospital, located across the river from the Houses of Parliament. The same phenomenon was happening all over the city: ten times the usual number of asthma attacks. Several emergency rooms ran out of equipment or drugs, or both. Many doctors called the fire services or the police, convinced that there had been a spill of toxic chemicals somewhere in London. What else could have caused such an epidemic of asthma?

The answer, when it later emerged, surprised everyone: it was the thunderstorm that had passed over the capital that evening. Following careful investigations by medical scientists in both Britain and Australia—where similarly dramatic episodes have occurred—we now know that summer thunderstorms, right in the middle of the grass pollen season, can wreak havoc with the airways of hay fever sufferers.

Exactly why these thunderstorms provoke such a spate of asthma attacks is the big question—and there is no consensus on this point yet. Some blame a downdraft of cold air preceding the storm for bringing down pollen from the upper atmosphere and producing a massive concentration of pollen at ground level. Others say there must be more to it than that, and suggest that electrically charged particles generated by the storm made the pollen more likely to irritate the airways.

Another school of thought is that the sudden rainfall (following several dry days with an unusually high pollen count) moistened the pollen in the air and so produced a bumper release of tiny allergen particles from the pollen grains. These smaller particles are much more likely to reach the airways than pollen grains themselves, so are more likely to provoke asthma.

Perhaps all these different factors played some part in the process. Or maybe there is some other asthma-inducing factor in thunderstorms that we just don't understand yet.

So far, there are no records of such thunderstorm-related incidents in the United States or Canada, but there is no reason why one shouldn't happen: the conditions that provoked these incidents in Britain and Australia are not unique.

If you should feel unusually breathless and tight in the chest during a thunderstorm, get to an emergency room but don't panic—of the 640 patients who went to the hospital that June night in London, none died, and only a hundred or so needed to be admitted.

Note that the hay fever sufferers affected by the London storm generally reported having had severe hay fever in the previous few days, undoubtedly due to the high pollen count that preceded the storm. The moral of this is: Treat your hay fever, and don't hesitate to step up the treatment when symptoms are more severe. A nerve reflex between the nose and the airways (see pages 19–20) explains why inflammation of the nose can provoke narrowing of the airways—conversely, treating the nose keeps the airways happy.

If you already have pollen asthma, make sure you have a steroid inhaler (or other preventive treatment) during the pollen season, and use it regularly to keep the inflammation of the airways under control. That way you are much less vulnerable to difficult asthma-provoking conditions.

ESCAPING DURING THE POLLEN SEASON

If you are not too tied down by family or work commitments, and if your hay fever symptoms are severe, you might like to consider getting away from your home area at the height of the pollen season. Obviously, this is practical only if the season is relatively short.

For those with ragweed allergy, a vacation in Alaska, northern Canada, or anywhere beyond the shores of North America is recommended. If you are heading for Europe, remember that, although this troublesome plant is not a native, there are a few areas of introduced ragweed, most notably in Hungary and other parts of eastern Europe (see page 130). Grass pollen is more difficult to avoid, since grasses grow almost everywhere in the world, but you can use appendix 1 to find vacation destinations where grasses pollinate either later or earlier than in your home area.

It is not always necessary to leave the country to escape the pollen season. Coastal regions with an onshore breeze generally have low pollen counts because the wind pushes the pollen inland. Mountain and moorland regions have stronger winds and the grasses found there tend to pollinate less prolifically, so pollen counts may be lower. You cannot rely on mountain regions being better, however, and inversions in mountain valleys (see "The Invisible Enemy" at the beginning of this chapter) can create pollen traps where the pollen count is very high. This is known to happen in the Swiss Alps, for example.

HAY FEVER AND VACATIONS

Apart from coming down with dysentery or yellow fever, nothing can spoil a vacation as thoroughly as having severe hay fever. Many plants with allergenic pollen have a worldwide distribution—grasses in particular. Birches too are naturally widespread, occurring throughout the northern hemisphere, and are often planted in gardens in the southern hemisphere as well. Ragweed, once confined to North America, is now spreading across wasteland and farms in many parts of the world. Cypresses are common worldwide, either as wild species or as garden shrubs and hedges.

Before planning a vacation, always check whether your problem pollen occurs at your destination and find out when it is airborne there; the times of year will not necessarily be the same as those at home. Appendix 1 gives pollen seasons for the major allergens in all the most popular vacation destinations of the world.

Another point to consider here are potential cross-reactions (see chapter 11). For example, many people with cypress sensitivity show a reaction to Japanese red cedar, and vice versa. A tourist with hay fever or asthma due to cypress pollen would be well advised to avoid Japan in spring.

If you are going to a warm climate, where pollen seasons are often very long and not entirely predictable, it is a good idea to take a supply of your usual hay fever medicine with you. This may prove useful in case of local quirks in pollen production or unexpected cross-reactions.

ELIMINATING THE POLLEN—COMMUNITY ACTION

Since the 1930s, a unique program of community action has been under way in the area around Montreal. At the instigation of a geography professor from the University of Montreal, people began an attempt to eradicate two species of ragweed from fields, pastures, and wasteland throughout the area. The program has continued ever since, with poster campaigns and organized ragweed-pulling by schoolchildren. There have been renewed efforts in the past 20 years, and research into different control methods has been carried out at Montreal's Botanic Garden. Researchers there have found that while hand-weeding is the most effective method of reducing pollen production, it is also the most expensive if paid labor is used. Mowing, on the other hand, is fairly cheap, and if done with the mower blades set 4/5 inch from the ground, it is highly effective, reducing pollen production by at least 88 percent and sometimes preventing it altogether. While ragweed has not been eliminated, the number of plants has certainly been reduced. Researchers have found that these efforts can cut the pollen count to about half the level it would otherwise reach, a significant achievement that brings relief to many hay fever sufferers.

Not all hay fever–causing plants are suitable candidates for this treatment. Grasses, for example, are vital to agriculture (although farmers might be induced to grow species with less prolific or less allergenic pollen). Birch

CROSSING THE LANGUAGE BARRIERS

Hay fever can be an embarrassing traveling companion. If, despite your plans and precautions, you are stricken by hay fever when abroad, you may feel the need to explain the explosive sneezing and red-rimmed eyes to the locals. You are more likely to get a hotel room if they know it's not infectious. (Explaining your problem will also be necessary if you have to buy drugs for your hay fever, but the best course is to purchase these at home and take them with you.) Because "I have hay fever" does not feature in many phrase books, these are the words you need around the world:

Bulgarian	*Stradam ot senna hrema.*
Danish	*Jeg har hofeber.*
Dutch	*Ik lijd aan hooikoorts.*
Farsi	*Tabé yonjeh.*
Finnish	*Minulla on heinanuha.*
Flemish	*Ik heb hooikoorts.*
French	*J'ai le rhume des foins* or *J'ai la fièvre des foins.*
German	*Ich habe Heuschnupfen.*
Greek	*Eecho anoixiatiki allerghia.*
Hungarian	*Szèna I àzam van.*
Italian	*Soffro di febbre da fieno.*
Japanese	*Kafunshō desu.*
Norwegian	*Jeg har hoy feber.*
Polish	*Cierpię na katar sienny.*
Portuguese	*Eu tenho asma dos fenos.*
Russian	*U menya sennaya likhoradka.*
Spanish	*Padezco de alergia al polen.*
Swahili	There is no expression for hay fever in Swahili, and most people will not know of the disease. *Nina makamasi yaletwayo na mavumbi ya nyasi na majani* means "I have catarrh brought on by the dust of grasses," which should be reasonably well understood. Pollen is *chanuva* in Swahili, but the word is not widely known.
Swedish	*Jag har hosnuva.*

trees and Japanese red cedar form vast and beautiful forests that few would wish to see eliminated. However, there may be some other weeds that are as unloved and as dispensable as ragweed, and they could be tackled with similar methods. This would be worthwhile only for those that are a major cause of hay fever among large numbers of people.

There is certainly a case for tackling ragweed—one of nature's most allergenic plants—in those parts of the world where it has become an unwelcome immigrant. These include parts of France (notably around Lyon), Hungary, Czechoslovakia, the regions that were formerly Yugoslavia, the eastern part of Austria, the lake regions of northern Italy, and parts of Russia, Switzerland, and Japan. In general, ragweed seeds have arrived with grain imported from the United States. Hay fever in response to ragweed pollen is spreading in all these countries, and it seems clear that numbers will grow as the weed spreads, causing another hay fever epidemic. If the people of Montreal can make such an impression on ragweed on what is essentially its "home ground," then areas where it is an invader should be able to achieve far more. The sooner this problem is tackled the better, for as any gardener knows, a weed problem simply grows worse with every passing year.

Ragweed-sensitive visitors to Britain will probably be told that ragweed doesn't grow there, because of the cool climate and short summer season. In fact ragweed can often be found on wasteland, especially near seaports and sometimes in gardens (it is believed to originate from birdseed in these cases). Although the plants rarely set seed and thus don't form thriving colonies, ragweed pollen sometimes turns up in noticeable amounts over London and East Anglia. There is no sign of the counts increasing from one year to another, but this could change if global warming becomes a reality, and if it produces warmer springs and summers, allowing ragweed to spread by seeding.

In some countries, particularly those with warmer climates, certain introduced trees (such as she-oaks and cypresses) are a major source of allergenic pollen. Where these trees are simply being planted as windbreaks, as in parts of Florida, for example, and another species would do just as well, it would seem sensible to discourage any further planting of the offending trees.

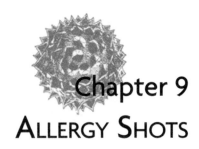

Chapter 9
ALLERGY SHOTS

There is something very satisfying about tackling a problem at the source—mending a broken pipe, for example, rather than just putting out a bucket to catch the drips. That may be why allergy shots for hay fever (more correctly called hyposensitization, desensitization, immunotherapy, or specific immunotherapy, or SIT) are so popular, since they apparently tackle the underlying problem, the malfunction in the immune system.

Treatments with allergy shots are far more expensive, at least in the short term, than most medicinal drugs and are certainly more time-consuming for both the patient and the doctor. There is no guarantee of success, and the treatment must be repeated every year at the outset. Nevertheless, many people choose allergy shots because they like the idea of turning off the allergic reaction, rather than trying to reduce it with drugs.

For some people, allergy shots may be the only viable treatment, since they have severe hay fever that is not helped by any of the drugs currently available. Other people use allergy shots in conjunction with drugs, since they find that the combined effect is far better than using one treatment alone. In every case, some sort of pollen avoidance will be valuable as well, reducing the allergen load so that the treatments have less to battle against.

Today there are two other forms of therapy with allergy shots, both of which are still hovering on the fringes of conventional medicine. One is known as **neutralization therapy,** the other as **enzyme-potentiated desensitization (EPD).** We will look at each of these three methods in turn.

ALLERGY SHOTS: THE CONVENTIONAL TECHNIQUE

This treatment uses injections of pollen extract just underneath the skin. A series of injections are given, with each one employing a more concentrated allergen extract than the one before. For the first injection, an extremely dilute solution is used, containing only the most minute quantity of allergen.

The dose is then increased gradually, which allows the body to learn to tolerate the allergen.

The treatment originated more than 80 years ago, when hay fever itself was still something of a novelty. Dr. Leonard Noon noted that hay fever was unheard of in those with the greatest exposure to pollen: farmers and farm laborers. (This is no longer the case today.) This observation led Dr. Noon to think that he might cure hay fever by exposing the patient to gradually increasing doses of pollen.

In Dr. Noon's original version of the treatment, the patient was given between 10 and 20 injections usually at the rate of 2 a week. Similar treatment schedules are used by some doctors today, although most draw the line at 15 injections and would not go up to 20 unless there were special difficulties.

Alternatively, there are now some much shorter courses, where the pollen extract is combined with another substance that speeds up the process. These shorter courses use only three or four injections, given at weekly intervals. While they can be helpful for some, the evidence available suggests that fewer patients benefit. Unpleasant side effects, such as asthmatic attacks and anaphylactic shock (see the box "Anaphylactic Shock" later in this chapter), may also be more likely.

Another approach is to use a large number of injections but to give them at daily intervals, known as **rush desensitization.** There are also experiments with speeded-up immunotherapy, called **ultrarush techniques;** at the outset, injections are given at hourly intervals or even more frequently (in a hospital, of course, where severe reactions can be dealt with immediately). Doctors have found that they can induce a remarkably rapid tolerance of the allergen in this way.

This long reeducation of the immune system has to be completed well before the pollen season arrives. An interval of at least a month is recommended between the last injection and the pollen onslaught. Some careful advance planning is therefore needed.

Time should be built in for possible setbacks. If an injection produces an allergic reaction (other than itching and redness at the injection site), it is clear that the treatment has progressed too quickly, so the allergist administers the same dose for the next injection or even goes back to a lower one. Infections make people more reactive to the injections, so if a cold or flu strikes during the course, the concentration will be lowered or kept the same until it has passed. Setbacks such as these obviously lengthen the whole process.

It is vital that appointments be kept throughout the course of injections because missing a couple of weeks can wipe out all the benefits so far accrued.

The treatment course may then have to start again, right from the beginning, and there will probably be insufficient time to complete it before pollen season.

To allow for hitches in the schedule, a few extra weeks are added to the total time needed for the course. If things go smoothly, this means that the course finishes well before the pollen season. In such circumstances, the allergist usually gives a weekly maintenance dose, equal in concentration to the last dose injected, until one month before pollen season.

Some allergists continue giving maintenance doses (but at a lower concentration) at monthly intervals throughout the pollen season. This seems to help sustain the good effects of the treatment. (At one time, allergy shots were carried out during the pollen season for those who had forgotten to start them in advance, but these have now been abandoned because they showed few good effects.)

To be sure of leaving enough time for the treatment, you should consult your doctor or allergist about allergy shots well in advance. Make an appointment to discuss the treatment six months before you expect the pollen season to begin.

If the treatment with allergy shots is carried out well, at least 80 percent of those treated will probably benefit to some extent. While they may not lose all traces of hay fever, they will be far less reactive to pollen and need smaller doses of drugs to keep their symptoms under control. The success rate seems to depend very much upon the technique used and the care with which it is carried out. Don't be afraid to ask the doctor or allergist about his or her success rate before you decide on taking the treatment.

You may be able to judge in advance if allergy shots are likely to help you. Observations by various doctors suggest that certain types of hay fever patients will not benefit from this treatment. They are the people whose symptoms do not come on immediately when they are exposed to the allergen and who take a long time to recover when pollen clears from the air. Suppose, for example, that you are grass-sensitive, but you know that walking through long grass in flower will not produce symptoms immediately—this is unusual for hay fever patients and indicates a slower type of response. If a rainy day during the pollen season does not clear your symptoms and it takes three days of rain to bring any relief, this too is a sign of unusually slow reactions. People in this group tend not to experience their worst hay fever symptoms when outdoors in the evening, but wake up the following morning with a bad attack—a belated response to the previous evening's dose of pollen.

Those who recognize this pattern of response in themselves are unlikely to do well with allergy shots. Research shows that such people frequently respond well to a treatment that is, unfortunately, not readily available in the United States at the moment, enzyme-potentiated desensitization, or EPD (discussed later in this chapter). In general, those who have tried conventional allergy shots without experiencing much improvement have a good chance of success with EPD: the two seem to have different effects on the immune system.

Conventional allergy shots are often continued for four to five years and then stopped. About 60 percent of patients who found the treatment helpful continue to show positive effects without the annual course of injections. A great deal of research has been done into how allergy shots work, and some answers have been obtained (see "Controlling IgE" in chapter 3).

When carried out with proper care, the treatment rarely has adverse effects. With most patients, any adverse reactions will appear within 30 minutes, and most can be dealt with promptly by an injection of epinephrine. Resuscitation equipment is rarely needed.

If you are having allergy shots, you can help to ensure your own safety. Inquire about the facilities for emergency care before you start the treatment. Once it begins, be sure to tell the doctor or nurse giving the injections:

- If you experienced any adverse reaction after the previous injection

- If you have an infection at present (this can alter your reaction to the treatment)

- If you develop asthma, either during a course of injections or between one year's treatment and the next; asthma may express itself as wheezing, tightness in the chest, shortness of breath (especially in cold air, or when exercising), or a persistent cough

Research is currently taking place on new and safer extracts for use in treatment with allergy shots. Various methods are being tried, all of which aim to change the allergen in some way, so that it activates the suppressive arm of the immune system without being able to fire off mast cells (see pages 139–140).

LIMITATIONS OF IMMUNOTHERAPY

Needless to say, if you are having allergy shots with extract of ragweed pollen when you are actually sensitive to mold spores, the treatment is not going to work. Accurate diagnosis is therefore essential. Before the treatment begins, you will be given a skin-prick test to confirm the diagnosis, but remember that the test can produce a false positive (see chapter 6).

ANAPHYLACTIC SHOCK

One of the drawbacks of allergy shots is the risk of **anaphylactic shock,** a massive allergic response affecting the whole body. Anaphylactic shock occurs when a large number of the body's mast cells discharge their mediators at once.

One effect of mast-cell mediators such as histamine is to make blood vessels wider and more leaky (for more details on mast-cell behavior, see chapter 3). This effect is beneficial during local infections, when it occurs in a restricted area of the body, but during anaphylactic shock it occurs *throughout* the body. With the same amount of blood coursing through a greatly enlarged set of channels, there is far less blood available to fill the vessels, and the blood pressure falls to a dangerously low level. Often, the patient's pulse becomes very weak.

Anyone suffering from anaphylactic shock is seriously ill and needs immediate hospital treatment. There is a very real danger of death if treatment is delayed, especially if the person is asthmatic, because the bronchi also become severely narrowed during the attack.

Resuscitation equipment, of the kind available in hospitals, may be needed to deal with the attack. Epinephrine and antihistamine (sometimes with corticosteroids as well) are injected to counteract the effects of the massive histamine release. (Anyone at risk of anaphylactic shock can carry a syringe that is preloaded with epinephrine. These are made available to anyone with a strong reaction to bee or wasp stings and to those with severe food allergy.)

With allergy shots, anaphylactic shock occurs if the patient's immune system has not "kept up" with the gradually increasing concentrations of allergen. Instead of steadily becoming less sensitive to the allergen, the immune system suddenly takes a violent objection to the increased dosage. Often there is a warning that this is about to happen—the preceding treatment session will produce some sort of adverse reaction, such as a very large local swelling or a minor bodily reaction. The cautious allergist should always take note of such reactions and either reduce the next dose or keep it the same.

You can save yourself, and the doctor, a lot of time by not embarking on a series of injections with the wrong allergen. Read chapters 6 and 12, then consider whether the skin-prick test result agrees with the other facts, such as when and where you experience symptoms.

The other major limitation of the technique is that there are only a certain number of extracts available commercially, and if you happen to be allergic to yak sweat or passionflower pollen, you will be out of luck. Assuming your allergen has been identified, and can easily be collected, some allergists may be prepared to make the extracts themselves.

ENZYME-POTENTIATED DESENSITIZATION

This desensitization method is said to rely on the ability of an enzyme (see the box "Understanding Proteins" in chapter 1) to enhance the desensitizing effect of a pollen allergen. The enzyme in question is called (ß-glucuronidase. The enzyme is mixed with the pollen extract and then injected into the skin (an intradermal injection). Alternatively, the skin can be scratched and the pollen extract plus enzyme applied to the area in a small plastic cup. This latter method is safer for people with violent allergic reactions because the extract is not injected into the skin and therefore should not provoke an anaphylactic reaction. (It has never yet done so, despite years of use with some very sensitive patients.) This degree of caution is rarely needed in hay fever, but it might be appropriate for some people with pollen asthma who are at high risk of anaphylaxis, and it is also useful for people with immediate-onset food allergies: both conditions are regarded as too dangerous for conventional allergy shots to be used. The scratch method of enzyme-potentiated desensitization (EPD) is also suitable for children who are afraid of injections, and in the hands of an expert the method is safe for quite small children.

An unusual feature of EPD is that a standard mixture of pollen allergens is used rather than individual pollen extracts, so each patient is treated with all the common allergenic pollens. However, a diagnostic skin-prick test is still used before the treatment, and where there are other sensitivities, such as to dust mites and mold spores, the appropriate allergen extracts can be added to the pollen mixture.

Careful scientific testing of EPD has been carried out several times in both Britain and Italy, and these trials have shown that it works work well for grass, olive, and pellitory pollen. Ideally, the method should be scientifically tested with other pollen allergies as well, but until this is done we must rely on the general observations of doctors using the method. These suggest that EPD is successful with many different pollen sensitivities.

Approximately 80 percent of patients are helped by EPD, with 40 to 65 percent being a great deal better than before. When compared directly with conventional allergy shots, using the same assessment methods, the two techniques produce equally good results, with EPD having far fewer adverse reactions and therefore being safer. It is also much less time-consuming, needing just one or two injections a year in most cases, compared with a series of 10 to 15 injections for conventional allergy shots.

Those who do not benefit at all from EPD are usually helped by conventional allergy shots, and the reverse is also true. This suggests that the two techniques work by fundamentally different mechanisms.

The EPD treatment should be given before the hay fever season begins, preferably about three weeks before. Some patients benefit from having a second injection in late autumn, which improves the response in the following year. The treatments will need to be repeated annually for three to five years, but after this period many patients find that they are free of hay fever.

Doctors are often suspicious of techniques that work by unknown means, and tend to reject both EPD and neutralization therapy (see below) for this reason. Yet the conventional technique, allergy shots, was in use for many years before anyone understood how it worked. Even now, no one can say exactly how it works in each individual who benefits from it (see "Controlling IgE" in chapter 3).

Enzyme potentiated desensitization is not currently available in the United States (except on a personal importation basis) due to a ruling by the FDA. There are hopes that this may change at some point in the future.

PROVOCATION-NEUTRALIZATION TECHNIQUE

This is also known as intradermal neutralization therapy, or the Miller technique, after Dr. Joseph Miller, of Alabama, who spent many years developing it and investigating its applications. The treatment can be given in two ways— either using injections of allergen extracts under the skin or giving the extracts in drops under the tongue, known as **sublingual drops.** With treatments for hay fever and other forms of rhinitis, sublingual drops are often used.

In both cases, the doctor must first discover which allergens are involved, by using a skin-prick test (see chapter 6). Once the problem allergens have been identified, the next step is to establish the **neutralization dose.** This is the concentration of each allergen extract that is necessary to desensitize the individual patient to that allergen—different concentrations are required for different individuals.

To test for the correct dose, intradermal injections, which put pollen extracts into the skin, are used. These go deeper than the skin-prick tests, but are not especially painful. A tiny amount of the allergen extract is used.

If the concentration is too low to produce any significant reaction in the skin, the injection simply results in a small raised area, known as a wheal, which begins to go down soon afterward. If the body does react, then the wheal grows slightly and takes on a characteristic appearance, becoming white, hard, and raised, with a sharp edge. This is known as a positive wheal.

When a positive wheal is obtained, the dose is then reduced for the next injection, and repeatedly reduced, step by step, until a concentration is reached that fails to produce a positive wheal. The highest concentration of extract that fails to produce a positive wheal is the neutralizing dose. As well as producing desensitization, it can, for some patients, actually "turn off" hay fever symptoms that have already begun.

Testing for the neutralizing dose can take one or two hours per allergen. Someone who is allergic to just a few pollens can have his or her neutralizing doses established in an afternoon, but for someone sensitive to several different allergens, a day or two of testing could be needed. Some practitioners speed up the process by using mixed pollen extracts and establishing a neutralizing dose for the mixture, but this does not give such good results as does testing with individual pollen types.

Testing for the neutralizing dose is best done a month or two before the pollen season, but if necessary it can be carried out at any time of year.

Once the neutralizing dose has been established, it can be self-injected by the patient, or taken as drops whenever needed. Most practitioners suggest a daily injection for the first week of the pollen season, then every other day for a few weeks. After that, the patient can experiment to find his or her own dosing regimen—as often as necessary to keeps the symptoms under control. The drops are used two or three times a day at first, then as often as needed.

How neutralization therapy might work is not known. It is possible that, when the neutralizing dose is used, the pollen allergens are bound to skin cells inside the wheal for a long period of time, allowing them to exert a particular influence on the immune system. Perhaps they act by stimulating T suppressor cells (see "Checks and Balances" in chapter 3), which could then reduce the immune response to pollen in the nose and eyes.

From a practical point of view, neutralization is less bothersome than allergy shots in that the tests for the neutralization dose can probably be carried out in a single day, rather than involving repeated visits to the doctor's office. Compared to EPD, it is rather more time-consuming because of the testing process required. Furthermore, the neutralization point may change, so that the vaccine stops working as well. If this happens, you will need to go back for retesting. On the plus side, testing for the neutralization dose can be carried out during pollen season and therapy begun then, and while it may not be as effective as treatment begun earlier in the year, most patients will probably reap some benefits.

Ensure that the practitioner uses a skin test to determine the neutralization dose. Once the neutralization dose has been established, the drops (or injection vaccine) are relatively inexpensive. Most practitioners retest for the neutralizing dose every year.

Doctors experienced in this technique have found that it is important to neutralize for all the pollens (or other allergens) that give a positive skin test. If only one or two allergens are dealt with, even though these may be the major allergens for the patient, the results will be less satisfactory.

NEW FORMS OF DESENSITIZATION

Medical researchers continue to experiment with different approaches to desensitization. Instead of injecting the allergen extract, some doctors are now giving it to their patients in capsule form, to be swallowed. Others are giving it as a liquid, to be placed under the tongue and held there for a few minutes, then spat out. Both these methods are developments of the basic technique developed for allergy shots and involve gradually increasing doses of the allergen, given over a period of time. Scientific trials show that both methods work well, at least with certain allergens. Surprisingly, some trials show that when allergens are held under the tongue, they are not absorbed into the bloodstream, but rather simply stay stuck to the surface of the mouth—somehow exerting an effect on the immune system in this way.

Much research is now focused on developing modified forms of allergens **(allergoids)** that could be used in allergy shots and could induce tolerance without any risk of a bad reaction.

To make an allergoid, scientists carefully alter the allergen so that IgE antibodies no longer recognize it (eliminating the risk of a bad reaction to the shot itself). At the same time, enough of the allergen is left unchanged for it to still interact with T helper (Th) cells. What makes this possible is the fact that one part of the allergen molecule interacts with antibodies while a different part interacts with Th cells.

An allergoid made from ragweed allergen and injected into someone with hay fever could teach ragweed-specific Th cells not to give the "go ahead" signal for a reaction to real ragweed pollen.

The safety of allergoids may allow a very fast schedule of allergy shots. Some experimenters claim that their allergoids can work with just a single shot.

A far more radical approach being developed by researchers in Belgium is to make a vaccine by extracting pollen-specific antibodies from the blood of hay fever sufferers and then combining them with pollen allergens. When allergen and antibody combine, they form a complicated tangle that includes many molecules of each type. This is known as an **immune complex.** Having made their immune complexes, the researchers inject them into the skin of hay fever patients, and this appears to produce a beneficial desensitizing effect. In trials carried out so far, there were no side effects at all. If future trials are equally successful, this treatment may become available in the next few years.

Another radical approach is to shift the immune system away from allergy altogether by altering the balance of Th1 cells and Th2 cells (see page 36). Given the new discoveries about hygiene (see chapter 4), researchers decided to try making a vaccine from soil bacteria and using it to treat adult asthmatics. It worked—at least one third of the asthmatics showed far less reaction to inhaled allergen after receiving the vaccine.

Chapter 10

ALTERNATIVE TREATMENTS
FOR HAY FEVER

Conventional medicine has some powerful weapons against hay fever, as described in chapters 7 and 9, but many people still turn to other forms of treatment. This chapter looks at all those that we have come across and tries to assess whether or not they may help you.

You will, no doubt, meet people who have "found the cure" for hay fever. There are two things to bear in mind when considering such claims. One is that most people grow out of hay fever as they get older, usually before the age of 30. So the friend or colleague who claims that his hay fever cleared up as soon as he cut down on beer, stopped disco dancing, or started having a milky drink at bedtime is probably just reporting a coincidence. The second point to consider is the **placebo effect,** a phenomenon well known to medicine, whereby any new treatment will have some positive effect for most people. The placebo effect can operate with pills or capsules, a visit to a helpful and reassuring doctor or therapist, a dietary supplement, a special diet, or a change in lifestyle. In all cases, belief that the treatment will work is the crucial element.

For example, in a trial of dust-proof mattress covers used for asthma, the control group of patients, who were given mattress covers that let through the dust-mite allergen, showed a small improvement in their symptoms. This is why scientific trials always include a control group—a set of patients who are given a similar but ineffective treatment. To separate the placebo effect from the real effect, the results observed in these patients can be deducted from the benefit seen with the real treatment.

The placebo effect works for everyone, not just the gullible or dim-witted, and it seems to work by harnessing the body's own potential for self-healing. We all have far more control over our bodies than we are aware of, and a placebo (originally the name for ineffective sugar pills dispensed by baffled doctors) somehow taps into that inner power and makes it work in our favor.

Placebo effects are part of any medical treatment—they give a boost to the benefits available from medicinal drugs, for example, and to the good effects of desensitization. But with these conventional treatments, scientific trials have been carried out to verify that there is also a *real* effect from the treatment itself. With unconventional treatments, such as herbs, this is generally not the case: they have not been tested and compared with a control group to see if they are any more effective than a placebo. Thus, the claim that such remedies "relieve hay fever symptoms" may be quite honestly made, yet the apparent benefits could be nothing more than a placebo effect.

If the placebo effect works, then why worry? This is a valid argument, but the placebo effect from a new treatment lasts only a short while. Once a person's initial enthusiasm about the treatment wears off, the placebo effect ebbs. Furthermore, the effect of a placebo will rarely match that of a genuinely effective drug or treatment. You may as well spend your money on something that really works.

Before leaving this subject, we should briefly mention **negative placebo effects.** These are seen, for example, when patients in the control group of a scientific trial—those taking a harmless placebo—report side effects. Here it seems that some people *are* far more susceptible than others. Those who have had bad reactions to a drug in the past may suffer negative placebo effects from a new drug, particularly if they are worried about side effects.

TREATMENTS TO UNBLOCK THE NOSE

A blocked nose can best be unblocked by means of corticosteroid nose drops, preceded if necessary by a brief treatment with sympathomimetic nose drops (see chapter 7). For those who do not wish to use such drugs, there may be other ways of easing the congestion.

The traditional treatment used for colds—inhaling steam—can also be very effective in hay fever. Use a mixing bowl from the kitchen, pour in boiling water, put a towel over your head and shoulders, and sit with your face over the bowl so that you are inhaling the steam. The longer you continue with this, the more effective the treatment will be. You may need to replace the water as it cools.

Menthol, eucalyptus, and other essential oils with a decongestant action are sometimes added to the hot water to improve its effects. They can be bought from most health food stores or pharmacies. You could try adding these, but stop using them if there seems to be any irritation to the nose.

There are now various steam-inhalation devices for sale (see appendix 3) that achieve much the same thing as the old-fashioned bowl of hot water and towel treatment.

Saltwater nose drops can also be useful in relieving congestion a little and soothing the irritated membranes of the nose. Sterile saltwater (or saline) solution can be purchased at any pharmacy. You can also buy a dropper bottle, the lid of which contains a dropper for placing the saltwater drops in the nose. Fill the bottle with the salt water and change it every few days. Use the drops as often as you feel you need them.

Nose drops containing vitamin C have been tried out by doctors in Israel, who tested them against placebo drops. They noted that the secretions of the nose are normally very slightly acidic, but that during a bout of rhinitis they become very slightly alkaline. It therefore occurred to them to try reversing this effect using a mildly acidic solution of vitamin C. About three-quarters of the patients tested experienced some benefit from these drops. Unfortunately, the concentration of vitamin C used in these tests was not reported. If you would like to try this treatment, start with a very dilute solution—a quarter of a teaspoon of pure vitamin C powder in a pint of water. Should there be no beneficial effect, slightly increase the amount of vitamin C used—but if it stings, the solution is too concentrated. The water used should be boiled for at least 20 minutes beforehand to kill bacteria. Alternatively, buy purified water from a pharmacist. As with saltwater drops, buy a small dropper bottle to contain the solution you have prepared and refill with fresh solution every few days. The drops should be used three times daily. Stop using the drops if you have a cold or other infection in the nose.

TREATMENTS TO REDUCE THE ALLERGIC RESPONSE

Research has shown that breathing hot humid air doesn't just help unblock the nose (see "Treatments to Unblock the Nose" beginning on the previous page), it also reduces the reaction that occurs when an allergen enters the nose. Exactly how it does this is unknown, but scientists have found out that just warming up the membranes of the nose has a good effect, making the nose far less sensitive to its allergens.

So how do you warm the membranes in your nose? Well, it might sound strange, but you put your feet in a bowl of warm water. Medical scientists at the University of Chicago had one group of hay fever sufferers sit with their feet in hot water for 5 minutes; another group sat with their feet in water that was at room temperature. Then they inserted pollen allergens into their noses (it wasn't pollen season at the time). The ones with warm feet sneezed only half as much and produced far less mucus than the others.

What on earth would make scientists try such a weird experiment in the first place? In fact, they already knew that warming the feet increases the temperature of the blood in the nose without substantially increasing overall body temperature.

If you have ragweed allergy, the idea of putting your feet in a bowl of hot water on a sweltering August day probably isn't that appealing, but people with allergies to tree pollens, which get airborne in early spring, might just find this esoteric piece of research useful. Of course, you can't sit with your feet in hot water all day, but you could buy some thermal socks or fur-lined boots and see if the spring sneezes abate.

Rather less bizarre are the findings of medical researchers in Spain, who tried simply flushing pollen out of the nose with salt water. Hay fever sufferers were asked to irrigate their noses three times a day, for 4 to 5 minutes each time, using a special device called a Water Pik, which forces a pulsating stream of salt water into one nostril and out of the other. They continued with this for eight weeks, throughout the grass pollen season. Rather than asking the patients how they felt, the researchers actually looked at the levels of IgE (the allergy antibody) in the blood to see what effect the nose-wash treatment was having. Sure enough, with the onset of the grass pollen season, IgE levels began to rise steeply in the control group (no treatment apart from their usual drugs) while those using the saltwater treatment (plus their usual drugs) showed a much more modest increase in IgE.

DIETARY SUPPLEMENTS

One treatment worth trying is to take cod-liver oil (two teaspoons a day). This contains certain natural oils that affect the production and control of **prostaglandins,** chemical messengers produced by the body that have a subtle influence on the inflammation process.

By favoring the production of some prostaglandins over others, fish oils reduce the tendency to inflammation in the body, which is why they are often recommended for rheumatoid arthritis. Recent studies have shown that they are also valuable in asthma and possibly in hay fever. Since it is an inexpensive treatment, it is worth a try. Never take too much cod-liver oil, as it is a rich source of vitamin A, which is toxic in excessive doses. The effect of cod-liver oil on the prostaglandins takes about three months to become fully established, so do not expect any immediate benefits. To maintain the effect, you need to keep taking the oil.

Evening primrose oil is likewise used for rheumatoid arthritis and has also been suggested as a useful supplement in hay fever. No one has yet carried out any tests to see if it really is effective, but it could be useful because it too has an impact on the prostaglandin balance in the body. It can be used in addition to cod-liver oil, and may augment the effects. Again, it takes about three months to build up its protective action.

High doses of vitamin C were once proposed as a treatment for hay fever, but medical trials have shown that they are not effective. Ginseng and cider vinegar have also been suggested, but there is no evidence for these either. Scientific trials with ginseng in healthy individuals have shown that it can have unpleasant side effects when taken for a prolonged period, such as diarrhea.

Eating honey in a honeycomb has also been suggested as a treatment, because it contains some pollen. There are no trials of this treatment but it does not seem likely to work. The pollen in honey will rarely be the sort of pollen that hay fever sufferers react to (see "Bees or Breeze?" in chapter 1). We all swallow quite a bit of pollen during the spring and summer anyway, as it catches on the saliva in the mouth. So if eating pollen could cure or prevent hay fever, nobody would develop this annoying disease in the first place—there would be an unseen remedy all around us.

IONIZED AIR

Air ionizers work as cleaning devices, removing particles from the air (see appendix 3). It has also been claimed, by some hay fever sufferers, that the stream of ions coming from the ionizer has a direct therapeutic effect. By facing the ionizer at close range, and so allowing the ions to flow over their face, they apparently experience relief from existing symptoms of hay fever, such as itchy eyes and a streaming nose. One German manufacturer has even produced a portable air ionizer, to be worn around the neck, that emits ions over the face.

There is nothing known about ions to suggest how this might work, and most doctors and scientists are dismissive of such claims. To the best of our knowledge, no one has tested the direct effects of ions on hay fever symptoms. However, claims of substantial improvement in hay fever have been made repeatedly, and there is probably no harm in trying the effects of ionized air, if you feel inclined to do so. Stores that specialize in selling ionizers often have a demonstration model running, so you can try it out—the effects are supposed to come on within a few minutes. Some ionizers may produce a small amount of ozone (see appendix 6), which you could inhale if at close range. Should you experience any coughing or irritation of the nose or airways, then turn off the ionizer immediately.

HYPNOTHERAPY

A scientist in the United States has looked at the effect of hypnosis on relieving congestion of the nose in hay fever sufferers. He classified the patients studied into "high hypnotizable" and "low hypnotizable" subjects.

The "high hypnotizable" set showed considerable benefit from hypnotherapy sessions aimed at reducing their congestion. However, they also did well on sympathomimetic drops (see chapter 7) and on placebo drops. Compared with "low hypnotizable" patients, they did much better on all three treatments, and still showed the benefits a month later, when they had fewer hay fever attacks and were using their medicinal drugs less often.

It seems that "high hypnotizable" subjects are more susceptible to placebo effects (discussed earlier in this chapter), although other studies of placebos have not found this link.

The practical conclusion from all this is that if you respond to hypnosis, you will respond equally well to any treatment that you believe in, so hypnotherapy is probably a rather expensive option. Self-hypnosis might be worth trying if you are keen on totally natural cures. There are various tapes available that teach self-hypnosis—inquire in health food stores or try the Internet.

HERBAL MEDICINES

There are various herbal medicines on sale that claim to alleviate hay fever and perennial allergic rhinitis. The following ones have been tested:

Butterbur *(Petasites hybridus)* may be a very effective treatment for hay fever. It was recently compared to an antihistamine and did just as well in controlling hay fever symptoms, but did not produce drowsiness. This plant contains substances that are known to affect the immune system, and it has also been used to treat asthma.

Stinging nettle *(Urtica dioica)* was thought to be as good as, or better than, previous hay fever medications by half of the patients tested. The dose used was two 300 mg capsules taken whenever symptoms were experienced. This is not a conclusive study, but it does suggest that stinging nettle might be a useful treatment. It is probably a safe herb.

Ginkgo *(Ginkgo biloba)* may decrease the body's reaction to allergens. (For those with pollen asthma, it could also help by calming the inflammation of the airways.)

Luffa complex (also marketed as Pollinosan) contains extracts of several different plant products, including the sponge cucumber. (Also called a luffa or loofah, this is better known as a scratchy cylinder used to scrub the skin while showering.) Unpublished results of a trial carried out by the manufacturer suggest that 75 percent of hay fever sufferers find benefit from this mixture. Needless to say, a published trial from an independent research team would be more convincing.

Grape seed extract has been tested with hay fever sufferers and showed no benefit.

Quercetin is found in red wine, apples, onions, and other foods and is therefore likely to be safe as long as you don't overdo the dose. It has been tested in the laboratory with mast cells taken from the noses of people with allergic rhinitis (mast cells are responsible for starting off the allergic reaction). Exposure to quercetin made the cells less likely to respond to allergen. That is impressive, but it is not known if this translates into real benefits when quercetin is swallowed by hay fever sufferers—there are all kinds of unknowns involved. When absorbed from the stomach, does it reach the nose intact? Does quercetin affect the mast cells in the same way when they are in the nose rather than in a test tube? If you want to give quercetin a try, in spite of these unknowns, the dose usually recommended is between 250 mg and 600 mg, taken 5 to 10 minutes before meals.

Perilla 6000, which is marketed as a treatment for hay fever and other allergies, contains *Perilla frutescens,* a Chinese herb with a long folk tradition of treating allergy, plus *Coleus forskohlii.* The latter has been tested for asthma and has definite benefits, but it can also cause unpleasant side effects: soreness in the mouth and nausea. Perilla itself has been tested only in animals, but did show promising results in blocking allergic reactions. (Unfortunately, this mixture also contains alfalfa, which is harmful to some people with autoimmune diseases such as systemic lupus erythematosus.) Perilla 6000 is not yet sold in the United States, but can be ordered from suppliers in the United Kingdom or Australia, who can be found via the Internet.

Before taking any herbal medicine, consider the possibility of allergic reactions, particularly if you suffer symptoms in the mouth from certain foods. Proceed very cautiously (see "Herbal Medicines" on page 167). Remember that something as apparently innocuous as chamomile could cause potentially fatal asthma attacks in a few susceptible hay fever sufferers (see the box with Jack's story on page 168).

Toxicity is also a possibility to bear in mind. The idea that something must be safe because it is "natural" is obviously mistaken—hemlock is natural and so is belladonna, both deadly poisons. Most plants are not this lethal but would still make you ill if you ate them. Why else do we warn our children, when out on rambles, not to eat leaves, berries, or fungi, other than the few that we know are safe?

The other great myth about herbal medicines is that they must be safe "because people have been using them for centuries." The fact is that side effects that are slow to appear, or affect only a minority of people, will not necessarily be traced back to their true cause. Dozens of cautionary tales can be told about substances (not just herbal medicines, but also local foodstuffs and ceremonial substances such as tobacco) that had been used for eons and seemed unimpeachable, but were actually very damaging. Their toxicity went unrecognized for centuries, even millennia, just because the bad effects were variable and didn't come on immediately.

It is also true, with substances derived from food plants, that they might be safe at the levels normally consumed but dangerous when taken at high dose in purified form. This has proved to be the case with beta carotene, a pigment and antioxidant found in carrots, apricots, mangoes, and many other fruits. When taken in high dose by smokers, it actually increased the risk of lung cancer rather than decreasing it, as was hoped.

If you are thinking about taking a particular herbal medicine, you could try writing to the manufacturer to ask if it has been tested for safety according to modern standards. Unfortunately, very few have, so you must be on the lookout for side effects when taking herbs. Notice any changes in your health, especially the signs of liver damage (yellow jaundiced skin, yellowing of the whites of the eyes, pale feces, dark urine, nausea, and pain). Deaths due to herbal medicines have generally been the result of either liver damage or kidney damage.

Herbal medicines can also interact with conventional drugs, in the same way that one drug can interact with another drug. The following herbs have unfavorable interactions with drugs that you may be taking for allergies:

- Kava-kava can increase the typical side effects of antihistamines: drowsiness and poor coordination.

MADELEINE

Madeleine was very sensitive to several pollens, including silver birch, plane tree, various grasses, plantain, and nettles. She suffered from asthma as well as hay fever, and because so many pollens affected her, she had to endure the symptoms from early spring right through to the autumn. Although she tried antihistamines, they did not help much, and as she disliked taking drugs anyway, she gave them up.

After four years of "summer misery," Mad-eleine decided to try alternative treatments and found that the most successful one for her was acupuncture. The treatment is carried out each spring, with two 20-minute sessions. Sometimes these are enough to protect her from symptoms for the entire summer, but occasionally she needs a booster dose later. Most hay fever sufferers find that they need more treatment sessions than this, usually five or more.

- Ginseng, buckthorn, aloe vera, cascara sagrada, and senna all interact with steroid tablets.

- Pheasant's eye, rhubarb root, squill, and lily of the valley interact with one particular steroid: *betamethasone.* They will increase both the desired effects of the drug and its side effects.

ACUPUNCTURE

This is a system of medicine originating in China that involves stimulating specific sites on the body known as the acupuncture points. Stimulation of these points is generally done with tiny needles, but there are many different versions of acupuncture treatment, some using needles that carry an electrical current, others using suction cups.

According to traditional Chinese theory, the acupuncture points all lie on **meridians,** channels that allow vital energy (called *chi* or *qi* in Chinese—you pronounce it "chee") to flow around the body. Illness occurs when the flow of qi is blocked. Western science can't measure qi and can't find anything significant at the acupuncture points, although quite a few of them are over deep pressure receptors or near major nerve endings. Some of the meridians run roughly in line with particular blood vessels or nerves, but they don't follow them exactly. On the other hand, there are observable and measurable effects from acupuncture, such as the release of endogenous opioids—the body's homemade painkillers.

Bear in mind that, just because the techniques are effective (or partially effective), this doesn't necessarily mean the traditional theory should be believed. This is true of any system of alternative medicine, not just acupuncture. It could be that the techniques were developed through trial and error, and the theoretical framework, although it was constructed in an attempt to explain how the techniques work, is not the true explanation.

Few would deny that acupuncture is an effective system of altering bodily responses—its dramatic effects in producing local deadening of the nerves, so that surgeons can operate on a fully conscious patient, are convincing evidence that this is a powerful form of treatment. Whether acupuncture effectively treats all the ailments for which it is offered is another matter.

Scientific trials are difficult to carry out with acupuncture, given that it is essentially an individualized treatment—a good acupuncturist tailors the treatment to you, not your disease. The usual basis of a scientific trial is that everyone has the same diagnosis (e.g., hay fever or allergic asthma) and everyone in the treatment group is given the same treatment. This may not give acupuncture a fair trial.

We know of only one trial using acupuncture for hay fever, and the placebo group (whose needles were inserted away from any acupuncture points) improved to about the same degree as the treatment group. The results with asthma are more promising—it seems that acupuncture can help open up the airways a little and may even reduce the inflammation of the airways, especially if an individualized treatment approach is used.

Where acupuncture works, it usually seems to do so by affecting nerve impulses in some way.

Because there are nervous reflexes that control the production of mucus and the swelling of blood vessels in the nose (see the box "Nerves in the Nose" in chapter 13), it is not implausible to suggest that acupuncture could help in reducing hay fever symptoms. During the 1980s, scientists in the United States also discovered tiny nerve cells that lie alongside mast cells (see page 30) and may influence their action. This unexpected discovery offers another route by which acupuncture could affect an allergic reaction such as hay fever—and affect it at a more fundamental level.

Acupuncturists are adamant that they can help people with hay fever, and many patients do report good effects. Most acupuncturists say that five or six treatments are generally needed during the pollen season to maintain the good effects. Some patients are helped by just two treatments in the spring, but this is unusual.

HOMEOPATHY

Homeopathy is a form of treatment first devised by a German doctor, Samuel Hahnemann, at the end of the 18th century. Hahnemann was appalled by the drastic effects of some of the remedies then used by doctors—such as blood-letting, emetics, and cathartics—and in this he was undoubtedly right. Hahnemann abandoned the medical techniques he had been taught and devised his own system based on the idea that "like cures like."

Homeopathy uses a substance—animal, vegetable, or mineral—that produces the same symptoms as those it aims to treat. The substance used is called a **similium.** The similium is ground up in alcohol, or a mixture of alcohol and water, and the extract is then diluted, 1 drop in 99 drops of water, alcohol, or both. A single drop of that mixture is taken and diluted with another 99 drops. This process is repeated many times, and each time the dilution is made the mixture is **succussed** or **percussed.** This means repeatedly hitting the container against "a hard but elastic object, such as a leather-bound book" (to quote Hahnemann). The dilution process might be repeated as many as 30 times, producing a **30C (or 30X) potency.** According to homeopathic ideas, the power of the extract to treat the patient *increases* with each dilution, so that one diluted 20 times (a 20C potency) is *less* effective than one diluted 30 times.

Having made the 30C potency, this is then "impregnated" into tablets made of lactose, the sugar found in milk. Homeopaths take a bottle of "blank" lactose tablets, add a few drops of the potentized solution, then shake the bottle. The drops of potentized solution fall on only a few of the tablets near the mouth of the bottle, and most of the tablets are untouched by them. Yet all the tablets in the bottle are said to acquire the same therapeutic power. Other homeopaths may give the liquid itself.

One of the reasons that scientists are so skeptical about homeopathy is that they can calculate, approximately, the number of molecules of the active substance (the similium) in the first drop of extract used. They can then calculate how many there are in the first dilution, the second dilution, and so on. Quite early on in the process, there are only one or two molecules of the similium left. By the 30th dilution, there is unlikely to be even one molecule left. *The 30th potency contains none of the similium.*

Homeopaths argue that, during succussion, the similium somehow imposes an "informational structure" on the water, alcohol, or water-alcohol mixture and that this is what makes homoeopathic medicines active. But substances such as alcohol and water are extremely simple chemically, and very well understood by science (far better understood, for example, than the subtle workings of the human body). Chemists can state fairly confidently that there is nothing in the alcohol or water that can take on a "structure," and certainly no way in which that structure could be passed on with successive dilutions, becoming more potent each time. Even if there were such a "structure," how could it be communicated to lactose tablets at the bottom of the bottle, where no drop or splash of the 30C potency is felt? Such explanations seem to be invoking something akin to magic.

Despite all this, there are people who are convinced that homeopathy cured them of hay fever. How can this be explained? First, it could be the placebo effect (discussed earlier in this chapter), and some experts think that homeopathy has a particularly powerful placebo effect for certain historical reasons (see below). Second, they might have been growing out of hay fever naturally, as many people do, and this spontaneous recovery happened to occur during the period of homeopathy treatment. This explanation is obviously more plausible if they have been using homeopathy for some time than if they just tried it for a short period.

Notice, too, that there is a "reporting bias" in relation to alternative medicine: people who have had success with an alternative therapy are keen to tell others about it, whereas those who don't have good results rarely mention their experience. If you make a point of asking your friends and colleagues, you'll hear comments such as "I must admit homeopathy has never done a thing for my allergies." But people don't usually volunteer this information, which helps create the impression that alternative therapy is far more effective than it actually is. (Why the reporting bias? Our guess is that there is a strong desire to believe in alternative medicine among many people, and those with negative experiences don't like to spoil things for others.)

This kind of "reporting bias" also affects research, unfortunately. When you read in a health magazine that "a new trial shows that homeopathy works for hay fever," you can be pretty sure that, over the previous year or two, there have been other trials showing no effect for homeopathy—but these won't get the same coverage. Some of these negative trials will not be published at all; others will appear quietly in a research journal but never be mentioned in the popular magazines.

In order to get a true picture of how effective a therapy is, it is necessary to look at all the published trials, collect details of trials that were never published, weed out the trials that are not truly objective, and then consider all the results together. This arduous process is called a "meta-analysis." One such meta-analysis of homeopathy trials—covering all the trials carried out between 1966 and 1995—was published in 1997. It found 119 trials that had been done with sufficient care to be worth considering. Some of these showed less benefit from homeopathy than placebo, some showed a greater benefit, and some showed the same level of benefit. Pooling the results from all these trials showed that there was slightly more benefit from homeopathy over-all—although it was only a small difference.

There were seven trials involving hay fever in this meta-analysis, and most of them showed greater benefit than placebo but—and it is important to remember this—the additional benefit was small. The remedies involved were of two different kinds: a homeopathic dilution of grass pollen in some trials and a dilution of Galphimia (a standard homeopathic remedy) in others. You can easily get the Galphimia remedy, and the grass pollen remedy is also available from some homeopaths.

Looked at rationally, the results with Galphimia and grass pollen don't suggest that any homeopathic remedy for hay fever will work. The variety of starting materials used for different homeopathic remedies, and the huge differences in the preparation techniques (see above), means that you can't necessarily extrapolate from these trials to the homeopathic tablets on the shelf in your local pharmacy or to the remedies that your own homeopath dispenses. That would be the same as saying, "Well, trials have shown that antihistamines work, so all other conventional drugs for hay fever must work as well." You would want, quite rightly, to see separate tests for the different kinds of drugs, and there is no reason to apply different criteria to homeopathic remedies.

So should you try homeopathy for your hay fever? If you have a strong belief in homeopathy, or are just curious about it, there is no reason not to do so. But keep an open mind, and don't spend a lot of time or money on it if it isn't helping. We honestly believe that you would be better off putting your faith in something that has a sound basis to it, and a good research record, such as immunotherapy (see chapter 9). You may think, given the results of the meta-analysis, that we are being excessively hard on homeopathy, because we would probably take such positive results at face value if they concerned another type of treatment. But the sort of logic being applied here is one that any sensible person uses. If someone tells you that he saw a dog in the garden yesterday, you will probably accept that he is telling the truth. If he says he saw a lion, you might be a little doubtful, and would want further evidence. If he says he saw a unicorn, you are going to be profoundly skeptical. The claims made by homeopaths about succussion, dilutions, potencies, and "informational structures" are definitely in the unicorn league.

Medical historians suggest that homeopathy acquired a good reputation early on because doing nothing was infinitely better for patients than subjecting them to the horrors of the conventional medical treatment of the time.

Many recovered naturally because the body has its own healing powers that simply need time to work—plus a healthy diet, clean air, and rest are all part of the traditional homeopathic treatment. But because they were being treated by a homeopath, their recovery was attributed to homeopathic remedies. We believe that this good reputation, passed down from generation to generation, gives homeopathy a "super placebo effect," which continues to work wonders today.

Where the patient visits a homeopath (rather than buying over-the-counter homeopathic remedies), there is the additional benefit of a long consultation with a sympathetic therapist, which is helpful for almost any medical complaint, especially one where some psychological factors are involved. Homeopaths ask a lot of questions about diet and lifestyle, and may often give useful advice. This, rather than the homeopathic remedies, is probably the source of their success. In the case of hay fever, however, psychological factors are of minimal importance, so this holistic dimension of homeopathy will not confer much benefit.

Chapter 11
UNDERSTANDING
CROSS-REACTIONS

None of us is perfect, and that goes for our antibodies as well. In theory, they should bind to just one type of antigen, but they can mistakenly bind to something that has a very similar chemical feature or epitope. In the fight against disease this can sometimes have advantages, but for people with hay fever, cross-reactions may multiply their problems by making them sensitive to other pollens, to foods, and even to cosmetics, insecticides, timber, or wood pulp.

CROSS-REACTIONS AMONG POLLENS

In forming antibodies to pollens, we are true individualists—each of us makes the antibodies by our own unique (and entirely random) process (see "The Fight Against Disease" in chapter 3). The antibody's binding site may fit the epitope like a tailor-made glove if you are lucky, but it might fit it only like a mitten—which would leave plenty of scope for that antibody to fit on to another, similarly shaped epitope. This is what causes a cross-reaction. Thus, two people who are sensitive to the same pollen do not necessarily show the same cross-reactions. Those with pollen-specific antibodies like tight-fitting gloves will probably have few cross-reactions, while those with the mittenlike antibodies may cross-react with several other pollens.

Bear this in mind when looking at the lists below. The fact that a cross-reaction is listed here simply means that it is *possible* and affects quite a few people. It does not mean that you will automatically suffer from it.

CROSS-REACTIONS AMONG GRASSES

Grasses belong to the family Poaceae (formerly called the Gramineae). Within that family there are many different species, and these are not at all closely related. Despite this, there appears to be a great deal of similarity among grass pollen antigens.

All grass pollens seem to have the potential to cross-react. Thus, someone from North America with grass pollen allergy could react to the pollen from an African species of grass even though he has never been previously exposed to it. There are more cross-reactions among grasses than in any other plant family.

Even with grasses, however, not everyone cross-reacts. A Danish study showed that three quarters of grass-sensitive patients reacted to timothy grass, a major allergenic pollen, but the remaining quarter did not. Taking four common grasses (timothy *[Phleum pratense]*, meadow fescue *[Festuca pratensis]*, false oat grass *[Arrhenatherum elatius]*, and couch grass *[Agropyron repens]*) 95 percent of grass-sensitive patients react to one or more of them, but that leaves 5 percent of patients who are allergic to some other grass and show no reaction to any of these four.

Reeds and sedges (Cyperaceae) sometimes cross-react with grasses, and so may rushes (Juncaceae) and reed-maces or cattails (Typhaceae).

CROSS-REACTIONS AMONG TREE POLLENS

The Birch Family

Birch, alder, and hazel all belong to the same family, the Betulaceae. Birch produces the most allergenic pollen of the three, and many people are allergic to birch alone. However, quite a few people with birch hay fever show a cross-reaction to alder or hazel or both. Hazel and alder begin pollinating very early in the year, so those showing this cross-reaction may suffer symptoms up to two months before the birch pollen season begins.

Hornbeams are usually put in a separate family, the Carpinaceae, but they are closely allied to the Betulaceae. People who are sensitive to birch may also react to hornbeam pollen.

Birches, Oaks, and Beeches

A variety of cross-reactions occur among trees in the order Fagales. These include the oaks, beeches, and chestnuts; the hornbeams, plus all members of the birch family—birches, alders, and hazels.

In Scandinavia, 90 percent of people who react to springtime pollens are sensitive to birch pollen, and it seems likely that this is the pollen that began their hay fever, with reactions to other pollens developing subsequently.

There may also be cross-reactions between birch and the pollen of unrelated trees (discussed later in this chapter).

Willows and Poplars

Willows, poplars, and aspens all belong to the same family, the Salicaceae. Cross-reactions among different trees and shrubs in this family probably occur quite frequently. Sallows and osiers are also forms of willow.

Cypresses, Junipers, Thujas, and "Cedars"

Cypresses and junipers belong to the family Cupressaceae, along with the trees known as thujas. There seem to be extensive cross-reactions among the pollens in this family. If you have a problem with cypress, always check the label before planting evergreen shrubs in the garden. Some cypresses and junipers have common names such as "mountain cedar," so it may not be obvious from the common name that they are part of this family. Check the scientific name: if it begins *Cupressus, Chamaecyparis, Cupressocyparis, Juniperus, Thuja, Thujopsis,* or *Fitzroya,* it is a member of this family.

There is a possibility of cross-reactions with some trees in the next group, the Taxodiaceae.

Redwoods, Bald "Cypress," and Japanese Red Cedar

Japanese red cedar belongs to the same family as the sequoias and redwoods of North America, the Taxodiaceae. Swamp "cypress" or bald "cypress," *Taxodium distichum,* is also a member of this family. Cross-reactions among the different trees are possible but not yet shown.

Cross-reactions between Japanese red cedar and true cypresses *(Cypressus)* have been found by several researchers, so it seems that this family has pollen allergens similar to the Cupressaceae (see above). Whether those with allergy to redwood or swamp "cypress" pollen also cross-react with true cypresses is unknown.

Olive, Ash, and Privet

These three species belong to the same family, and there is some cross-reactivity among them. The only one whose pollen contains powerful allergens is olive, which grows in warmer parts of the United States, such as California. Those who are sensitized to olive may then react to ash, which is a heavy pollen-producer but rarely causes hay fever of its own accord, being only mildly allergenic. People who are sensitive to olive can also show a reaction to privet. Privet is insect-pollinated, yet its pollen grain is small and quite large numbers become airborne.

RELATIONSHIPS OF LIVING THINGS

The more closely related two living things are, the more likely they are to have allergens that are chemically similar.

For the purposes of allergy studies, it is usually assumed that all members of a single **species** share the same antigens. A species is a group of animals or plants, all of which can potentially breed with each other. We are usually aware of species as creatures that we can recognize and put a name to because they all look similar: a tiger, for example, or a giraffe, or a silver birch.

Groups of related species, such as silver birch, downy birch, yellow birch, and paper birch, are grouped together in the same **genus.** When the scientific name of a plant or animal is given, the first word is always the name of the genus. In the case of birches, it is *Betula.* Silver birch is *Betula pendula,* downy birch is *Betula pubescens,* yellow birch is *Betula lutea,* while paper birch is *Betula papyrifera.*

For the most part, species in the same genus seem to share chemically similar allergens, so doctors describe someone as being allergic to "ragweed," even though there are several different species of ragweed. The ragweeds are referred to collectively as "*Ambrosia* spp." (spp. is shorthand for "species"), *Ambrosia* being the name of the genus. The same goes for nettles (*Urtica* spp.), docks and sorrels (*Rumex* spp.), plantains (*Plantago* spp.), pellitories (*Parietaria* spp.), and sagebrush (*Artemisia* spp.).

Related genera (the plural of genus) are grouped together in a **family.** At the family level, there may still be enough in common among the different species for them to cross-react, but they will not necessarily do so. Some families, such as the grass family, show extensive cross-reactions among the many different members, even between species that belong to distant branches of the family and are not closely related. In other families there may be few shared allergens: nettles and pellitories belong to the same family, for example, but cross-reactions have never been observed between them.

Related families are grouped together in an **order,** and while few cross-reactions occur at this level, there are some. The only well-known ones are within the order Fagales, a collection of trees that includes birches, alders, hazels, hornbeams, beeches, and oaks.

There is an exception to most rules, and the domestic dog provides one here. Although this is a single species (yes, a Chihuahua *could* still mate with a Great Dane, given a stepladder), there are substantial differences between the allergens of some breeds. This has become apparent because a few people show an allergic response to *only one breed of dog* and not to others.

However, this highly selective response to dog breeds is rare. Most people who are allergic to dogs respond equally to all the different breeds.

CROSS-REACTIONS INVOLVING "WEED" POLLENS

Ragweeds and Their Allies

Ragweeds belong to the daisy family, the Compositae (also called the Aster-aceae). Cross-reactions with other members of this family do occur for some ragweed-sensitive patients. The most commonly reported cross-reactions involve:

Bur ragweed, slender ragweed, or false ragweed *(Franseria)*

Marsh-elder or poverty weed *(Iva)*

Burro-bush or burrobrush *(Hymenoclea)*

Cocklebur *(Xanthium)*

Groundsel bush or tree *(Baccharis)*

Sagebrush, mugwort, wormwoods, saltbush "sage" *(Artemisia)*

Feverfew *(Parthenium)*

Goldenrod *(Solidago)*

Boneset or thoroughwort *(Eupatorium)*

Sunflower *(Helianthus)*

Dandelion *(Taraxacum)*

Broom weed *(Xanthocephalum)*

Goldenrod illustrates the question of cross-reactivity perfectly. In Britain it is grown as a garden flower, a fact that amazes U.S. visitors sensitized to rag-weed. Here goldenrod is regarded as a noxious weed, along with ragweed itself, since 30 percent of ragweed-sensitive people are also allergic to golden-rod. Clearly, goldenrod causes such problems (or causes them on a grand scale) only if ragweed pollen has set the stage for it to do so. The same is true for dandelion pollen.

Many other members of the daisy family show cross-reactions with rag-weed, but far less frequently than those listed above. They include several garden flowers such as asters, chrysanthemums, dahlias, various daisies, cone-flowers *(Dracopsis* and *Rudbeckia)*, marigolds, African daisies *(Arctotis),* and zinnias. Among wildflowers, thistles, knapweeds, brittle bush, chicory, rosin-weed, sneezeweed, rabbit brush, coltsfoot, and ironweed are all implicated occasionally.

Chamomile flowers, when used in teas and cosmetics, have caused cross-reactions for ragweed-sensitive people, The allergens concerned are found in the chamomile pollen, which in theory could cause hay fever, but this has never been reported. Perhaps there is too little of the pollen becoming airborne.

The daisylike flowers of *Pyrethrum* can also show some cross-reactions with ragweed pollen. It is these flowers that are used to make **pyrethroids,** a type of insecticide and acaricide (mite-killer) that is often marketed as "natural" and safe. In fact, most pyrethroids used today are synthetic ones, made in a laboratory but based on the chemicals found in the flowers. Like their natural counterparts, they can cross-react with ragweed pollen. This does not happen often, but a few ragweed-sensitive patients do react badly to pyrethroids.

Sagebrush

Sagebrush, mugwort, and other members of the genus *Artemisia* belong to the daisy family along with ragweed. There are reports of cross-reactions between ragweed and mugwort, but cross-reactions between mugwort and other members of the daisy family have not been reported. It would seem that mugwort and sagebrush are not such potent sensitizers as ragweed and have fewer shared antigens with others in their family.

Lamb's-Quarters and Pigweed Families

There are often cross-reactions between the plants in these two closely related families. The plants most often implicated are:

Lamb's quarters or goosefoot *(Chenopodium album)*
Mexican tea *(C. ambrosioides)*
Goosefoot *(C. berlandien)*
Russian thistle *(Salsola pestifer* or *S. kali)*
Mexican firebush or burning bush *(Kochia scoparia)*
Saltbush or scale *(Atriplex* species)
Silverscale *(A. argentea)*
Wingscale *(A. canescens)*
Lenscale *(A. lentiformis)*
Spearscale *(A. patula)*
Allscale *(A. polycarpa)*
Redscale *(A. rosea)*
Wedgescale *(A. truncata)*
Sugar beet *(Beta vulgaris)*
Pickleweed *(Salicornia ambigua)*

Red glasswort *(S. rubra)*

Winter fat *(Eurotia lanata)*

Smotherweed or bassia *(Bassia hyssopifolia)*

Greasewood *(Sarcobatus vermiculatus)*

Russian pigweed *(Axyris amaranthoides)*

Alkali blite, sea blite, or seepweed *(Suaeda americana)*

Pigweed *(Amaranthus* species)

Palmer's amaranth or carelessweed *(A. palmeri)*

Redroot pigweed *(A. retroflexus)*

Spiny pigweed *(A. spinosa)*

CROSS-REACTIONS AMONG UNRELATED POLLENS

When cross-reactions occur between pollen and food, plant relationships are frequently irrelevant, as we shall see. This raises the possibility that there are also cross-reactions between pollens from unrelated plants. It is a topic that has not been studied a great deal as yet, except in the case of birch pollen.

The one well-documented case relates to birch pollen cross-reacting with apple pollen. The fact that birch pollen and apple fruit cross-react so often (see "The Links between Pollens and Foods" later in this chapter) inspired researchers to see if the same could occur with apple pollen, and it did.

Birch appears to show other cross-reactions of this kind, as with sweet gale, a wild shrub that is in an entirely separate plant order. Over 80 percent of those sensitive to birch pollen give a positive skin-prick test to sweet gale.

Skin-prick tests of Swedes with birch-pollen hay fever reveal that they frequently react to pollen from a wide range of other plants, including many that are not close relatives, such as elder and horse chestnut. Whether these are true cross-reactions remains to be proved. It could simply be that the allergic reaction to birch pollen makes the nose more easily sensitized to other pollens that are airborne at the same time of year.

Could the pollen of other plants, besides birch, produce cross-reactions to the pollen of unrelated plants? At present, this is a question that researchers have not even begun to look at.

CROSS-REACTIONS TO FOOD

Only a minority of hay fever patients are affected by cross-reactions to food, and if you are one of the select few, you will probably know about this sensitivity already. It usually causes symptoms in the mouth only, generally itching or tingling. This is often known as **Oral Allergy Syndrome, or OAS.** There can also be hay fever–like reactions in the eye and nose that usually pass quite quickly, along with the symptoms in the mouth.

More severe allergic symptoms can occur, however, including a swelling of the tongue, lips, and throat; an outbreak of itchy urticaria (hives) all over the body; and an asthma attack. In the most serious cases, there can be a reaction affecting the whole body, known as **anaphylactic shock** (see the box in chapter 9). Such reactions can be life-threatening because the throat swells so much that the airways become blocked, or because there is a prolonged and severe attack of asthma, or through the effect of anaphylactic shock on the blood vessels, which makes the blood pressure fall to very low levels.

If you do not suffer from cross-reactions to food at present, there is *no point whatsoever* in worrying about them—the chances are they will never occur, and if they do, they will be mild and transient.

The only people who do need to be cautious, even though they have never reacted to food before, are those with asthma. As the case of Jack, described later in this chapter, makes clear, a cross-reaction can be very dangerous. If you are asthmatic and you begin to feel odd after eating a food (e.g., with tingling or itching in the mouth or lips), then stay close to a telephone for an hour at least, so that you can summon help if necessary. In most instances the symptoms will wear off and nothing further will happen. In this case there is no cause for concern, but do avoid eating that food in the future. Should any further symptoms appear (see the box "Taking Care with Food Allergies" later in this chapter), do not hesitate to seek medical help.

It must be emphasized that for the majority of hay fever sufferers, cross-reactions to food are very mild and affect the mouth only. Such reactions should be regarded as a warning, and the food avoided as much as possible, but there is no need for scrupulous avoidance in most cases. By "scrupulous avoidance" we mean never consuming the food under any circumstances, which can involve considerable vigilance when eating away from home.

The exceptions—those instances where the food should be avoided altogether—are as follows:

- If you have asthma (see above)

- If the food concerned is celery, since this is particularly likely to provoke a swelling in the throat that can lead to suffocation if not dealt with promptly

- If peanuts or any other type of nut is involved; these tend to provoke severe reactions

- If the symptoms you experience on eating the food have been getting progressively worse

- If you have ever experienced swelling of the tongue, lips, or throat; difficulty in breathing; or urticaria (hives) all over the body

- If you are taking the drugs known as ß-blockers (beta-blockers), used for a variety of heart conditions; these increase the risk of a severe anaphylactic reaction

- If you have ever collapsed after eating a food (anaphylactic shock); under no circumstances should you eat it again or eat any food that has been in contact with it

Of all hay fever sufferers, those most often affected by allergies to foods are children. Quite often there is a sign of an impending reaction because the child instantly dislikes the smell or taste of the food. Of course, children often react like this to new foods, so it is hard to judge when the child's objection

TAKING CARE WITH FOOD ALLERGIES

Anyone who has had an allergic reaction to food in the past should be aware that a further exposure can sometimes precipitate a worse reaction. Even a relatively mild reaction, such as localized urticaria in response to a food, can be the foretaste of something much more serious, and it is vital that such warnings be heeded.

An initial test that can be done at home is to apply a small amount of the food to the face, making sure that none of it goes anywhere near the mouth. If this produces a rash, then the food should not be eaten. If it does not, you can try applying a tiny amount to the outer lip. Should that test pass uneventfully, then the food may be safe to eat, but there is no guarantee—talk to your doctor before actually eating the food. He or she may be able to arrange for you to try it under medical supervision.

For those who have had a severe anaphylactic reaction to food in the past, it may be advisable to carry a syringe containing emergency medication in case the food is inadvertently eaten again. The syringe can be used only once. It contains epinephrine, which counteracts the effects of histamine and other mast-cell mediators by causing the blood vessels to contract. It is still necessary to avoid the food, of course—the contents of the syringe will be effective only if a very small amount has been eaten.

An inhaler containing epinephrine (Asma Haler Mist) can be issued to those who have suffered severe swelling of the throat or an asthma attack in the past, in case they unintentionally eat the food again. Your doctor should be able to prescribe either the injection or the inhaler.

Do not delay in using the syringe or inhaler if you begin to experience a severe reaction to food. In this situation, a wait-and-see attitude could be disastrous. The sooner you use the epinephrine, the more effective it will be, and you will avoid the possibility of lasting, irreversible damage to the body. Having used the syringe or inhaler (and you can safely use both, as long as you don't have a heart condition), contact your doctor or go to a hospital quickly, because you will probably need further treatment. The epinephrine injection should be repeated every 15 or 20 minutes until you are fully recovered. Tell the doctor if you have been taking corticosteroids, as these may suppress your body's normal ability to produce its own corticosteroids, which are needed in this crisis situation. Extra corticosteroids can be given to counteract this.

Not all anaphylactic reactions come on immediately. They can sometimes take an hour or even two hours to develop. There are usually some initial signs that things are amiss, such as itching or swelling in the mouth, nausea, and stomach pains. If the food is affecting the throat, hoarseness or a lump-in-the-throat sensation may be the first sign. Should this be followed by more generalized feelings, such as itching all over, sneezing, runny nose, diarrhea, and weakness, a serious anaphylactic reaction may be developing. Other odd sensations that may accompany this stage are a feeling of warmth and a peculiar sense of dread or apprehension. Incontinence, disorientation, and abdominal pains may also be experienced.

If there are any signs such as these, **do not delay in getting medical help.** Go to the emergency room and make sure you are seen quickly.

Anyone who has had a severe reaction in the past should consider wearing a medical-information bracelet or pendant with the relevant information on it. (You can find out how to obtain such a bracelet from your doctor or pharmacist.) If you were to eat your culprit food by mistake while away from home and were found unconscious, it could save your life. Without it, you might not get the correct medical help.

should be taken seriously and when it should be ignored. In general, however, if a child with hay fever strongly dislikes a fruit or vegetable, you should not insist on it being eaten, nor try to present it in a disguised form.

THE LINKS BETWEEN POLLENS AND FOODS

Not all pollens are involved in cross-reactions with foods. The prime offender here is birch pollen, which causes a great variety of reactions with different fruits, nuts, and vegetables. Mugwort, grasses, and pellitories are also linked to some cross-reactions.

One or two of the cross-reactions make sense in terms of plant relationships, such as grass hay fever and wheat sensitivity, and pine pollen and pine nuts. But these are the exceptions, and most of the cross-reactions cannot be explained in this way. It seems that some fruits and vegetables just happen to have substances in them that are similar to pollen allergens. In the case of birch, which has been studied far more than the others, some of the shared allergens seem to be "heirloom" molecules, like profilin (see "Cross-Reactions" in chapter 3), which were found in ancestral plants and have been retained by many different plant families.

These are the known cross-reactions, with the most commonly implicated foods listed first for each pollen:

Pollen	Food
Birch	Apple, Carrot, Cherry, Pear, Peach, Plum Fennel, Walnut, Potato, Spinach, Wheat Buckwheat, Peanut, Honey,
Mugwort	Celery, Carrot, Spices, Melon, Watermelon, Apple, Chamomile tea
Grass	Melon, Tomato, Watermelon, Orange Swiss chard, Wheat
Pellitory	Cherry, Melon
Ragweed	Melon, Chamomile tea, Honey, Bananas Sunflower seeds
Pine	Pine nuts
Hazel	Hazelnuts, Filberts, Cobnuts

There are a number of other fruits and vegetables that may cause symptoms in people with hay fever, but these are not strongly linked with any particular pollen.

The last example does not involve a pollen, but we will include it here for completeness. It is probably the strangest cross-reaction of all—between dust mites and kiwi fruit. This is a true cross-reaction due to an entirely coinciden-tal similarity in the epitopes. Occasionally people with dust-mite sensitivity react badly to kiwi fruit the very first time they eat it. There are reports of the same cross-reaction between dust mites and papaya fruit (papaw).

Sensitivity to foods can sometimes be so pronounced that they do not have to be eaten to produce symptoms. For example, some patients with birch pol-len hay fever cannot even peel or scrub potatoes without reacting to them. One woman with grass pollen hay fever suffered asthma, red eyes, and a streaming nose at the smell of boiling Swiss chard.

Very often the allergen in the food is destroyed by cooking, or even by storage, so it is worth some cautious experimentation with cooked, canned, or frozen and defrosted versions of the culprit food. Cooked apples are almost always tolerated by apple-sensitive people.

You can always apply some of the food to your face first, before eating it, to see if it produces a rash—this will warn if a severe reaction is likely (see the box on page 163).

Treatment of hay fever symptoms is rarely of any help in clearing up responses to food. But some research suggests that patients receiving allergy shots for hay fever may experience a lessening of their Oral Allergy Syndrome.

ECZEMA, HAY FEVER, AND FOOD REACTIONS

Do you have **eczema** (also called **atopic eczema** or **atopic dermatitis**) as well as hay fever? And are you sensitive to birch pollen, which causes symptoms in April and May?

If you answer "yes" to both these questions, then you may be interested in some research carried out by doctors at Hannover Medical University in Ger-many. They decided to study a group of adult patients with birch pollen hay fever and persistent eczema. They chose patients who had never experienced any reaction in the mouth to foods such as apple, carrot, celery, and hazelnut—the foods that are known to affect some patients with birch allergy.

Initially, the patients were given a diet that excluded all these foods for four weeks. Then they were given one of these foods—apple, for example—in a disguised form on two successive days, and the state of their eczema was observed for the rest of the week.

About half of these patients reacted badly to certain foods, their eczema getting substantially worse within 48 hours of eating apple, carrot, celery, or hazelnut. Because the reaction to the food was so delayed, none of them had previously suspected that his or her eczema was related to food.

By avoiding these foods thereafter, these patients were better able to con-trol their eczema.

CROSS-REACTIONS TO OTHER ITEMS

A beautician who suffered from hay fever in late summer, brought on by ragweed pollen, found that she was developing a congested nose all year round, along with itchy hands that grew worse when she was at work. A resourceful allergist looked into the cosmetics she was using and discovered that they contained chamomile, a member of the daisy family, like ragweed. Switching to other brands of cosmetics cured the hands and the stuffiness in her nose, although her hay fever still came back every year as expected.

Chamomile is found in a great many different items, from shampoos and face creams to teas and herbal remedies. Fortunately, only a tiny minority of those with ragweed hay fever are sensitive to chamomile, but if you are, you should read labels on cosmetics with care.

Insecticides containing pyrethrum or synthetic pyrethroids can also cross-react with ragweed pollen (discussed earlier in this chapter).

Those sensitive to cypress pollen sometimes react to the wood of cypresses or other conifers. This type of cross-reaction may well occur with other pollens from coniferous trees. Wood pulp, used for making paper, is also reported as causing allergic reactions in some hay fever sufferers, perhaps as a result of a cross-reaction.

Just occasionally there can be allergens in the stuffing used for furniture. In former times, furniture-makers sometimes used Spanish moss (*Tillandsia*) to stuff their settees and armchairs, and those sensitive to the pollen of this plant (found in the air in some southern states) may react to the furniture as well. (Similarly, old sofas stuffed with horsehair will almost certainly contain microscopic flakes of horse skin as well, and this could provoke symptoms in someone who is highly allergic to horses.) Allergy to kapok, a soft plant fiber used for stuffing toys, is also known.

HERBAL MEDICINES

Herbal medicines, naturopathic remedies, and the like could well contain plant materials (e.g., feverfew) that cross-react with certain types of pollen. Before taking these, you should check that you are not likely to be sensitive to them. Find out the ingredients, if possible, and see whether any of these belong to the same plant genus or family as your problem pollen (you may need the help of a plant field guide). Reject any medicines that contain closely related plants. Proceed cautiously with others, testing some of the medicine on your face first. If this provokes no reaction, try a very small dose of the medicine and gradually build up to the recommended dose.

JACK

Jack was 6 years old and had suffered from hay fever since he was 5. Skin-prick tests showed him to be sensitive to a wide variety of pollens, including ragweed and mugwort. The doctor gave Jack allergy shots, which were successful, and Jack continued with them for two years.

One spring evening, when Jack had just completed his second annual course of injections, he began to cough, and later became breathless and wheezy. His mother suffered from asthma herself, so she knew the signs, but she did not take Jack back to the doctor immediately. The nighttime coughing and wheeziness continued, and one evening, when Jack could not sleep, his mother decided to give him a cup of chamomile tea, which she thought would be soothing.

Jack drank a few sips of the tea but didn't like it and refused the rest. A few minutes later he began wheezing violently and was obviously having difficulty breathing. He began scratching himself hard, as he felt itchy all over, and complained of a terrible pain in his stomach. Soon afterward, Jack was sick and he then became very pale, began sweating violently, and collapsed. His terrified mother had by now telephoned for an ambulance. The doctors in the emergency room at the hospital were equally alarmed—Jack was clearly close to death. However, they were well versed in the treatment needed for such a case, and quickly injected the boy with epinephrine, antihistamine, and corticosteroid. The color began to return to his cheeks a few moments later, and within an hour and a half he had regained consciousness. Tests later showed that the IgE antibodies (see chapter 3) he produced to ragweed and mugwort pollen could also react with an antigen in chamomile flowers—it is the flowers that are used to make chamomile tea.

Chamomile belongs to the same plant family as ragweed and mugwort, the daisy family (Compositae or Asteraceae). Shared antigens are quite common among related plants, although they rarely cause such a violent reaction to a food as they did in Jack's case. In fact, a cross-reaction to chamomile tea is remarkably unusual, considering how common ragweed allergy is. However, anyone who is ragweed-sensitive would be wise to approach this herb tea with some caution.

Chapter 12
WHAT'S IN THE AIR? ALLERGENS AND IRRITANTS OTHER THAN POLLEN

"You can't live on fresh air" is an old saying, but it is not entirely true. The air around us actually contains millions of tiny particles, both animal and vegetable, that would provide a good balanced diet, full of protein, vitamins, and minerals—if only you could filter out enough of the particles.

Many of these airborne particles are only a few thousandths of a millimeter in diameter, but they can be seen even without a microscope. Look at any landscape (or any landscape painting) and you will notice that the distant hills or trees are bluish in color, more blurred and less colorful than items in the foreground. This is the result of particles in the air scattering light. Distant trees are viewed through a far thicker "layer" of air than trees close to, and this changes their color from green to blue. (On a damp misty day, when there are minute droplets of water in the air as well as the usual particles, the effect is even stronger.)

We are breathing a veritable zoo—there are particles from insects, spiders, and mites; scales from the wings of butterflies; flakes of skin from people, dogs, cats, and other animals; and tiny fragments of feathers. In addition to the "animal," there is plenty of "vegetable"—pollen grains, plant hairs, and particles; volatile molecules from plants; and the spores of fungi. Finally, there is also a fair amount of "mineral"—particles of rock and soil dust. And, of course, there are bacteria and viruses.

Those are just the *natural* airborne particles. Small wonder that, in the course of evolution, we acquired noses, whose job is to filter from the air all this junk destined for our lungs.

When human ancestors discovered fire, about 1.5 million years ago, a new kind of particle joined the natural ones in the air—man-made smoke. We have been adding new synthetic particles ever since, and at increasing speed in the past 200 years.

169

The nose that originally developed to cope with natural particles has proved fairly adept at handling the new synthetic particles as well. But among the hundreds of different particles that we now breathe, several can cause bad reactions in the nose—reactions similar to hay fever including sneezing and a runny nose or a blocked nose.

These reactions are covered by the general term **rhinitis,** meaning inflammation of the nose. (Sometimes you may also hear doctors use the word **rhinopathy,** a broader term meaning something wrong with the nose that might or might not involve inflammation, or **rhinorrhea,** which just means a runny nose.) Strictly speaking, "rhinitis" should be used only when there is genuine inflammation—that is, an immune response in the nose. In practice, the term is often used rather more loosely than this.

Those particles that cause rhinitis through an allergic process (see chapter 3) are called **airborne allergens.** Those that cause rhinitis or rhinopathy in other ways are generally referred to as **airborne irritants** and are dealt with at the end of this chapter.

Of all the microscopic items that we inhale, only a very few can act as allergens. Even those that *can* act as allergens do not necessarily do so. Most people never react to any allergens, and even severely allergic individuals do not react to *all* potential allergens. This is an important point to remember; otherwise, the thought of the airborne "zoo" that sweeps into the nose with every intake of breath may induce a feeling of panic!

The six major groups of airborne allergens (other than pollen) are:

- Dust-mite droppings

- Mold spores

- Fragments of animal skin

- Proteins from the saliva or urine of animals

- Fragments of feathers

- Particles of insect bodies, or their droppings

Of these, most can cause either rhinitis or asthma, or both. They do not cause symptoms in the eye as readily as pollen does, but eye symptoms certainly can occur. Symptoms are usually present all year round, but they can be seasonal in some people (see "Seasonal Allergies from Allergens Other Than Pollen" at the end of this chapter).

Other allergens may be encountered at work, such as wheat flour and wood dust in the air. These are dealt with in chapter 12 (see "Allergens and Irritants at Work").

HOUSE DUST

House dust is the major source of airborne allergens after pollen. Dust itself is largely a human product—flakes of dead skin that we shed unknowingly every day of our lives. Mixed in with the skin flakes are hairs, human and animal, and tiny threads from clothing and upholstery. Not a very appetizing mixture, you might think, but to some animals that dusty corner behind the sofa is a land flowing with milk and honey; those animals are dust mites, which feed mainly on skin particles. There are several different kinds, the most common being known as *Dermatophagoides,* or "skin-eater."

Skin is made of a protein called keratin, and to a microscopic creature such as the dust mite a discarded human skin flake must be like a large, tough, dried-up piece of steak—chewy but very nutritious. Part of the difficult job of digesting these skin flakes has already been done, however. Like a piece of well-aged game, they are already colonized by microorganisms such as molds, yeasts, and bacteria long before the dust mites eat them.

If dust mites did not produce allergies, we would all get along with them quite happily. Quentin Crisp, the English eccentric and writer with a famous aversion to housework, once observed that "after the first four years the dust doesn't get any worse"—no scientist has ever investigated Mr. Crisp's observation, but perhaps, when four undusted years have passed, the dust-mite population reaches a peak level and the mites promptly devour all newly arriving dust. Unfortunately, if you are allergic to dust mites, you cannot take Mr. Crisp's sanguine view. Dust and dust-eaters alike have to be kept to a minimum. There will be further details on how to achieve this later in the chapter.

One point to emphasize here is that many people with an allergy to dust mites are quite unaware of the source of the problem because they may not feel any worse in a house that is apparently very dusty nor much better in a house that is spick-and-span. This is because our main exposure to dust mites comes from mattresses, sofas, armchairs, and other upholstery. However clean these might seem on the outside, they will contain our skin flakes within, and conditions there are ideal for the dust mite. There are often huge and thriving populations of mites, and whenever we roll over in bed or flop into an armchair, a blast of air rich with mite allergens is expelled from within the mattress or upholstery. The older the mattress or armchair, the more mite allergens there will be.

Most allergens are proteins, and in the case of the dust mite, the main allergen is a digestive enzyme that the mite produces to break down the skin proteins (see chapter 1). This enzyme and other mite proteins are found on the mite's droppings or fecal pellets. Thus, the inhaled particle that affects the nose of the rhinitis sufferer is not the mite itself, but its droppings. These are much smaller than the mite and can become airborne easily and stay airborne for a long time (see "The Size of Airborne Particles" later in this chapter).

Some people, however, react to allergens found on the mite itself, while a certain number react to some other component of dust, not to the dust mite or its products. Some of these individuals react to molds or mold spores in the dust. Others are allergic to cockroach particles in the dust or to fragments of other insects, such as houseflies and carpet beetles. More rarely, someone may be reacting to tiny fibers of sheep's wool, a difficult allergy to diagnose. All of these allergens are discussed later in this chapter. A few people react to a different mite, one that preys upon *Dermatophagoides* (without, unfortunately, reducing its numbers very much). A tiny minority of patients are allergic to human skin itself.

Although dust mites mainly favor houses, substantial populations can also

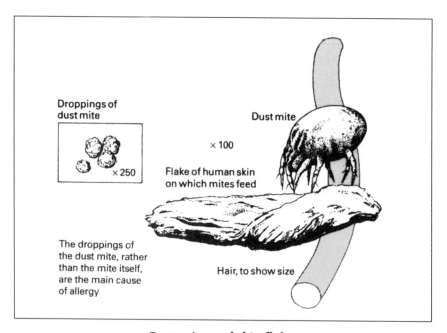

Dust mite and skin flake

be found in cinema seats (the older the better) and fabric-covered car seats. The sort of dust encountered on building sites or in factories does not cause any problems. There are rarely many dust mites in offices either, because the harsh cleaning fluids used tend to kill them off. However, recent reports have identified high dust-mite levels in some offices and linked them to outbreaks of "sick building syndrome" (discussed later in this chapter). Hospitals generally have very few mites, which is a large part of the reason that asthmatic children recover when in the hospital, dust mites being the major allergen in asthma.

Identifying Dust-Mite Allergy

An allergy to dust mites can produce rhinitis or asthma or both, and when it produces rhinitis in children, this is often accompanied by glue ear (see the box on page 175). It can also cause eczema and, much more rarely, stomach cramps, vomiting, or diarrhea. Even nasal polyps (see chapter 13) can be due to dust-mite allergy.

It is possible for dust-mite allergy to coexist with pollen allergy, resulting in year-round symptoms that get worse during the pollen season. Alternatively, someone may be allergic to both, but not sufficiently sensitive to dust mites for them to cause symptoms on their own. Such people will experience hay fever in the usual way, but also have a reaction to dust during the pollen season—this reaction may or may not be noticeably linked with dust exposure.

Researchers in Japan have found that people who are already allergic to dust mites tend to have a far stronger reaction if they then develop hay fever. For this reason alone, it is worth trying to prevent sensitivity to dust mites in children (see chapter 14).

How do you know if dust mites are responsible, or partially responsible, for your symptoms? For some people, the reaction is so obvious that the diagnosis is not in doubt, particularly those who have to do housework and are afflicted by symptoms when dusting, vacuum cleaning, or making the bed, activities that stir up the mite allergens and make them airborne. For others, sneezing attacks that occur only in bed or first thing in the morning are a tell-tale sign—the allergens coming from the mattress are to blame. (Bear in mind, though, that feather allergy is also a possibility, since pillows and duvets are often stuffed with feathers. However, feather allergy is not as common as dust-mite allergy.) People with house-dust allergy may notice their symptoms are far worse in some houses than others, even though the houses seem clean and free from dust. A cozy home with wall-to-wall carpets and plenty of armchairs and cushions is dust-mite heaven, as there are millions of well-protected crannies where skin flakes can collect and mites can hide within upholstery and among the fibers of the carpet. Apart from wall-to-wall carpeting, another modern improvement has proved highly congenial to dust mites: tightly fitting windows and doors, intended to provide total draft-proofing. While this may save on heating bills, it increases the moisture in a house by sealing it in, so that fewer mites perish through desiccation now. In the draftier conditions of unimproved, old-fashioned houses, the air is drier and many mites die a thirsty death, which helps to keep down the numbers. Molds also grow more slowly in drier conditions, making the skin flakes less digestible for the mites.

Houses that are damp, such as those built near rivers or near the sea, usually have many more dust mites than houses in drier conditions. Symptoms are likely to be worse in such houses, but this could also indicate mold allergy, and you would need a skin-prick test to determine which was important.

There is another clue, but it is not a very reliable one. Seasonal variations in symptoms are possible because damp weather favors the mites, and in some houses they tend to be more numerous during autumn and winter. (Note that molds may give the same sort of seasonal pattern, however—see "Seasonal Symptoms from Allergens Other Than Pollen" later in this chapter.) This clue is unreliable because, according to a study carried out in Germany, not all houses are affected by the outside climate. Some are so sealed off from the outside world that the dust mites are affected only by the houses' internal conditions. Allergy symptoms that begin, or get much worse, when the central heating first comes on in the autumn may be caused by dust-mite allergy.

Finally, shampooing carpets stirs up the mites and their droppings, producing an unusually heavy load in the air for some time afterward. This can provoke a severe attack of symptoms, especially in children playing on the newly cleaned carpet.

If you think that house dust may be your problem but are not sure, ask your doctor to carry out a skin-prick test. You should be given tests for both dust mites and house dust. If both are negative, you can be fairly sure you are not allergic to dust mites or anything else in dust, but there is a remote possibility that the result is a false negative and you really are sensitive to dust. In this case, you will need a nasal provocation test (see chapter 6).

A positive result should be interpreted carefully, as quite a few people give a false positive skin-prick test to dust mites—that is, the skin test is positive but they actually show no symptoms when they encounter the allergen. Before you set about reducing dust-mite allergens in your home, you should be sure the diagnosis is correct.

GLUE EAR

Rhinitis can lead to **glue ear,** particularly in children. This is especially likely when there is allergy to dust mites but can also happen with other forms of rhinitis. Glue ear arises when there is so much buildup of mucus in the nose that it works its way up into the Eustachian tube (see "The Ear" in chapter 2) and blocks it off. (The proper medical name for this condition is **chronic secretory otitis media.** Not surprisingly, even doctors prefer to call it glue ear.)

Once the Eustachian tube is blocked, air can no longer get into the middle ear, so pressure on either side of the eardrum cannot be equalized. This may cause pain and "popping" in the ears. In time, the air that was already in the middle ear is gradually displaced by a thick, sticky liquid exuded by the ear. Part of the function of the healthy Eustachian tube is to let this treacly stuff drain away, but now there is nowhere for it to go. Eventually it fills the cavity, gumming up the three tiny bones that are a crucial part of the hearing apparatus. This impairs hearing and may produce an uncomfortable feeling in the ears.

A baby or toddler with glue ear may be too young to complain of earache or popping in the ears, but there are other signs that can alert you to the problem. Often children scratch at their ears or shake their head repeatedly in an unusual way. Deafness is usually obvious, although it is sometimes mistaken for simple disobedience. Occasionally the first sign that anything is wrong is that a baby does not begin talking as soon as it should, because it cannot hear properly. (There can, of course, be many other reasons for delayed talking.)

Glue ear becomes a serious problem for some children, and sorting out the problem is vital because impaired hearing can interfere with their intellectual development and success at school. If nasal drops do not relieve the symptoms, then the condition is usually treated by inserting small tubes, called grommets, into the eardrum. Where allergy to dust mites or some other airborne allergen is the underlying problem, treating the allergy can often avoid the need for grommets.

Children with recurrent glue ear and adenoids sometimes turn out to be suffering from an allergic problem, even though there is no obvious sign of allergic rhinitis. Some children suffer glue ear as a result of food intolerance (see chapter 13).

Dealing with Dust Mites

The measures needed for adults and older children are described here. Babies and toddlers need a slightly different approach, described later in this section. The recommendations largely refer to cool climates. In hot and humid climates the mites will thrive even more, and ventilation will not help much in controlling them.

People vary greatly in their sensitivity to dust mites. Some remain well unless confronted with a massive amount of the allergen. In their case, the only thing causing problems may be an old armchair or mattress, one that has housed generation upon generation of dust mites and is now loaded with their allergens. Replacing this item may be all that is needed to put a stop to their symptoms, although it is also advisable to seal a new mattress so that mites do not move back in. It is also possible, rather than replacing a mattress entirely, to use a treatment that kills the mites and then to seal the mattress. (Both options are discussed later in this section.)

Other sufferers need more thorough measures that substantially reduce the dust-mite population in the rooms they spend most time in—the bedroom and living room. Others must go further, but only the most sensitive individuals need to reduce the dust-mite population to a bare minimum throughout the home. This involves quite a lot of effort, so the obvious thing to do is to start with minimal changes and gradually work your way up.

First you should deal with your mattress. The best thing is to replace your mattress with a new one and then seal it immediately in a cover that acts as a barrier to dust-mite droppings, to skin flakes, and to the mites themselves. The cover prevents dust mites from repopulating the new mattress: research has shown that they usually colonize new bedding within three months. The cheapest way to seal a mattress is with a cover made of plastic

JUNE

At five o'clock every morning, June woke with a volley of sneezes. Once her husband decided to count them and the total was 53. During the summer, the sneezing and streaming nose were not as bad, so June was clearly not suffering from hay fever.

Her problems had begun two years earlier, when they had first moved to Britain from the south of France. The family had been forced to live in temporary accommodations, for a while, and the apartment they rented was very damp. Although her symptoms had improved since moving into a house, they were still troublesome.

It was apparent to June's doctor that an allergy to dust mites or mold spores was the most likely cause: both are favored by damp conditions and both are worse in autumn and winter. However, the fact that June's symptoms peaked when she had been in bed for a few hours pointed more strongly toward dust mites. Mites thrive in mattresses.

As it turned out, June was sensitive to both these allergens: the doctor used skin-prick tests to discover this. Before prescribing any drugs, the doctor asked June to try simply reducing these allergens in her house. June bought a plastic mattress cover and improved the ventilation in the house to reduce any dampness. Later, she bought a dehumidifier for the bedroom. These measures improved her symptoms considerably and she decided against any further treatment.

sheeting, either homemade or a ready-bought one. (The sort of cover used for small children who wet the bed will also protect against dust mites, as long as it has no holes anywhere and the seams are reasonably airtight. You could make it more airtight by sealing the seams, or any holes, with packing tape.) This sort of smooth plastic cover can create a problem in that the mattress pad and bottom sheet tend to slip off, but a few small strips of double-sided sticky tape between the mattress and the bedding can help to solve this.

These plastic covers have been superseded by a much improved product made of **microporous material.** Such material lets water vapor through while acting as an impenetrable barrier to mites and their allergens. (Water vapor is the gas produced by the evaporation of water; under warm conditions water can become water vapor, while in colder conditions water vapor turns into water again, the process known as condensation.) With the older, completely impermeable plastic covers, a drop in temperature could produce condensation on the inside of the cover from water vapor leaving the mattress and might result in mold growth. With the new microporous material, this will not occur. The material is not as slippery as the cheapest plastic covers, so it has an additional advantage in that the mattress pad and bottom sheet stay put. Similar covers are also sold for pillows, duvets or comforters, and the box springs. Covers made from tightly woven Egyptian cotton will also do the job effectively and have certain advantages over microporous covers. See appendix 3 for additional information on all these products and a list of suppliers.

In the past, those with dust-mite allergy were often advised to choose a foam mattress rather than the traditional interior-spring design, since foam—or so it was claimed—harbors fewer skin particles and therefore fewer mites. Pillows filled with synthetic materials were also said to be better than feather pillows. Recent research has failed to confirm this (in fact, feather pillows harbor *fewer* dust mites than synthetic ones because the fabric of the covers is more tightly woven), and it is now widely accepted that allergen-proof mattress covers, pillow covers, and, possibly, duvet or comforter covers are much the best measure that can be taken against dust mites. With these covers on, it does not matter what the pillow or mattress is made of. Duvets or comforters that can be washed regularly to kill mites (details follow) are also useful instead of the allergen-proof covers.

Another recommendation often made in the past was to vacuum-clean the mattress regularly, but this is now considered far less valuable than sealing the mattress in a cover. There is also the possibility of increasing the level of mite allergen in the air while vacuuming, unless you have a specialized type of vacuum cleaner with a filter (see below).

If a new mattress is out of the question, there are ways of reducing the number of mites in an existing mattress prior to sealing it in an allergen-proof cover. One is to spray the mattress with an **acaricide,** a chemical that kills mites and ticks. There are certain doubts about the safety of long-term exposure to this spray, and the spray will not reach mites inside the mattress anyway, so it is probably not a good idea except as a short-term measure. Another option is to treat your mattress with a special high-temperature process that is designed to kill dust mites inside mattresses and upholstery (see appendix 3). This process is expensive but might be worthwhile if you have a mattress that would be costly to replace.

In both cases, the treatment needs to be followed by thorough vacuum cleaning, because killing the mites is only half the battle—you also need to remove their old droppings and their tiny corpses since these can release allergens as they decompose. Once the vacuuming is done, you can seal the mattress into its new cover.

Why go to all this trouble if the mattress is going to be enclosed in an allergen-proof cover? It might seem just as effective to cut out the mite-killing treatment and vacuuming, but this is not generally recommended. If enclosed by a cover, the mites will be locked in with their food supply and will continue to feed and breed. Allergens will build up inside the cover and if it then develops a small hole, the allergens will seep through and begin to cause trouble again. (There could also be some seepage around the seams of the cover, depending on how these are constructed, although most manufacturers do their best to prevent this.) Similarly, if the allergen-proof cover has to be removed for any reason, the allergens will flood out.

EIGHT LEGS OR SIX?

Mites are often referred to as insects, but in fact they are related to spiders. The most obvious difference is in the number of legs: insects have six, spiders and mites have eight.

Mites, along with their close relatives the ticks, make up the zoological order called the Acari. The chemicals that kill mites and ticks are therefore called **acaricides.**

Note that an insecticide will not necessarily act as an acaricide, although some do, notably **permethrin** and those based on **pyre-throids.** For this reason, flea sprays, fly killer, and other household insecticides will not necessarily affect dust mites. Some acaricides, including benzyl benzoate, are specifically mite-killers and do not work against insects. The potential hazards of using acaricide sprays to combat dust mites in carpets, mattresses, and bedding are discussed on pages 183–185. With so many other options now available, using these sprays really should be unnecessary.

However, if you are aware of these drawbacks and watch the cover carefully for holes, then this shortcut method could work just as well. If the cover has to be removed at some point, make sure the allergy sufferer is out of the room and remains out of it for a whole day, during which time the room should be thoroughly vacuumed and dusted.

Where acaricides do have a role is in treating clothes, curtains, and other fabrics that cannot be washed at 131°F (58°C) or higher. Benzyl benzoate laundry additive (see appendix 3) will kill the mites during a low-temperature wash and is then rinsed out afterward, so no residue remains in the fabric. Check that laundry additives really do contain benzyl benzoate before you buy—read the claims being made carefully, and don't fall for laundry additives that do nothing more than remove allergens.

At the same time as treating or replacing your mattress, you should deal with your pillows. Replacing them with new ones is a good idea, but as with new mattresses, it is vital to put an allergen-proof barrier over a new pillow, underneath the pillowcase, to prevent recolonization by mites.

Blankets and duvets should be replaced with new ones if at all possible, or washed. Some launderettes have machines large enough to wash a whole duvet or comforter. A wash temperature of at least 131°F (58°C) is needed to kill the mites. Lower temperatures will wash out the droppings and their allergens but leave many live mites to replenish the stocks. Dry cleaning will kill some mites and remove some of their allergens but is less satisfactory than washing at high temperatures. Duvets and comforters should be aired outside for a day after dry cleaning. If these measures are difficult because you have no other bedding available, simply putting the comforter, dry and unwashed, into a tumble-dryer and keeping it hot and dry for a couple of hours should kill off many of the mites, and may also **denature** (see the box "Washing at the Right Temperature" on page 180) some of the allergens.

One of the advantages of buying a new duvet is that there are some special ones available (see appendix 3) that separate into two layers. This allows them to be washed in an ordinary washing machine at home, one layer per wash. They are also suitable for laundering at 131°F (58°C).

Maintaining Low Dust-mite Levels

Once the changes to your mattress and bedding have been made, a little extra effort every week will help to keep down the mite population. The bedding should be shaken outside and hung in the sun at regular intervals—dust mites, like vampires, have an aversion to sunlight. If this is impossible, a long spin in a hot tumble-dryer is valuable. Sheets, pillowcases, and blankets should be washed

WASHING AT THE RIGHT TEMPERATURE

If you are aiming for a wash that will kill dust mites, you need a temperature of at least 131°F—preferably 140°F—but your washing machine may not give an exact temperature for the washing water. The temperature of the hot water depends on the kind of hot-water heater you have in your house (and if you're at the laundromat, you're at the mercy of its water heater).

Choose the hot wash/warm rinse setting for your washes. To check what temperature you are getting, set the washer on "hot" and fill the basin, then test the temperature with a candy thermometer. If it's not hot enough, turn up the temperature on your hot-water heater until the washing water is the right temperature.

If you have an "on demand" hot-water system, you can try turning up the temperature setting, but that still may not do the trick. You may be able to overcome this problem by turning down the valve for the washing machine water intake until the flow of incoming water is reduced. This slower flow will produce hotter water from the system than when the flow is fast.

once a week at 131°F (58°C) or higher. If there are problems in washing blankets, you could just place them on a radiator once a week, making sure that they get good and hot for a while. This will kill the mites but not remove the allergen, so it is a measure that is useful only if they have been washed at least once.

Always make sure that beds are aired thoroughly before they are made because the body produces moisture at night, which penetrates all the bedding. The duvet or blankets should be pulled back and left for at least an hour before the bed is made. As an additional measure, an electric blanket can help to reduce the moisture in the bed, creating hot, dry conditions that dust mites dislike. (This can be useful as a temporary measure if you cannot afford mattress covers.)

Needless to say, while these activities are going on, the level of allergen in the air will rise dramatically. The allergy sufferer should not have to dust, vacuum, sweep floors, or make beds if there is anyone else in the household who can do the work or if it is possible to pay someone to do the cleaning.

Think hard about the options here—if you are a homemaker with dust-mite allergy, perhaps you can spend the time you would normally spend cleaning on a part-time (dust-free) job that would bring in enough to pay for a cleaner. It might not make sense in purely economic terms, but if you factor in the improvement in your health (and reduction in medication expenses, perhaps), then the benefits probably outweigh the costs.

If you really must do the cleaning yourself, then wear a good-quality mask throughout (see appendix 3). This won't give you absolute protection from dust-mite allergen, but it will decrease your exposure substantially.

PUTTING ALLERGENS OUT OF ACTION

An allergen can act as an allergen only as long as it keeps its particular chemical features—the ones that make it recognizable to allergy-producing antibodies (see chapter 3). If those features are changed in some way, the allergen no longer binds to the antibody, and there is no allergic reaction.

Most allergens are proteins. Proteins can be **denatured**—have their shape changed—in various ways, and such changes often stop them from acting as allergens.

One way to denature a protein is to heat it to a high temperature. Heating to the boiling point of water (212°F, 100°C) will denature one of the main dust-mite allergens (Der p1) but not the other one (Der p2).

Another way to denature proteins is to treat them with certain chemicals. One that is widely sold is **tannic acid.** Tannic acid is assumed to be safe, since it is found in tea and red wine at concentrations only a little lower than those in the sprays. Thorough vacuuming is essential after use of the spray, and this is said to remove most of the tannic acid (which dries to a powder) anyway.

However, there have been no tests involving close contact with tannic acid for long periods of time and it is just possible that residues left in a carpet could act as an irritant to the skin of a baby or toddler playing there regularly, especially if that child has sensitive skin.

Tannic acid can be used on carpets, mattresses, and all upholstery, and the formulations sold are said not to stain fabrics.

Another type of treatment inactivates allergens by sticking to them, rather like microscopic cotton candy, thus preventing them from becoming airborne and being inhaled. These sprays use polysaccharides, cellulose, or some other large molecules to glue together the allergen molecules. The same caveats about safety apply as with tannic acid—these sprays are probably safe, but nobody has ever looked at the long-term effects of daily exposure.

With both types of spray, other allergens will also be inactivated, so these treatments could be helpful for those allergic to pets or cockroaches. (However, if most of the allergen exists as very small *airborne* particles, as it does with cat allergen, these will have limited usefulness.) Treatments need to be repeated every three to four months. Suppliers are given in appendix 3.

Note that allergen-inactivating treatments are *not* acaricides—they do not kill the mites. However, they destroy the reservoir of mite allergens. Although these build up again with new mite droppings, it apparently takes at least three months for the allergens to reach the sort of levels that generally cause symptoms.

If you are reluctant to use acaricides, and cannot afford superheated steam cleaners or a powerful dehumidifier that will kill mites, then an allergen-inactivating treatment may be a good option for carpets and furniture (see appendix 3).

The most important measure of all (assuming that you don't have an air conditioner) is to increase the ventilation in your bedroom and in the rest of the house. As long as it is not raining outside, opening a window will reduce the amount of moisture in the air, making conditions far less congenial for mites. Airing the room at the same time as you air the bed makes excellent sense. Try to get a good blast of air through the whole house every day.

Tackling Dampness in the House

Anyone living in a house that is clearly damp should take steps to combat this, as the mite problem is bound to be worse in such conditions. Many of the measures described later in this chapter for combating molds are relevant for dust mites as well. You should try to reduce the dampness coming into the house and the moisture being generated indoors. However, measures aimed solely at reducing condensation on walls and windows are not relevant to controlling dust mites.

Taking Additional Steps

Reducing nighttime exposure to dust-mite allergens is enough for many people. We spend an average of eight hours a day in bed, far longer than in any other single place, which makes the bed a happy hunting ground for mites, as we shed a lot of skin while sleeping. Being in bed also gives us a prolonged exposure to the plentiful mite allergens found there. By reducing the allergen load experienced at night, many people reduce the sensitivity of their nose or bronchi, which makes them less likely to suffer symptoms at other times.

If symptoms are still experienced after dealing with the mattress and bedding, then you should turn your attentions to the rest of the bedroom, particularly the carpet if there is one. Mites in a wall-to-wall carpet can rapidly recolonize the bedding, and if there are enough of them, they could undermine your efforts at keeping the bedding mite-free.

The major problem with carpets is that dust mites cling to the fibers for dear life using eight tiny suckers, one at the end of each leg. When a vacuum cleaner zooms overhead, a few of the mites may be caught unawares and sucked up into the mouth of the roaring monster, but most hang on to the fibers around them and live to fight another day. A research team found that even if a carpet was vacuumed thoroughly three times in quick succession, 65 percent of its mites still remained. Where vacuuming *is* effective is in removing the mites' droppings, but because each mite produces about 20 fecal pellets a day, the surviving mites soon replenish this source of allergen.

There are three things that can be done about this problem. One is to use a specialized mite-killing steam cleaner (the kind that produces super-heated steam—see appendix 3). The second is to banish wall-to-wall carpets and use area rugs. The third is to use a dehumidifier to kill the mites (see appendix 3).

If you choose the first option, make sure you buy a steam cleaner that is right for the job. It should produce superheated steam—that is, steam at a temperature above the boiling point. It does this by means of high pressure. This inactivates the main dust-mite allergen (Der p1) at the same time as killing the mites. Ask whether the machine has been tested for its effects on dust mites. Don't accept test data based on a different brand of machine; as you can see by comparing the results with the two machines that have been thoroughly tested (see appendix 3), a small difference in technical specifications can make a big difference in mite-killing performance. (Note that most products described as "steam cleaner," and most commercial carpet-cleaning processes described as "steam treatment" are using nothing more than hot soapy water. These can make your mite problem a whole lot worse.)

Knocking out both the mites and their main allergen in a single treatment makes this type of special steam cleaner a very powerful ally in the fight against mites. You can use it on upholstered furniture and curtains as well as on carpets. Ideally, the steam treatment on bedroom and living room carpets should be repeated once a month.

What about using acaricides (mite-killing sprays) to treat your carpets? Various sprays are available, some containing benzyl benzoate, others containing permethrin and pyrethroid compounds, still others with disodium octaborate tetrahydrate (or DOT).

Permethrin and pyrethroid are quite powerful chemicals, with the potential to cause allergic reactions in some individuals and toxicity in almost anyone if the amount absorbed is sufficiently high. We really don't think you should expose yourself to these, unless there is no other way of tackling a particular mite problem. Even then, you should use them only on a very short-term basis. Note that pyrethroids were originally derived from chrysanthemum-type flowers, and advertisements may describe them as "natural." Don't be seduced by this—natural poisons can be just as poisonous as man-made poisons.

Benzyl benzoate is relatively safe—indeed, it is used to treat scabies, caused by mite infestations, and is applied directly to the skin. But it can occasionally cause sensitivity reactions when so used, and many doctors feel concerned

VACUUM CLEANERS

Most ordinary vacuum cleaners have tiny pores in the bag that are large enough to let dust-mite droppings escape—so as you vacuum up dust, many of the allergenic particles are spewed out again through the bag, leaving the vacuum cleaner via the exhaust. This can triple the amount of dust-mite allergen in the air.

Special vacuum cleaners, designed for those with dust-mite allergy, are now available (see appendix 3 for suppliers). These use better bags, which help retain the particles, backed up by a high-quality filter (a HEPA filter) that cleans the exhaust before it leaves the machine. Their suction power is generally greater than an ordinary vacuum cleaner, so they pick up more dust. One model can be fitted with a dust-detection device to show that an area of carpet has been vacuumed fully and all dust removed.

If you suffer from symptoms during or after vacuuming (the particles can take several hours to settle from the air), one of these vacuum cleaners could be the answer.

Someone who suffers from dust-mite allergy should not change the bag on a vacuum cleaner, even on one of these specialized models, as the potential for spillage of dust and high exposure to allergens is always there.

If this is absolutely unavoidable, wear a high-grade face mask (see appendix 3).

A more radical solution is to get rid of carpets entirely, and for those with severe dust-mite allergy this may be the only solution. The great advantage of area rugs is that they can be hung up outside, beaten to remove dust, and then left in the sun. This purges dust mites far more effectively than any amount of vacuuming. Try to give all the rugs this treatment once a week. If buying rugs, avoid those with foam backing or a thick pile.

The floor itself can be wooden boards, vinyl flooring, cork tiles, or linoleum. Cork tiles are the warmest to the feet, and sealed cork tiles, with a thin coat of vinyl on them, are now available and easily kept clean. Whatever the surface, it should be vacuumed regularly to remove dust mites from the crevices. On a bare floor, vacuuming removes about 80 per cent of the mites.

If you use a dehumidifier to kill mites, thorough vacuuming is very important; otherwise the allergens will remain in the carpet. You should invest in a new vacuum cleaner, one that retains all the dust mites and their droppings within its bag.

about the idea of using it regularly around the home, year in, year out. Its safety, when used in this way, has never been tested. The effect on babies and small children is especially uncertain; they have a lot of close contact with carpets and are bound to pick up far more of the substance than an adult would. (The same goes for spraying bedding with acaricides or buying bedding already impregnated with them. The amount absorbed with regular nightly contact is worrying—this goes for both adults and children.)

A newer anti-mite product is disodium octaborate tetrahydrate, or DOT. This is not a new product in itself—it has been used for years for termite control in buildings—but marketing it for dust mites in carpets (under the brand name Dustmitex) is a new development. Is it safe? Scientific tests have shown that very little DOT is absorbed by intact skin, though these tests were done with adults rather than children. There is concern that it would be absorbed across skin that is scratched, grazed, or eczematous—and you cannot prevent your children from playing on the carpet whenever their skin is not in perfect condition.

So what would the consequences be of a significant absorption of this compound? It is relatively innocuous but, according to the manufacturer's own safety data, "absorption through large areas of damaged skin could cause nausea, vomiting, and diarrhea, with delayed effects of skin redness and peeling." We believe that if you have children in the house, especially small children, you should look for other ways of dealing with dust mites in your carpets.

With so many other safe and effective options now available, there is little justification for using acaricides to combat mites in carpets, except as a short-term measure.

Dust in the Living Room

If reducing your exposure to mite allergens in the bedroom has helped only a little, you should tackle the carpet and upholstery in the living room.

Armchairs and sofas should be vacuumed, especially the areas where the arms and head normally rest. This treatment, like the thorough vacuuming of the carpet, should be repeated weekly with a high-quality HEPA vacuum cleaner (see the box "Vacuum Cleaners" on the previous page).

Those who are still suffering from symptoms may need to treat the carpet with a special mite-killing steam cleaner (discussed in the previous section).

A very elderly sofa or armchair can also prove resistant to treatment. The living mites may be killed, but there are seemingly inexhaustible reserves of allergen within the upholstery.

There are various options here. First, you could buy a new sofa and armchairs. If you decide to do this, choose something that will not become infested with dust mites. Leather or vinyl-covered furniture is one possibility.

Alternatively, buy a futon sofa with a wooden frame and full-size futon pad. This pad is the same size as a double-bed mattress so you can cover it with a standard allergen-proof mattress cover (see pages 176–177). The decorative cover that comes with the futon can be put on over the allergen-proof cover; try to find one that is washable. You can wash the decorative cover periodically in cool water with a laundry additive containing benzyl benzoate to remove mites (see appendix 3 for suppliers). Make sure that the pillows you use on this couch are equipped with allergen-proof covers.

There are matching futon armchairs with small, shaped futon pads, and you can order custom-fitted mite covers for these from certain allergy companies (see appendix 3 for suppliers). This is obviously more expensive than just buying a standard allergen-proof cover for the futon sofa, but not totally out of reach, and creates an armchair that doesn't poof out mite allergen every time you sit down.

Another option will be possible when the heat treatment known as "Diathermic Envelope" (appendix 3) becomes available in the United States and Canada. This treatment inactivates mite allergens deep inside upholstered furniture.

Having taken care of the carpet and upholstery, you may need to undertake a general "spring cleaning." Needless to say, the person doing the cleaning becomes exposed to a higher level of dust while at work, so it is preferable if the allergy sufferer goes out for the day and someone else does the work. Paying someone to clean the house may be worthwhile, but make sure it is understood that the work needs to be done very thoroughly. If the cleaning has to be done by the allergic person, the mouth and nose can be protected with a dust mask (see appendix 3 for the type of mask needed). Another useful tip is to use a damp cloth when dusting to minimize the amount of dust going into the air, rinsing out the cloth in water at intervals. (To prevent staining of polished wood, rub off all the moisture immediately with a clean, dry cloth.) Even if someone else does the cleaning, damp dusting is a worthwhile measure. There are now special dust cloths that retain the dust by an electrostatic charge, so that very little becomes airborne (see appendix 3).

Picture rails, moldings, and door tops should all be dusted, and again a damp cloth should be used. Long-handled feather dusters are obviously out, because they simply scatter the dust in the air. A vacuum cleaner with dusting attachments can be useful, and the special models designed for allergy sufferers have these.

Relatively few people will need to go beyond these measures, but for the unfortunate sufferers who are ultrasensitive to dust mites, it may be necessary to treat all fabrics with a superheated steam cleaner (see discussion earlier in this section), give them a hot wash or a wash with benzyl benzoate added (see appendix 3 for suppliers), or—as a last resort—use an acaricide spray.

Alternatively, remove as many fabrics as possible. This means doing without curtains where possible, or choosing thin, smooth materials. Textured materials and those with a pile, such as velvet, can harbor dust. All curtains should be washed every month or two. Any fabric items in the bedroom should be removed unless really essential. Hang clothes elsewhere if possible, and remove soft toys, bathrobes, armchairs, and cushions. Overcoats and sweaters should be dry-cleaned or washed because these can contain many mites.

As a last resort, you could move to a new house! Old houses, particularly if they are damp, are absolutely infested with dust mites. A newly built house, or one that has been stripped and thoroughly refurbished, is largely free of mites, and it takes about five years for the numbers to reach their normal level. Timber treatment for woodworm is likely to kill dust mites as well, if it uses **permethrin** or **pyrethroids** (see the box "Eight Legs or Six" earlier in this chapter).

Pros and Cons of Mite Control

One of the drawbacks to controlling mites in the home, apart from the effort and expense involved, is that allergy sufferers may become preoccupied with the problem of dust mites, and perhaps become "prisoners" in their own home, feeling unable to venture into other people's houses for fear of the hordes of mites lurking there. This fear is largely unfounded, because reducing your exposure at home will mean that your nose (and your bronchi if you have asthma) are not being constantly irritated by an allergic reaction. They are in far better condition generally and not likely to be upset by a brief dose of dust in someone else's home. (Sleeping on an old and untreated mattress in someone else's house is a different matter, however.)

Before you begin, consider the other options. If you simply have rhinitis, you could well use drugs to control the symptoms or some form of desensitization. The information about antiallergy drugs, given in chapter 7, and desensitization, in chapter 9, is as relevant to dust mites as it is to pollen. Understanding the other options fully can help you to decide on the best way of tackling your allergy. For those who have asthma and are allergic to dust mites, some form of mite control is considered sensible.

Most people eventually find a mixture of treatments that is right for them. A balanced approach is to reduce dust exposure in bed by using allergen-proof mattress and pillow covers, and then to reduce exposure in other parts of the home as much as possible without excessive fuss. This minimizes the basic level of sensitization in the nose or bronchi, and drugs or allergy shots can then be employed to control any remaining symptoms.

To some extent, the decision made will be influenced by the severity of the symptoms. In this respect, asthma should always be taken more seriously than rhinitis because the bronchi, once sensitized, can become increasingly reactive to both allergens and irritants and sometimes to emotional stress. An asthma attack is alarming, especially for small children, and asthma can prevent children from getting enough exercise or developing a healthy independence as they grow up. All in all, any cleaning measures in the home that can prevent a child's asthma from getting worse are probably worth taking. (Bear in mind that irritants such as tobacco smoke also need to be eliminated.)

Mite Avoidance for Babies and Toddlers

For babies and small children, avoiding dust-mite allergens is basically a similar process, but with some changes in emphasis. An infant's mattress is probably sealed or coated with plastic anyway, to guard against bed-wetting, so the mattress is unlikely to be a major source of allergens. Pillows and bedding do need to be kept mite-free however, and allergen-proof covers are recommended. Make sure that you buy only products that are specifically designed for babies and children because there is a risk of suffocation with some covers designed for adult beds; if the cover is loose fitting, it might be possible for it to obstruct a child's mouth and nose. New bedding for a new baby is a good idea. Any bedding that cannot be covered with allergen-proof covers or washed regularly at 131°F (58°C) should be avoided.

There should be much more emphasis on carpets—babies and toddlers spend a lot of time at floor level, after all, and are close enough to breathe the allergens that they stir up while playing or crawling about.

Some quite difficult choices need to be made here. If you abandon wall-to-wall carpets and opt for area rugs, the level of dust-mite allergen will be greatly reduced but your child will have fairly cold hard floors to crawl and toddle on. Cork tiles are one solution to this, as is old-fashioned linoleum, both of which are fairly warm to the touch. Looking on the positive side, children brought up on a carpetless floor from birth will probably not know what they are missing, and will develop into hardy little individuals who won't mind the cold in the future!

If you hate the idea of bare floors, you could cover the floor extensively with area rugs, but have a smooth, bare surface underneath. The drawback with this option is that it creates a lot of housework because the rugs need regular airing and beating outside to keep them mite-free. In an area with an unpredictable climate, passing showers will make life doubly difficult. However, if you have a tumble-dryer, where the airing process can be carried out artificially, a large number of rugs (made of a heat-resistant fabric such as cotton) may be a practical proposition.

Another possibility is to stick with wall-to-wall carpets and buy a super-heated steam cleaner designed to kill mites and denature their allergens.

Another option is to increase the ventilation in the home by opening the windows every day so that moisture levels fall. Alternatively, you could use a dehumidifier to reduce moisture levels. This type of strategy will gradually reduce the number of dust mites over a period of months, but it won't make a dramatic difference straight away, and it won't remove the existing allergen. Once the house begins to dry out, you would need to begin a campaign of very thorough vacuuming (using a vacuum cleaner with a HEPA filter—see the box earlier in this chapter) to remove the dead mites and their allergens from the existing carpets. For quicker results, you could recarpet the house at the same time as improving the ventilation. This is expensive, of course, but would give you a clean start with fresh, mite-free carpets.

A third approach is to use a special high-powered dehumidifier that can get the air in a room so dry as to kill most of the mites outright (see appendix 3). This device is designed to be used when the room is unoccupied, and could be left on at night in the living room. You must follow up with intensive vacuum cleaning to remove the dead mites and their droppings—or start fresh with new carpets. With regular use of the powerful dehumidifier, the overall number of mites should steadily decline, so vacuuming will not be needed quite as often.

Special measures may be needed for the teddy bear or favorite soft toy—it's difficult to part a child from this source of comfort, even if it *is* home to a million mites! The best solution is to give the soft toy a "vacation" once a week, which it spends wrapped in a plastic bag in the freezer. Six hours of this treatment knocks back the mite population considerably, although it may not kill all of them. At the outset, it is advisable to wash the toy to remove the existing dust-mite allergens, then to dry it as quickly as possible, preferably in a tumble-dryer. (Be sure, first, that the eyes of the toy are not made from the kind of plastic that melts easily.) Two days on the clothesline in bright sun should follow. This treatment will reduce the mites to a fairly low level, and weekly sessions in the freezer should then keep the problem under control. If you have a tumble-dryer at home, you can follow the weekly freezer session by a hot spin for 45 minutes, which will demoralize the mites even further.

Bunk beds are not a good idea for children who may be prone to allergy—the child in the lower bed has dust-mite allergens showered on him or her from above, doubling the nightly dose. If you already have bunk beds and only one child with dust-mite allergy, he or she should sleep in the top bunk. However, both mattresses should have special allergen-proof covers to protect the other child from developing the same sensitivity. In general, where children share a bedroom, it is a good idea to treat all the mattresses in the room, not just the one belonging to the allergic child.

WHAT DUST MITES LIKE

There is a great deal of information and advice on dust-mite control now available. A lot of it comes from companies selling mite-control products, and while most of the information is excellent, some is contradictory or confusing. In particular, you are likely to read conflicting statements about the sort of temperature conditions dust mites like best. This is because their reaction to temperature conditions is quite complex. The story is roughly as follows.

What dust mites like best is a high temperature, 77 to 86°F (25 to 30°C), and very moist air with a relative humidity of 75 to 80 percent. (This means that the air is holding 75 to 80 percent of the maximum amount of water vapor it could hold at that temperature.) This is a high moisture level, unlikely to be encountered in a well-ventilated house except for brief periods. However, levels of 70 percent are found in many modern homes where draft-proofing has been enthusiastically applied and ventilation reduced to a minimum.

At high temperatures (86°F or 30°C), the lowest relative humidity a dust mite can tolerate is about 65 percent, which is commonplace in modern energy-saving houses. The humidity can also reach these levels quite easily in a mattress that is not aired regularly, and in a pillow, since this receives moisture directly every night from the sleeper's breath. Given these high temperatures and moist air, the dust mite thrives. Warmth makes all its life processes speed up—it lays more eggs, eats more food, and produces more droppings, which is bad news for anyone allergic to the little beast.

However, if the humidity is not allowed to build up in the house, high temperatures will produce dry air, and this can kill off many mites. Very dry air kills them directly, while moderate dryness keeps down mold growth, making the skin particles on which the mites feed tough and rather indigestible. This keeps the mite population at a fairly low level.

At cool temperatures, such as 59°F (15°C), the dust mite can tolerate much drier conditions. A relative humidity of 45 percent (which is considered low for a house and is the target for a standard dehumidifier) is tolerated well. Because the temperature is lower, the mites do not breed as fast, but they still produce a fair number of young. Each mite lives much longer, which partially offsets the lower breeding rate. Consequently, a cold empty room will have quite plentiful dust mites, while a vacation home that is left empty and unheated during the winter months will be developing a steadily growing population. This can precipitate a severe attack of rhinitis or asthma in a susceptible person at the start of a vacation.

Are Air Cleaners or Ionizers Useful for Dust-mite Allergy?

Air cleaners and air ionizers will remove particles from the air. Details of the different kinds and how they work are given in appendix 3. Whether they are of any use to those who are allergic to dust mites is debatable. They are certainly not recommended as a first step in reducing your exposure to dust-mite allergens, because the main sources of allergens are likely to be your mattress, your pillow, and your armchair. You have such intimate contact with these items that you are inhaling the allergens "at the source," and an air cleaner will make little difference. (The exception here is some special air cleaners fitted to the headboard of a bed that provide a stream of filtered air over the sleeper's face. These work quite well, but are not widely sold now, and encasing the mattress in an allergen-proof cover is a much cheaper alternative.) There is no point in trying an air cleaner if you have not:

- Put the mattress and pillow in allergen-proof covers

- Washed the other bedding regularly, or put it into allergen-proof covers

- Aired the bed and the bedroom regularly

- Dusted with a damp cloth, rather than a dry one, for at least the past two weeks

- Bought a good-quality vacuum cleaner with a HEPA filter, so that allergens do not become airborne during vacuuming

The first three measures will reduce the amount of allergen being breathed at the source. The last two will reduce the amount of allergen being made airborne by housework.

While there may still be plenty of allergen left lurking in your carpets and elsewhere, this will not create problems unless it actually becomes airborne in sufficient quantities. Allergens being generated at floor level by dust mites do not become airborne all that easily. In a quiet household, without much activity and air movement, the allergen will probably remain where it is, in which case an air cleaner will not serve much purpose.

If you have taken the five measures listed above and are reluctant to make further changes to the bedroom (e.g., treating the carpet with a superheated steam cleaner or removing the carpeting altogether), yet you still suffer from symptoms at night or first thing in the morning, then a filter might be worth trying. Suppliers are given in appendix 3.

In the living room, before considering an air cleaner, at least try:

- Cleaning the upholstered furniture with a vacuum cleaner equipped with a HEPA filter

- Wet dusting for a minimum of two weeks

You might also try spraying cushions and upholstered furniture with tannic acid (discussed earlier) as a way of rendering these sources harmless. If there are still symptoms when you are in the living room and you are unable to make further changes, then an air cleaner might be useful.

Only air cleaners with HEPA filters (see appendix 3) have been shown to have any beneficial effects for people with dust-mite allergy. Tests have shown no benefits from air ionizers, and in one study there was actually an increase in nocturnal coughing among asthma sufferers using ionizers, perhaps due to ozone (see appendix 3).

MOLD SPORES

Mold is familiar to us as the furry covering that develops on old fruit and vegetables or the green dust on last week's bread. Molds belong to the group of living things called **fungi,** which also includes mushrooms, toadstools, and puffballs. Fungi are neither plant nor animal, but a distinct life-form. (It used to be thought that they were descended from plants, but this is not the case.)

Fungi cannot make food for themselves, as plants can, so they feed on dead organisms (although some fungi are parasites and attack living things). In the wild, fungi colonize the discarded leaves of trees and plants, overripe fruit, or the wood of dead trees. In your fridge, molds are simply living the same sort of lifestyle, digesting forgotten bits of food, just as they would digest fallen leaves and berries in a forest.

But how did the molds get into your fridge in the first place? The answer is that they went in as spores, minute specks, visible only with a microscope, that can each grow into a new mold. Those spores are on the surface of every fruit and vegetable we buy, and on most other things as well. *There are more mold spores in the air than anything else.* In a damp climate there can be as many as 160,000 per cubic meter of air, whereas the record pollen count is only 2,800 per cubic meter. Fortunately, mold spores are not particularly allergenic.

A spore is to a fungus what a seed is to a plant, but very much smaller. To maximize the chance of some spores reaching a favorable spot, molds produce millions upon millions of them. Most come to nothing, but a few hit the jackpot and land on a spot where they can grow into an adult mold that then produces spores itself. Like pollen, mold spores are very light, so they disperse easily and remain airborne for a long time.

There are many different species of mold, each feeding in a different way. Some can make do on the most meager diet, scraping out a living on damp paintwork or glass, or on the rubber seal of a refrigerator door. You may wonder what food supply these molds can possibly have, and the answer is that the abundant food found in "fresh air," as described at the beginning of this chapter, is keeping them alive. Ironically, the proteins released by pollen grains when they land on a damp surface (see page 9) may be an important part of the diet for these molds. (Wallpaper paste on a damp wall is an absolute bonanza for them, but it usually contains fungicides to prevent mold growth.)

Fungi can also feed on wood, and those well-known pests dry rot and wet rot, if they have infested the timbers of a house, can both produce spores. While not everyone who is mold-sensitive will react to them, some will.

Detecting Mold-spore Allergy

An allergy to mold spores can produce symptoms all year round, especially in a damp house, but most sufferers find that their symptoms are seasonal, occurring mainly in the late summer, autumn, and early winter. In temperate climates, this is when the air is damp and there is plenty of food available in the form of rotting fruit and vegetation—"mists and mellow fruitfulness" are exactly what molds like best. The release of spores is generally timed to coincide with these most fungus-friendly seasons of the year.

Some mold spores are present in the air all year round, however, such as those of the blue-green *Penicillium* mold, often seen on bread and oranges. One mold, *Cladosporium herbarum,* begins spore production in June in temperate climates and can roughly coincide with the grass pollen season. Allergy to this mold can easily be mistaken for hay fever (see page 218). If there is doubt, a skin-prick test (see page 77) should reveal whether pollen or mold spores are the culprit.

In the case of molds, however, the skin-prick test is unlikely to include all the possible mold allergens. More than 20 different molds are known to produce allergic reactions. The allergic person may be sensitive to several different molds or just to one, and if that one is not included in the extract used for the skin-prick test, no reaction will occur, even though the person is sensitive to some mold spores. This will not happen often, but it is a possibility.

Fortunately, mold allergy can usually be identified by the circumstances in which symptoms arise or in which they get worse. Compost heaps are alive with molds, and handling compost, leaf mold, or fallen leaves may well bring on symptoms. Greenhouses, conservatories, cellars (molds do not need any light), old damp houses, churches, and church halls are often full of spores. Damp straw or hay breeds molds, as do grass clippings if not collected. In the latter case, mowing the lawn again will stir up the molds on the old clippings and release a cloud of spores, so this may be the moment when symptoms arise. (However, a reaction on mowing the lawn can also indicate grass pollen allergy; see pages 22–23.) Houseplants and bowls of potpourri around the house may be breeding molds, and so may humidifiers and air-conditioning systems, which then pump out the spores into the air. Molds that have been in a cold situation and then experience warm air are likely to release their spores suddenly, which is why Christmas trees often provoke symptoms—there are microscopic molds on their needles. Installing central heating in an old house can have a similar effect, warming up the molds and causing a major release of spores.

In the countryside, damp areas near rivers or lakes are likely to be rich in molds, and symptoms may begin when camping in such places. Forests in autumn and orchards that are carpeted with rotting fruit are also likely spots. In late summer, fields of grains or oil-seed rape can become infested with molds just before harvesttime, and this can cause symptoms in those living nearby or out on a walk. Any crop that goes moldy in the field can have the same effect. Mold spores are plentiful after the first frost of autumn, when they are released in large numbers by molds in the soil. Damp weather and ground fog will promote fungal growth, although rain itself will wash the spores out of the air.

Dealing with Mold Spores

Avoiding situations where molds abound (see above) is an obvious first step. Persuade someone else to rake up the fallen leaves, spread the compost, and cut the dead leaves from garden plants. The number of mold spores in the air is sometimes given along with the pollen count, mainly by telephone information services. If you are severely affected, you may wish to stay indoors on days with high spore counts.

Be very careful about where you choose to live, avoiding anywhere damp. Have an inspection done before buying a house to ensure that there is no dry rot or wet rot. If there is, have the problem thoroughly treated, and stay completely clear of the house until the renovation work is completed: huge numbers of spores will be released when old timbers or partitions are removed or floors pulled up. Spores are small and may take many hours to settle from the air (see the box "Particle Sizes" later in this chapter). It is probably wise to steer clear of any old house where extensive structural work is going on.

KEEPING DAMPNESS OUT OF THE HOUSE

Should the house you live in already be damp, there are various steps you can take to remedy this. If the house is old and built of stone or brick, it may have no moisture barrier, a horizontal waterproof layer, near ground level, that prevents moisture from soaking up into the walls from the soil. Houses built before about 1920 generally did not have a moisture barrier, but one can now be created, even in an old building, by drilling a row of small holes in all the outside walls, just above ground level, and injecting a silicone compound that hardens to form a waterproof layer within the wall. This acts as a barrier to rising dampness, and is not particularly expensive.

A thin, invisible layer of silicone can also be sprayed onto the outside of the walls, to prevent rainwater from coming directly through them. This may be useful around the corners of windows, where rain often penetrates, but it is not advisable to treat whole walls in this way. The advice of an architect or contractor should always be sought.

Within a house, if water is seeping up from the ground through the floors, a new floor can be laid with a layer of waterproof material incorporated. Most roofs now have a waterproof layer under their slates or shingles, but some older buildings may lack this. It can be a useful addition in making the house more watertight.

If these remedies are too expensive or troublesome, then dampness must be tackled in some other way. Any damp spot should be kept warm and well ventilated using electric space heaters, which are cheap to run. Fan heaters are not recommended because they churn up any mold spores in the vicinity. Silica crystals, which absorb water vapor and are then dried out in the oven for reuse, may prove helpful in a damp closet where heating is impossible. Dehumidifiers are another possibility, and air-conditioning units will also reduce moisture in the air.

Reducing Moisture Production Indoors

So much for moisture coming into the house from outside—that is only part of the story. Human activities within the house also generate a great deal of moisture. Steaming kettles, potatoes boiling on the stove, clothes drying in the bathroom, a hot shower or bath, liberally watered houseplants—all these are pumping moisture into the air. In addition, the average human being gives off about 2 pints (1 liter) of water in sweat every night, and more during the day. A family of four is estimated to produce 18 to 36 pints (10 to 20 liters) of water vapor every 24 hours.

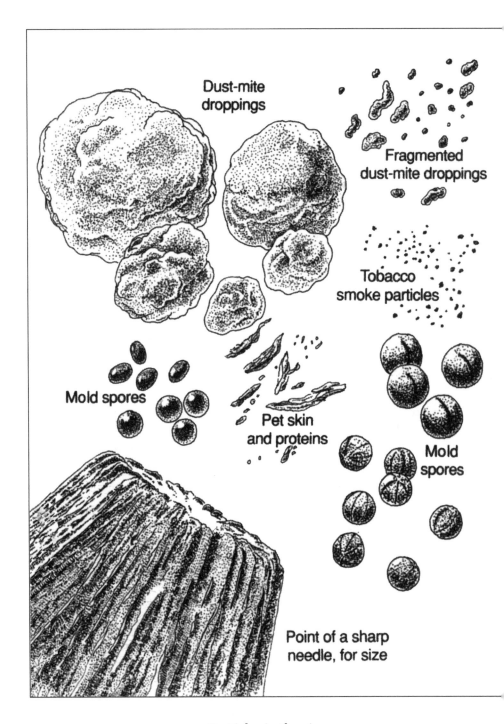

Dust-mite droppings

Fragmented dust-mite droppings

Tobacco smoke particles

Mold spores

Pet skin and proteins

Mold spores

Point of a sharp needle, for size

Particles in the air

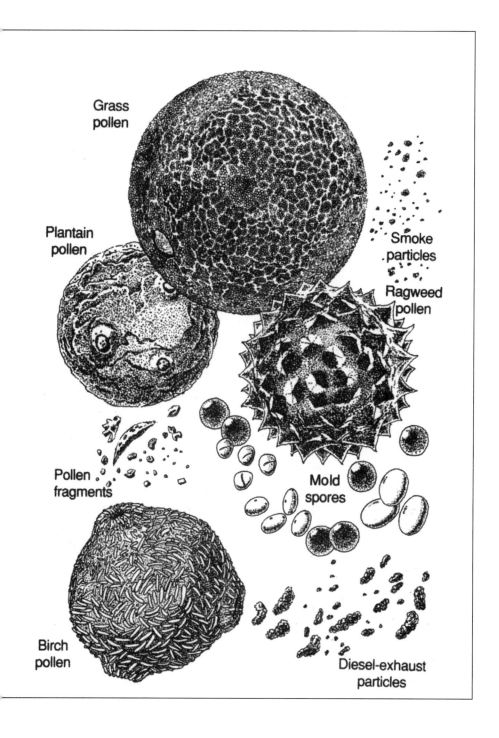

Grass pollen

Plantain pollen

Smoke particles

Ragweed pollen

Pollen fragments

Mold spores

Birch pollen

Diesel-exhaust particles

The problem will become visible as condensation, which occurs because warm air can carry far more water vapor than can cold air. The water vapor is a gas in the warm air, but as soon as the air cools it turns to water again—fine droplets of water that we see as steam.

The major part of the solution is to reduce the amount of water vapor going into the air by switching off the kettle as soon as it boils and using lids to cover pans of vegetables or other boiling liquids. Do not dry clothes indoors unless there is no alternative. If you can, get a tumble-dryer and make sure that the exhaust is vented outdoors.

Whenever the air is dry outside (hot and dry preferably, but cold and dry will do), give the house an airing. Open several windows and get a draft through. It is the lack of ventilation that creates much of the dampness in modern homes. By airing the house regularly (preferably every day), you will give the moisture a chance to escape.

Ventilation is particularly important in a newly built house or in one that has been renovated. A huge amount of water, up to 300 gallons (1,360 liters), is used in construction, mainly for plastering. This takes at least nine to twelve months to evaporate under normal conditions. A dehumidifier may be worthwhile during this period, especially if there is a lot of wet weather, and some high-capacity models are available for this specific purpose (see appendix 3 for suppliers). Beware of speeding up the process too much (e.g., by overheating the house), as this can cause plaster and concrete to crack and timber to warp.

Fighting Condensation

The other part of the solution, if you are sensitive to molds, is to combat condensation, because wherever there is condensation on a surface, molds will flourish. Condensation forms on any surface that is colder than the air around it, particularly cold windowpanes and cool walls in bathrooms and kitchens.

To combat condensation, you must remove temperature variations in the house as far as possible, keeping it warm throughout. Metal window frames, which are always cold, create a lot of condensation and should be replaced by wooden or PVC frames if at all possible. Double glazing is also helpful, as it makes the inner surface of windows warmer. Mop up any condensation that does occur on windowsills every day. Watch for black mold growth and remove it promptly if it appears.

Heat all parts of the house well, and do not leave any rooms permanently cold or unventilated. Check in closets and behind furniture for any damp spots. Attic insulation will help to keep ceilings warm.

Where some condensation is inevitable, as in bathrooms and kitchens, never make the walls or ceiling impermeable with vinyl wallpaper or gloss or eggshell paint. This will trap the condensation so that it runs down to the base of the wall, creating a wet area where molds will flourish. A permeable wall (one coated with ordinary wallpaper or emulsion paint) can absorb a certain amount of water and gradually "breathe it out" again, either to the outside air or back indoors again. Sometimes, for those with a serious mold problem, installing an extractor fan in the kitchen or bathroom is necessary. This is the only way to reduce condensation effectively.

Combating Molds

Having kept moisture out and reduced condensation within, the third step in the program is to combat molds directly. Any fabric or furniture that smells of mold or mildew must go. Although they may now be bone dry, that smell is indicative of old mold spores, millions of them, lingering within the article.

Clean the rubber seals around fridges and freezers with great care, going into all the crevices to get out the black mold that lives there. This process needs to be repeated regularly and should be done by someone other than the allergy sufferer, because exposure to spores will be high during the cleaning process. Shower curtains should be replaced entirely or thoroughly washed. If there is black mold on walls or window frames, it can be cleaned off with mineral spirits, which removes it without making the wall damp, and thus delays its regrowth. Alternatively, use a mixture of one part bleach to four parts water, with a little dish washing liquid added. Never brush off mold growth or tackle it with a dry cloth, as this simply disperses the spores into the air. Sprays are available to help control mold growth (see appendix 3).

Houseplants should be reduced to a bare minimum, and any that need to be wet all the time should definitely go. Learn to love cactuses if you can. The plants that remain should have their dead leaves and flowers removed regularly, and the top layer of the soil should also be scooped off occasionally and replaced.

Eat bread, potatoes, vegetables, and fruit promptly and do not leave ripe fruit about for long.

There may be a lot of mold spores in house dust, especially in an old house or in one that has been damp in the past. Anyone who is allergic to the spores should not have to dust, vacuum, sweep floors, or make beds. Wear a mask (see appendix 3) if this sort of housework is unavoidable.

Air Cleaners and Mold Spores

There have been no actual tests on the usefulness of air cleaners for mold-spore allergy. However, common sense suggests that they may be valuable in this context. Many mold spores are very small, and this means that they stay suspended in the air for several hours, rather than settling rapidly (see the box "Particle Sizes" on page 203). An air cleaner that is adequate for the size of the room (see appendix 3) should reduce the number of mold spores significantly. But you need also to substantially reduce any mold growth in the house.

Saying Goodbye to Your Humidifier. . .

The idea that central heating makes the air very dry, and that this irritates the nose and airways, is a popular one. Many people have bought humidifiers in an attempt to combat this supposed problem. In most cases, a humidifier is the last thing they need, since dry air is not the actual problem unless the heating is turned up high and the ventilation in the house is particularly good. The air in most modern homes is actually far too moist, and this has led to the upsurge in asthma (due to dust mites and mold spores) that all developed countries have seen in the past 20 years. Humidifiers add to the moisture in the air and, to make matters worse, can provide ideal breeding grounds for molds.

Scientific tests in which the humidity of the air was gradually decreased from 70 percent to 10 percent (a very low level) showed that people felt no ill effects, except for noticing a slight dryness in the mouth at the lowest levels. In another test, patients inhaled very dry air (only 9 percent relative humidity) for more than three days and nights. There were no changes in the membranes of the nose or the amount of mucus they produced.

If your nose feels uncomfortable when at home, try simply turning down the thermostat and putting on a sweater—it may be the heat that is affecting you. Another possibility is that "indoor pollution" is to blame. The scientific tests with dry air described above were carried out with very clean air, and it is conceivable that warm dry air *does* affect the nose if it is also polluted.

Most of us are subjected to far worse levels of pollution indoors than out (see "Airborne Irritants Indoors" later in this chapter), and reducing this is often remarkably easy. If your discomfort seems to be connected with having the heat on, it is possible that the radiators are very dusty and that the dust is burning off, producing irritants in the air. Clean the radiators thoroughly to prevent dust accumulation.

PETS AND OTHER ANIMALS

Pets are a frequent, and sometimes unsuspected, source of rhinitis. They can also cause asthma and eczema. For people who are highly sensitive, small amounts of allergen carried on the clothing of pet-owners may be enough to spark symptoms. In such cases, allergy shots (see chapter 9) may be the only solution. People with an allergic disposition who work with animals, such as vets, farmers, jockeys, animal breeders, and laboratory technicians are highly susceptible to developing allergic reactions. Again, allergy shots may be an option, but some find that they have to change their job because the symptoms cannot be controlled.

Cats

"Such clean animals," people say as they watch a cat carefully licking itself. Little do they know that this feline obsession with cleanliness fills the air with microscopic specks of dried saliva. The saliva contains a protein that is the main allergen for those affected by cats. It is absolutely everywhere in a house that has a cat, forming a coating on the walls, windows, and furniture, and staying airborne for hours.

The ubiquitous presence of the cat allergen means that people with an allergy to cats are usually well aware of it—their symptoms tend to appear promptly when they enter a house with a cat. The fact that cats are more likely to provoke allergies than are dogs may partly be explained by the constant presence of salivary proteins in the air.

Cat salivary protein can be found in houses where no cat has lived for many years, and occasionally there are traces of it in houses that have never had a cat at all—an observation that science has yet to explain, although the allergens may have been brought into the house on clothing.

Although salivary protein is the main cat allergen, skin particles from cats can also cause symptoms. The fur itself is not allergenic, although it can carry salivary proteins. Thus, a short-haired cat will not be less allergenic than a long-haired cat, contrary to popular mythology.

The allergic symptoms to cats can include rhinitis or asthma. Eczema is another possibility, especially in children.

In theory, eliminating cat allergens is very simple compared with dealing with something like pollen or dust mites—simply find a new home for your pet. Of course, this can be a very difficult decision, but it is the only sensible option, particularly if asthma is among the symptoms caused, or if the allergy sufferer is a child, whose problems could worsen with continued exposure to the allergen.

Think twice before replacing your lost pet with a dog, as cat allergens can cross-react with dog allergens (see the box "Cross-reactions Involving Airborne Allergens" later in this chapter). This may not happen in your case, but if it does you will be faced with another heart-wrenching decision about the new pet. Another animal, such as a hamster or guinea pig, is unlikely to provoke cross-reactions, but a new sensitivity could develop when it has been in the house for a while.

A thorough spring cleaning is needed once the cat is gone, with all curtains and other fabrics being washed, carpets shampooed, and walls washed down. If the carpets and armchairs are fairly old, and you have had a cat for many years, consider replacing them with new ones. When cleaning, pay particular attention to any areas where the cat used to sleep.

You don't need to wash fabrics at a high temperature to destroy cat allergen. It is not sensitive to heat but it does wash out, even in cool water, as long as a detergent is used. Don't fill the machine completely; leave plenty of space for good water circulation. Run the rinse cycle twice.

The allergy sufferer should be out of the house while this cleanup is in progress and for a day or two afterward. Alternatively, a mask can be worn, but it must be the right kind (see appendix 3) and should be kept on all the time, not just while cleaning, because the particles will remain airborne for a long time. As a minimum precaution, the allergic individual should wear a mask at home and sleep somewhere else. If this is impossible, omit cleaning the bedroom at first and keep the bedroom door closed during the cleanup. Clean the bedroom a week or two later, while the allergic individual sleeps in another room. If the cat has slept in the allergy sufferer's bedroom, tackle the problem the other way around: clean that first, while the patient sleeps in another room, preferably one where the cat rarely went. After a few days, the patient can go back to sleeping in the bedroom. The rest of the house can then be cleaned, keeping the bedroom door closed.

Even after a cleanup, some cat allergens may persist for a while, and it may therefore be a few months before symptoms subside completely.

As an additional measure, you could spray carpets and upholstery with tannic acid or another type of spray treatment to inactivate the allergens (see the box "Putting Allergens Out of Action" earlier in this chapter). In situations where a major cleanup is difficult, or it is impossible for the allergy sufferer to be elsewhere for a few days, an allergen-inactivating treatment could be used as a substitute for cleaning.

Cat allergen is not affected by heat, unfortunately, so a steam cleaner won't help you.

PARTICLE SIZES

The size of a particle makes an enormous difference to its role in causing allergies. Size affects how quickly particles settle, for example, and how easily they become airborne.

Particles larger than 40 microns (40 thousandths of a millimeter) settle from the air rapidly, so there are very few in the air that we breathe. (Pine pollen is an exception here, as it has air sacs that make it more buoyant, despite its large size.) If particles are not airborne in any great number, they are unlikely to cause allergies because too few are inhaled.

Particles of 30 microns, such as grass pollen grains, also settle relatively rapidly in still air (e.g., inside a house with doors and windows closed). But they are released from the grass plant when warm air currents will carry them skyward, and rising air often takes them high into the atmosphere, to rain down on the earth later. So there are plenty available to be inhaled.

Particles of 20 microns, such as ragweed pollen grains, take a little longer to settle, but in still air even they can fall 10 feet (3 meters) in just four minutes. An average room will be clear of the pollen in this time. However, if there are tiny fragments of pollen in the air (see page 21) these will take longer to settle.

At the lower end of the scale, settling times increase dramatically. For a particle 2 microns in diameter (which includes some mold spores, cat allergen particles, the smallest fragments of dust-mite droppings, and some pollen fragments), it takes a full six hours to drop 10 feet (3 meters). This means that the allergen load in a room with still air is unlikely to settle out except overnight. The particles may begin to settle in the daytime, but before they do so, the air is disturbed again.

With small allergen particles that are actively propelled into the indoor air (such as mold spores and cat saliva particles), this slowness in settling means that the air is unlikely to be free of the particles for long. However, good ventilation will rapidly blow these tiny particles out of the house, so they build up to problematic levels only in houses with extensive draft-proofing.

Small allergen particles that are not actively propelled into the air are less of a problem. Thus, the fragmented droppings of dust mites that are generated by mites in a carpet tend to stay at or near floor level, unless actively dispersed (by a standard vacuum cleaner, for example). However, a small child, whose nose is a lot closer to the ground, may be inhaling air containing far more of these allergenic fragments.

Particle size also determines how far the allergens penetrate the airways. Larger particles, when inhaled, are caught by the hairs and mucus in the nose, or by mucus in the windpipe, and do not reach the bronchi. This is the case for any particle bigger than 10 microns, although there is a reflex reaction (see pages 19–20) that can produce narrowing of the bronchi when large allergenic particles land in the nose.

Particles of between 4 and 10 microns can reach the bronchi and may provoke an asthma attack directly. Only those smaller than 4 microns are likely to go beyond the bronchi, into the lungs themselves. Here they can accumulate and eventually cause a more serious disease called **extrinsic allergic alveolitis** (see the box "Allergens Deep in the Lung" later in this chapter).

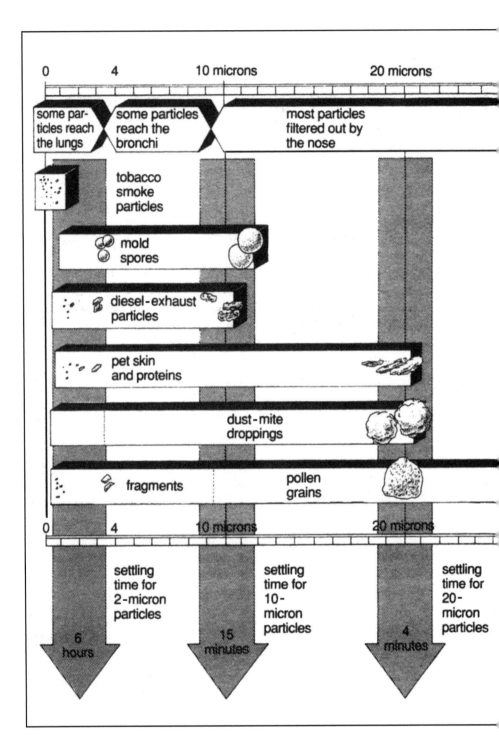

The sizes of airborne particles

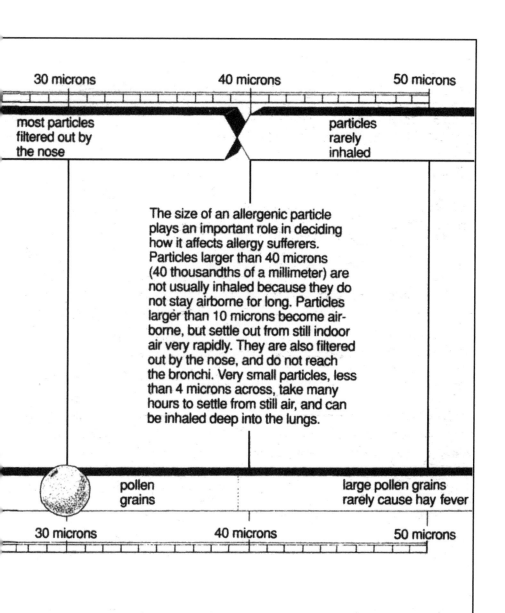

30 microns   40 microns   50 microns

most particles
filtered out by
the nose

particles
rarely
inhaled

The size of an allergenic particle
plays an important role in deciding
how it affects allergy sufferers.
Particles larger than 40 microns
(40 thousandths of a millimeter) are
not usually inhaled because they do
not stay airborne for long. Particles
larger than 10 microns become airborne, but settle out from still indoor
air very rapidly. They are also filtered
out by the nose, and do not reach
the bronchi. Very small particles, less
than 4 microns across, take many
hours to settle from still air, and can
be inhaled deep into the lungs.

pollen
grains

large pollen grains
rarely cause hay fever

30 microns   40 microns   50 microns

Settling time:
time taken for particles to settle
completely in a room with a ceiling
10 feet (3 meters) high

Research shows that a surprising number of people keep their cat despite the health problems it causes. Our emotional welfare and our physical welfare may make conflicting demands, and sometimes the emotions win. If you really cannot bear to part with your pet, then the allergen levels can be kept down in other ways.

First, the cat should be excluded from the allergy sufferer's bedroom at all times. If it has slept there in the past, all bedding should be thoroughly washed. Duvets or comforters on which the cat has slept should be washed or replaced.

Second, if the house is well sealed against drafts, you need to increase the ventilation. In houses with snugly fitting doors and windows, the tiny particles from a cat can build up to very high levels. Even a modest increase in the amount of air flowing through your home will help to blow away the cat allergens. For some people, these two steps may be enough on their own.

If regular ventilation to the outside is impossible, you could use a HEPA air filter instead (see appendix 3). However, research has shown that, with the very small particles from cats, the air currents set up by the fan in the air filter will churn up allergens from the floor and furnishings. This can partially offset its effectiveness in filtering the air. Placing the air filter well away from the floor will help, but a better solution is to clean carpets and furniture thoroughly at the outset, thus reducing the reservoir of cat allergen. (During cleaning, the allergy sufferer must go elsewhere or be protected from the allergen that is disturbed.) You should also remove as many cushions and upholstered items as possible, as this will reduce the surfaces that can act as reservoirs for cat allergens.

Third, try persuading your cat to spend more time outdoors. This will reduce the amount of allergen being generated in the house. Providing a warm and comfortable place to sleep outside, in a shed, porch, or garage, may be helpful.

The next step is a big one for you, and an even bigger one for the cat—give it a thorough wash with shampoo twice a week. This substantially cuts down the amount of allergen that is shed with its fur and skin and thus decreases the amount of allergen in the air. Some cats get used to this treatment in time; others decide that the house next door is more congenial after all. (If its affections seem to be wandering, you can try improving the food being offered.)

Make sure the cat's bedding is also washed regularly, at least once a week. Research shows that a well-used blanket can contain as much allergen as the fur of 70 cats.

You may see sprays and tablets for cats that claim to reduce the amount of allergen produced. Some scientific tests have shown that they don't actually work.

Cutting the cat's claws every week is also said to reduce the amount of allergen in the air, presumably because it sheds less skin when scratching. Unless you have a particularly docile individual, this is likely to be even less popular than the weekly shampoo.

If these measures are not enough to eliminate the symptoms, you could try replacing your wall-to-wall carpets with area rugs, vacuuming armchairs and sofas regularly, and using a high-quality air cleaner (see appendix 3). Research in the United States has shown that these measures, combined with washing the cat, will reduce the amount of cat allergen in the air considerably.

JERRY

Jerry suffered from hay fever in the summer, as he had done since his teens. On top of this, he had asthma attacks accompanied by a runny, congested nose all year round, particularly on the weekends. Skin-prick testing produced several positive reactions, making it difficult to know which ones were actually causing the symptoms, so the doctor began questioning Jerry about the pattern of his symptoms. It seemed that the asthma and rhinitis built up slowly over the weekend and then cleared when he returned to work. The doctor questioned Jerry closely and found that he had suffered from recurrent bronchitis as a child, which had ended abruptly when he was about 15. Knowing that the terms used for asthma had changed over the years, and that methods of diagnosis had changed too, the doctor suspected that this childhood "bronchitis" might actually have been asthma.

"Did you move to a new house when you were fifteen?" asked the doctor, "or did anything at home change?" The only thing Jerry could remember was that the family cat had died. It seemed irrelevant to Jerry, but the doctor was interested and asked whether there were any cats in his present house. "Yes, my girlfriend has two," Jerry replied. The cause of the weekend asthma and rhinitis now seemed clear, and a check with the results of the skin-prick tests showed that there had been a positive reaction to cats.

Jerry's doctor suggested ways in which cat allergens could be cut down—a thorough spring cleaning, followed by a weekly bath for both cats. In the meantime, Jerry was given an inhaler to help stave off the asthma attacks. Once the anti-cat-allergen measures were in action, Jerry was able to stop using the inhaler without ill effects.

Jerry is not typical of cat-allergic people, who generally know that cats cause their problem because the reaction to them is so dramatic and immediate. As Jerry's case shows, skin-prick tests are often only a rough guide, and some careful detective work may be needed to pinpoint the culprit allergen.

Buying a new vacuum with a HEPA filter or, less ideally, fitting a filter to your existing vacuum cleaner is advisable because the allergen particles could go through the bag and become airborne again (see the box "Vacuum Cleaners" earlier in this chapter).

Another approach is to designate the living room a cat-free zone, spray the upholstery and carpets with tannic acid or another allergen-inactivating spray, and install an air cleaner. This will keep the allergens in the air at a low level, but only as long as the cat stays out of the room. (With tannic acid sprays, the cat will probably collect quite a bit on its paws, which it will then lick off. No one has investigated the effect of this on the cat, but it may be detrimental, so you should not use the spray regularly on an area that the cat inhabits.)

Someone highly sensitive to cats should avoid buying a house where cats have lived in the past, because their allergens will linger on.

Dogs

Dogs are less likely to cause allergic reactions than cats, but they are a fairly frequent source of problems, particularly for children. Rhinitis, asthma, or eczema is the common symptom.

The allergens occur mainly in the skin particles and saliva. As with all animals, the fur is not allergenic in itself, but allergenic proteins can become attached to the hair. The urine and feces of dogs can also contain allergens. A few people react to one breed of dog only (see page 158), but most are allergic to all dogs and may react to cats too.

Parting with the dog is the best solution, but it can be heartbreaking, and many people prefer to live with the problem. Washing the dog thoroughly in a bathtub, using dog shampoo, will help, but you must do it at least twice a week because allergen levels build up again within three days.

Regular vacuuming of carpets and armchairs will be helpful in reducing the level of allergens in the air, and tannic acid or another allergen-inactivating spray (see the box "Denaturing the Allergens" earlier in this chapter) may also be useful. Replacing wall-to-wall carpets with rugs will reduce the reservoir of dog allergens in the house, provided you mop or vacuum the bare floors regularly and beat rugs outdoors to remove the skin particles.

The dog's bedding should be washed every week, and the animal itself should be strictly excluded from the allergy sufferer's bedroom. If it has ever slept on the bed, all the bedding should be washed thoroughly to remove the allergens, or replaced.

Small Animals

Any animal can produce an allergic reaction, and rabbits, guinea pigs, mice, hamsters, gerbils, and rats are no exception. Unfortunately, these allergies are often overlooked by doctors, who inquire about cats and dogs but forget to ask about smaller pets. An allergy to such a pet can be investigated with a skin-prick test, and you should ask for this test if it has not been carried out already. (People working with small animals can be similarly affected; see "Allergens and Irritants at Work" later in this chapter.)

Skin particles, or proteins from the animal's urine, are probably the allergen involved. Rhinitis or asthma may occur as a result of the allergy, and either can come on gradually, beginning some time after the pet has arrived in the home. The only real solution is to move the animal's cage outside, or at least onto a porch.

Where houses are infested with mice or rats, allergic reactions to these animals develop. As with cockroach allergy (see "Unsuspected Allergens?" in chapter 6), those most likely to be affected are those least likely to get the medical treatment they need. Recent research has shown that 18 percent of American children living in inner-city areas are allergic to mice. This allergy can contribute to asthma. A constant runny nose is very common in children living in poor housing and is often attributed to repeated infections. Anyone living in poor housing who has a "perpetual cold" should perhaps be tested for allergies to rats, mice, and cockroaches, particularly if he or she has shown negative results to tests for molds and dust mites.

Birds

Feather particles, or proteins from the droppings, are the main allergens in the case of birds. They can cause rhinitis, asthma, or a lung complaint known as bird-fancier's lung (see the box on page 211).

The particles are very small and therefore difficult to control. You could try keeping the cage in a room that the allergy sufferer does not enter, but this is unlikely to help, as the particles will be wafted into the rest of the house whenever the door is opened. The best solution is to find another home for the bird.

If this is impossible, a HEPA air cleaner (see appendix 3) would probably keep down the particle levels, but it must be sufficiently powerful for the size of the room. Even with an air cleaner running, the affected person will probably be unable to enter the room where the bird is kept.

Whether or not the bird is removed from the house, a general cleanup to remove the existing reservoir of allergens may be valuable. Follow the cleaning guidelines described earlier in the chapter for cat allergy.

Sheep's Wool

Until recently, the medical profession had been largely unaware that some people have an allergy to sheep's wool. A recent study, however, revealed that many people with an allergy to house dust but not to dust mites were actually sensitive to wool particles in the dust. It is not clear what the allergen is in this case, since fur and hair (of which wool is one form) are thought not to be allergenic. And there is another puzzle regarding wool allergy: for reasons that are not understood, very few of those affected give a positive reaction when skin-prick-tested with wool extract itself. However, they give strong reactions to a nasal provocation test (see chapter 6) with wool. Some are already aware of the source of their problems, as they experience symptoms (rhinitis or asthma) from sheepskin jackets and rugs, from woolen blankets and carpets, or when knitting with wool.

The obvious treatment for this allergy is to avoid woolen clothing, bedding, and carpets. A thorough spring cleaning may be necessary to remove the existing pool of wool fibers in the household dust. Unfortunately, avoiding wool can be difficult, as the fibers are almost everywhere. If medicinal drugs do not control the symptoms adequately, a desensitization treatment may be helpful (see chapter 9).

Horses

Few people have much contact with horses these days, yet these animals seem to cause reactions very frequently, suggesting that they produce powerful allergens. Fortunately, avoidance of horses is relatively easy. If you are very sensitive, you may find that antique sofas and armchairs stuffed with horsehair affect you. These should be replaced, as should any carpet pads made of horsehair. In some old houses, the plaster may contain horsehair. You can find out by removing electrical switch covers and looking closely at the plaster. If it does contain horsehair, you may be able to reduce the amount of allergen getting into the air by simply repairing all cracks and holes.

The clothes of someone else who has been riding may contain enough allergen to affect you, and in some cases *this source can sensitize a person who has no direct contact with horses themselves.* When one person in a family is a keen rider and another is allergic to horses, the best compromise is for the nonallergic person to change his or her riding clothes before coming indoors. He or she may also need to take a shower.

Insects

The discovery of insects as a major and widespread cause of rhinitis and asthma—that is, one affecting more than 10 percent of those with allergic disease—is a relatively recent development. Such allergic reactions have been found in a surprising number of countries, and the true extent of the problem is still unknown.

Widespread insect allergy generally comes to light only where it is specifically looked for, as with cockroach allergy (see "Unsuspected Allergens?" in chapter 6). More recently, both mosquitoes and cockroaches have been found to cause rhinitis and asthma in India. Silkworm moths are a problem in Japan and some parts of central Asia, while midges and caddis flies are also a cause of rhinitis in Japan. Around the Great Lakes in Canada, the molted skin of mayflies can cause asthma and rhinitis in the breeding season. The green nemitry fly of Egypt and Sudan causes widespread seasonal rhinitis and may aggravate asthma, mainly in the hot summer months. In several countries, allergies to maggots are found among fishermen using them as bait, and the symptoms may include rhinitis.

Looking at indoor insect pests other than cockroaches, there are well-documented cases of people who react strongly to houseflies or to carpet beetles. In the case of carpet beetles, the larvae (often called "fuzzy bears") are covered with tiny hairs. It is these hairs that are likely to provoke allergic reactions. There have also been occasional cases of allergy to daphnia (not insects, but

ALLERGENS DEEP IN THE LUNG

Very small particles that go deep into the lung can cause **extrinsic allergic alveolitis** (see the box "Particle Sizes" earlier in this chapter), but only if they are inhaled in large amounts. Farmer's lung and bird-fancier's lung are two examples of this disease, the first caused by mold spores from moldy hay and the second by feather particles or proteins from bird droppings. Cage birds such as parakeets can bring on this disease, but it is most often seen in those who keep pigeons.

The disease produces attacks of a flulike illness, with feverishness, pains in the limbs, breathlessness, and a dry cough. The symptoms tend to last a few days, then disappear, only to come back later. They may not develop immediately after exposure to the allergen, but rather many hours later, so the link is not obvious. The disease is produced in a different way from hay fever and other common allergies, and unlike them it carries a risk of serious long-term damage. If you have any symptoms of this sort, you should see your doctor immediately. (There is a widespread medical belief that you cannot suffer from rhinitis or asthma to an allergen *and* have extrinsic allergic alveolitis to the same allergen. Recent research shows that this is not correct.)

crustaceans) used to feed fish; inhaled particles from these can cause rhinitis or asthma.

Asian ladybugs, first introduced into the southeastern United States in the 1970s, often overwinter in houses and can cause allergic symptoms in the eyes and nose. In order to keep out the ladybugs, you need to caulk the outside of your home, sealing all the gaps. Repainting the house a very dark color is also worthwhile, because the insects seek out pale walls that resemble the light-colored cliffs where they overwinter in their natural habitat. You will need to clean up well indoors to get rid of the existing allergen.

With insects that infest houses, such as cockroaches, their droppings may carry the allergen. Alternatively, it can be hairs that they shed, bits of broken-off wing and skin, or tiny fragments of their bodies that have disintegrated after death. With largely outdoor insects, such as midges and caddis flies, it is hairs and body fragments floating in the air that cause problems. Bees, butterflies, and moths can also cause problems in this way, but allergies to these insects are very rare.

Treatment for insect allergy, where the insects are household pests, involves eradication. There are various commercial companies that can advise and assist with this. The eradication process could involve pulling away paneling (around baths or at the back of closets, for example) or removing carpets if they are heavily infested with carpet beetles. This will release a great deal of allergen into the air, and it is therefore vital that the allergy sufferer be out of the house at the time and for several hours afterward. (On one occasion, an asthmatic with cockroach allergy suffered a fatal asthma attack when cockroach allergens were released during an eradication treatment.) Insecticide sprays, or the solvents in which they are dissolved, can in themselves cause symptoms, and it is really best to leave the house for several days after spraying, particularly if there are children in the household. (This advice also applies to standard treatments for woodworm and dry or wet rot.)

According to a report in the scientific journal *Clinical and Experimental Allergy* in 2000, spider mites (family Tetranychidae), which live on the leaves of fruit trees and are major agricultural pests in fruit-growing areas, can also provoke allergic reactions. Those affected may suffer from asthma as well as allergic symptoms in the nose and eyes. Spider mites are common pests in the United States, especially in apple, pear, and citrus orchards.

Workers in the fruit-growing industry and their children are those most likely to be affected by spider mite allergy. However, research from Korea suggests that residents in fruit-growing areas who don't work in the orchards can also become sensitized. In the case of those living near pear and apple orchards, their symptoms are likely to get worse in summer and early fall, when the numbers of spider mites on the fruit trees peak. This sensitivity problem could easily be mistaken for hay fever, probably for ragweed allergy.

IRRITANTS IN THE AIR

A few of the items found in the air can act as irritants to the nose. If they affect the nose, they generally affect the bronchi as well, except for large particles that cannot reach the bronchi (discussed earlier in this chapter).

Anyone can be affected by these irritant particles or gases, not just those of an allergic disposition, but some people are more sensitive than others. Those with hay fever are often more susceptible during the pollen season. Someone whose nose is highly sensitive to a variety of airborne irritants but who has *no* allergic responses may be considered to have vasomotor rhinitis (see chapter 13).

The irritants may have their effect just by stimulating nerves in the nose, so that the parasympathetic nervous system (see the box "Nerves in the Nose" in chapter 13) reacts. Some irritants, however, do provoke genuine inflammation—a response that involves parts of the immune system. This is the case with sulfur dioxide, for example.

Most of the airborne irritants are man-made, but some are natural substances produced by plants or animals.

Irritants in Outdoor Air

Pine pollen may act as an irritant because of its large size, the enormous quantity inhaled, and certain chemicals carried on its surface. The tiny hairs produced by plane trees, which are scattered in spring and summer, irritate the eyes of some people. The hairs from peaches are also a major irritant and may affect anyone close to a peach tree in fruit; the symptoms are similar to those of hay fever.

Volatile substances produced by plants can also act as irritants, and certain plants, such as oil-seed rape, produce these in abundance (see the box "Smaller Than Small" in chapter 8). The scents of flowers can irritate the nose in some people.

Many man-made substances act as irritants, notably smoke. The smoke that we see consists of tiny unburned or partially burned particles, plus droplets of moisture in some cases. These particles and droplets act as irritants, but there are also many invisible constituents in smoke, including **acrolein,** a gas that is highly irritating to the airways. The more moisture there is in the material being burned and the less ventilation at the base of the fire, the more smoke particles and acrolein will be produced. A really hot fire produces no smoke at all. Garden bonfires, particularly those burning damp wood or leaves, are an unrecognized hazard, particularly for anyone with asthma. Plastics and other synthetic materials, when burned on a bonfire, can make matters worse by producing a variety of powerful irritants.

Ozone, a gas produced by the action of sunlight on car exhausts, is also irritating to the airways, and has been shown to aggravate both rhinitis and asthma. Nitrogen dioxide, which is produced by car exhausts, can also be an irritant when it builds up to sufficiently high levels. Both are discussed in detail in chapter 4.

A variety of gases produced by industrial processes and expelled from factory or power station chimneys into the surrounding air can act as irritants. Sulfur dioxide and sulfuric acid droplets (see chapter 4) are notable offenders. As with many irritants, those most affected will be asthmatics.

Advice on reducing exposure to outdoor pollutants can be found in appendix 6.

Airborne Irritants Indoors

One major indoor irritant is tobacco smoke, which can make both rhinitis and asthma worse. Some people are far more susceptible to this irritant than others.

The smoke produced by frying, particularly if the oil or fat is overheated, is also a powerful irritant to the airways. An oven that has not been cleaned for some time will produce a similar type of smoke when heated.

Nitrogen dioxide is produced by burning most fuels and is an irritant when it reaches a certain concentration in the air. With gas ranges and old-fashioned paraffin heaters, nitrogen dioxide may build up to high levels in poorly ventilated rooms (see page 57).

Many household products—such as polish, some cleaning fluids, paint, mineral spirits, turpentine, and bleach—can act as irritants to susceptible individuals, particularly those whose nose or bronchi are already inflamed by an allergic reaction. Air fresheners can irritate the eyes, nose, and chest.

Formaldehyde is an indoor pollutant of which people are often quite unaware. It can cause dryness and irritation in the nose and throat and may affect the eyes or the bronchi as well. Research shows that children exposed to high levels of formaldehyde, especially in their bedrooms, are more likely to develop allergic reactions. One source of this gas is injected cavity wall insulation. Some of the materials used in this process generate formaldehyde and will continue to do so for months after it has been injected. Particleboard is the other major source, but if it has been painted with gloss paint, this will keep the formaldehyde locked inside. Plywood gives off lesser amounts of formaldehyde. Other minor sources are foam rubber, new textiles and carpets, paper (including newsprint), photographs, leather luggage, antiperspirants, some cosmetics, and some shampoos. Mobile homes and caravans are often rich in formaldehyde, because plywood and particleboard are used extensively in making them. Modern buildings such as offices and hotels can also have high levels of formaldehyde in the air. Formaldehyde is also used to sterilize soil and greenhouses, and there may be an unhealthy level of exposure if these processes are not carried out carefully. There is a personal monitoring system that can show how much formaldehyde you are being exposed to (see appendix 3).

An interesting study from Finland shows that children living in houses with easy-clean wall and floor coverings, made from plastic materials, were more likely to develop asthma. Whether this effect is due to formaldehyde or to some other gas given off by the plastics is unknown.

Sprays used to kill dust mites (see "Dealing with Dust Mites" earlier in this chapter) have sometimes produced symptoms in those suffering from asthma. Advice on reducing exposure to pollutants in the home can be found in appendix 6.

ALLERGENS AND IRRITANTS AT WORK

Any particles that are inhaled all day in large quantities may affect the airways. Sometimes it is clear that the workplace is the cause of symptoms, particularly with irritants. With an allergen, however, late-phase reactions (see "The Late-phase Reaction" in chapter 3) are often important, and these can make the allergic reaction continue all weekend. This frequently obscures the source of the problem, although symptoms should clear up during a longer holiday.

With asthma, the symptoms may continue over the weekend, even though the substance responsible is merely an irritant.

Particles encountered at work that are known to act as allergens include wheat flour, rye flour, soybean flour or dust, castor-bean dust (see chapter 3), and tiny droplets of egg sprayed on to pies and pastries. Farmers may show an allergic reaction to wheat dust or to mold spores.

Some of the complex salts of platinum can also act as allergens, having first combined with proteins in the body, and workers in the platinum-refining industry are especially vulnerable to asthma.

Natural pyrethroid insecticides, and the flowers they are made from, can also produce an allergic reaction.

Mold spores can act as allergens (discussed in detail earlier in the chapter), and a variety of workers have a very high exposure to these, including farmers, builders and decorators (when stripping out fittings in old houses or in those with moisture problems), mushroom growers, and those working in breweries.

Sometimes wood dusts act as allergens, but they are more likely to be irritants (see below). Those with hay fever to a tree pollen may show a cross-reaction to wood dust or pulp (see chapter 11), but this is unusual.

Laboratory workers who look after rats, mice, and other small mammals can readily develop an allergy to the proteins found in their urine or to skin particles. Powered respirator helmets (see appendix 3) are sometimes used to protect such workers from the allergens.

Those working on maggot farms may become allergic to maggots, and people rearing locusts, fruit flies, silkworms, butterflies, stick insects, or bees can be similarly affected.

As already noted in chapter 1, anyone working closely with plants may become allergic to the pollen, even though it is a pollen that does not normally cause hay fever.

With all allergens, a skin-prick test can be used to confirm that this is indeed the cause of the problem. However, a negative skin-prick test does not entirely rule out an allergic reaction, as false negatives are possible (see chapter 6).

The potential irritants encountered in industrial processes are too numerous to mention here. The industries where large numbers suffer from symptoms in the airways include platinum smelting, electronics, plastics manufacturing, detergent manufacturing, the textile industry, and any industrial process using formaldehyde, toluene, diphylmethane, hexamethylene, naphthalene, phthalic acid, or trimellitic acid. For the majority of people, it will be obvious that something in the workplace is producing symptoms in the nose or bronchi. Sometimes, as in platinum smelting and electronics, there may be both irritants *and* allergens in the air, and a single chemical may even take both roles. The irritant effects will generally be known to other workers, trade union officials, the company medical service, or local doctors, who can advise on long-term effects. Everyone is different, and if a substance affects others far less than it affects you, this is no reason to ignore the irritation it causes. Taking the early signs seriously may help to avoid more significant long-term consequences.

In general, those with an allergic disposition should avoid going into jobs where there is high allergen exposure, such as in bakeries, or looking after animals. If asthma is already present, they should not work with known irritants.

With nonindustrial jobs, there is often assumed to be little or no hazard.

While this is largely true, there are certain problems that have been generally ignored in the past. For example, permanent-wave solutions can produce rhinitis in hairdressers, and hair spray can produce the lung disease thesaurosis. Carpenters and wood-turners may be affected by wood dust, as may goldsmiths who use wood dust for drying jewelry. Laser printers may occasionally affect the nose too, due to the styrene-butadiene toners used. Photocopying machines produce small amounts of ozone, and if there are several machines in a poorly ventilated area, this irritant gas may build up to a level where it can affect people with rhinitis or asthma.

Ozone can also be produced by electrostatic air cleaners, although this problem has been overcome with newer devices. If the electrostatic plates are left on over the weekend but the fans turned off, there can be a buildup of ozone, which then floods into the building when the ventilation system is switched on at the beginning of the week. This can produce severe symptoms of coughing and nasal irritation in a large proportion of the workforce. The problem is relatively rare, but it can occur in older office buildings. There are now companies that can investigate and remedy health problems caused by buildings (see appendix 3).

Sick Building Syndrome

This controversial problem, which often affects workers in large office buildings, probably has several different causes. One may be formaldehyde in the air, produced by office furniture and fittings. There may also be other gases in the air that act as irritants, gases that are slowly being given off by plastics and other materials used in carpeting or office fittings. The dryness of the air may make exposure to such pollutants more irritating to the nose. Ozone from photocopiers and fumes from laser printers (see above) can sometimes add to the problem, as can cleaning solutions such as bleach. Increasing the ventilation usually dispels such pollutants.

Another cause of sick building syndrome may be allergic reactions to mold spores. The molds are usually growing in the air ducts or water tanks and then being circulated around the office. More serious, mold spores and other microbes growing in water tanks can cause **humidifier fever** or **humidifier lung,** but this occurs only when there is a significant infestation producing large numbers of spores and microbes in the air. Anyone can be affected by this, not just those of an allergic disposition. The symptoms are fever, cough, a general feeling of malaise, tightness in the chest, and aching muscles. They develop within a few hours of starting work and are worse on Monday mornings when the ventilation system is turned on, releasing a large dose of spores and microbes that have built up in the system over the weekend. This disease is similar to **extrinsic allergic alveolitis** (see the box "Allergens Deep in the Lung" earlier in this chapter) and requires prompt treatment.

Tobacco smoke may also be a factor in sick building syndrome, and studies show that people vary greatly in their sensitivity to this pollutant. Occasionally dust mites turn out to be the problem (discussed in detail earlier in this chapter). Sometimes fluorescent lighting is at the root of sick building syndrome, but if this is the sole cause, the symptoms are unlikely to affect the nose. Psychological factors, including monotonous work and the feeling of being trapped in a building in which the windows cannot be opened or the heating system controlled, may contribute to sick building syndrome.

SEASONAL SYMPTOMS FROM ALLERGENS OTHER THAN POLLEN

If you appear to have hay fever but give no positive skin-prick tests to pollen, then there are other possibilities you should consider.

In temperate climates, one mold, *Cladosporium herbarum,* releases its spores from June to September. Someone who is allergic to this species and not to other molds may seem to have grass pollen hay fever, but his or her symptoms will be entirely out of step with the pollen counts. Another mold, *Alternaria,* sporulates mainly in July and August. Skin-prick tests that are specific for these molds and not for other types are available.

In cool climates, cockroaches may produce allergic symptoms only in summer (see "Unsuspected Allergens" in chapter 6). Similarly, houseflies will be much more common in summer. In both cases, symptoms will be worse indoors, unlike with hay fever.

Many outdoor insects such as midges, mayflies, and caddis flies will produce symptoms only in summer, and such symptoms could be mistaken for hay fever. These insects are more common in damp places and by water.

Mosquitoes are obviously more common in summer, and might produce symptoms indoors, outdoors, or both.

Mold-spore allergy, where the main source of spores is outdoor air, can produce seasonal symptoms, usually in late summer and autumn. (Indoors, winter is a more moldy time of year, because windows are opened less, people are at home more, clothes are dried indoors, and more hot meals are prepared. Dust-mite allergy often peaks in winter too, and cat allergy could get worse due to less ventilation—see "Cats" earlier in this chapter.)

Volatile substances from plants (see the box "Smaller Than Small?" in chapter 8) could also act as seasonal irritants, and some people may show a nonallergic reaction to pollen. Nonallergic seasonal reactions are considered in more detail in chapter 13.

UNEXPLAINED SEASONAL SYMPTOMS

If you have negative skin-prick tests for pollen and none of the other explanations for seasonal symptoms seems likely in your case, you could ask for a nasal provocation test (see chapter 6) with pollen. This may reveal a positive reaction when a skin-prick test has given a false negative.

It is well worth identifying such an allergy and having it properly treated, especially if you have asthma. Research among asthma patients in the Midwest has shown that being allergic to *Alternaria* greatly increases the risk of having a really serious asthma—the kind that lands you in the emergency room. Attacks of this kind are potentially fatal, of course. Medical scientists in

CROSS-REACTIONS INVOLVING AIRBORNE ALLERGENS

There are few cross-reactions between pollen allergens and the airborne allergens described in this chapter, although mugwort pollen can cross-react with the dust from wood of the spindle tree. It is possible that grass pollen might cross-react with inhaled wheat flour or wheat dust.

For those who are sensitive to dust mites, there are often cross-reactions to other mites, such as those found in stored grain and those that live as parasites on dogs, cats, or horses. There is also a most peculiar cross-reaction between dust mites and two fruits: kiwi and papaya (see pages 165–166).

For those sensitive to dog allergens, there can be some cross-reaction to cats and vice versa, because certain allergens are similar. However, these cross-reactions are unusual.

People who are highly sensitized to feather allergens or to protein from bird droppings sometimes develop a cross-reaction to egg proteins, and may react badly when they eat eggs. The same can be true, naturally enough, for those sensitized to inhaled egg droplets from working in the food industry. Those who are highly egg-sensitive sometimes react allergically to certain vaccines, notably influenza and measles vaccine, because these are often cultured in eggs or in cells taken from eggs and minute traces of egg protein remain. The risk is very low with measles vaccines, but discuss the matter with your doctor.

A few people with mold allergy show a cross-reaction to fungi found in some wines. Occasionally, people who seem to be sensitive to strawberries are actually reacting to the gray mold known as *Botrytis* that grows on them. A cross-reaction with edible fungi, such as mushrooms, is also possible.

Those allergic to horses may react to old mattresses, armchairs, or settees stuffed with horsehair, while anyone sensitive to birds may obviously react to feather stuffing in furniture, pillows, or duvets. (These are not true cross-reactions, just reactions to the same allergen from a different source.)

New Zealand have found the same thing, with *Alternaria* and *Cladosporium* being major culprits.

Other evidence also points to the deadly importance of mold allergy. Researchers in Chicago looking at the mold-spore levels during summer found that more asthma deaths occurred on days when the mold-spore count was high.

If you find that you are allergic to molds, you should make sure that your asthma is always well treated. Severe asthma attacks tend to happen when anti-inflammatory "preventer" medication, such as steroids or antileukotriene drugs, is neglected and the warning signs of deterioration (like needing your reliever inhaler every day) are ignored. Consider having immunotherapy (see chapter 9) for your mold allergy, and take steps to combat molds at home (see "Keeping Dampness Out of the House" earlier in this chapter).

Some doctors believe that asthmatics with allergy to *Alternaria* and *Cladosporium* should also learn to recognize the kind of days on which spores are likely to be released and then take extra care. Both these molds favor clear days with dry air and brisk winds. Faced with this kind of day, it might be wise to take an extra dose of preventer in the morning—having sought your doctor's agreement to this in advance. You could also wear a mask if you are outdoors for any length of time (e.g., on your way to work) just to reduce your exposure to the spores. Both molds have spores of about 4 to 10 microns in size, so a basic dust mask should do the job adequately—you don't need an expensive HEPA mask.

Chapter 13
OTHER FORMS OF RHINITIS

So far we have looked at pollen and the various other allergens and irritants found floating in the air. These have direct access to the nose and are prime suspects when symptoms occur there, but there are several other ways in which problems in the nose can be caused.

INFECTIONS

The most frequent cause of problems is, of course, infection. Indeed, the common cold, produced by a viral infection, brings most of us a short sharp dose of **rhinitis** (inflammation in the nose) each winter. Here the immune reaction that causes inflammation (see chapter 3) is doing its proper job—fighting off infectious microbes. That is why you should never use corticosteroid drops (see chapter 7), which you may have been prescribed for hay fever, when suffering from a cold or other infection—they will reduce your resistance to the microbe.

Colds generally last less than a week, and if one continues for more than three or four weeks, you should see your doctor. Asthmatics should see the doctor if their attacks become more frequent or more severe during a cold, as they frequently do.

INFECTION-PLUS-ALLERGY

Very rarely, patients develop a damaging allergic reaction against certain infectious bacteria in the nose. This causes a prolonged rhinitis, with a great deal of unpleasant mucus coming from the nose. Because the condition is rare, your doctor may not recognize it at first. Antibiotics are needed to kill off the bacteria, and allergy shots (see chapter 9) to control the allergic reaction.

Allergic reactions to infectious fungi are also possible, and can sometimes cause rhinitis. This is known to happen with the fungus that causes athlete's foot, *Trichophyton*. As well as infecting the skin, the fungus can sometimes make its home in the nose, and an allergic reaction there then causes rhinitis. Occasionally, asthma is due to an allergic reaction to the same fungus. For more detailed information, see *Asthma* by Jonathan Brostoff, M.D., and Linda Gamlin (Healing Arts Press, 2000).

REPEATED INFECTIONS

A long succession of infections in the nose can leave its delicate inner structure damaged, with the membranes thickened and the blood vessels congested. This will produce a constant stuffiness in the nose and may impair the sense of smell. The condition is known as **hypertrophic rhinitis.** Surgery may help but is used only for the more severe cases.

PROBLEMS IN THE NOSE CAUSED BY DRUGS

Certain drugs can affect the nose badly, and the rather pompous Latin term **rhinitis medicamentosa** is used to refer to the problems they can cause. The most common culprits are decongestant nose drops containing **sympathomimetics** (see chapter 7), to which the nose readily becomes addicted. To avoid this problem, such drops should not be used for more than a few days. Cocaine, when "snorted," has a similar effect to sympathomimetics, and can therefore produce rebound congestion in the same way. Cocaine can also cause problems simply by acting as an irritant.

Very occasionally, sympathomimetics taken by mouth (e.g., *pseudoephedrine, phenylephrine,* and *phenylpropanolamine*) can have the same effect, but the doses used in tablets that combine a sympathomimetic with an antihistamine (see pages 96–98) are low enough to be very safe. Certain drugs used to lower blood pressure can cause rhinitis, although this again is rare. Ask your doctor or pharmacist about this possibility.

Nose drops containing **corticosteroids** can also cause problems such as crusting, dryness, and nosebleeds (see chapter 7). Much more rarely, contraceptive pills can cause a mild rhinitis (see below).

HORMONAL EFFECTS

The female hormones estrogen and progesterone can affect the nose, causing runniness or congestion. This can create problems for a minority of women during pregnancy. All the usual treatments for rhinitis have been tried, but nothing seems to help in this situation. As soon as the baby is born, however, the rhinitis disappears.

This hormonal interference with the nose can also affect women taking contraceptive pills or going through menopause, although these effects are most unusual.

People with underactive thyroid glands may also suffer a blocked nose until they are treated.

FORMS OF RHINITIS WITH NO OBVIOUS CAUSE

The diseases dealt with so far in this chapter (and in earlier chapters) are those where the factor causing the problem has been identified and largely understood. From this point on, we are entering much murkier waters, where the cause of disease is not fully understood by the medical profession. Nevertheless, doctors can identify certain types of disease on the basis of characteristic features, and they can often provide quite effective treatments.

In trying to understand sickness and find cures for it, classifying diseases and naming them is all-important. When a field of medicine is still evolving, the classifications tend to change rather often, as doctors realize that what they previously thought of as one disease is actually two quite different ones. Several changes of this kind have happened in nonallergic rhinitis in recent years, and if you were diagnosed as having vasomotor rhinitis several years ago, that diagnosis may no longer be considered appropriate for your condition. Medical science may have caught up with you, and can perhaps offer more appropriate treatment than before, so it might be worth seeing a specialist again. If your vasomotor rhinitis is still being treated with a sympathomimetic-antihistamine mixture (see chapter 7) or with sympathomimetics alone, then this is almost certainly the case and you should see your specialist again. You can look up the name of the drug you are using in appendix 4, and this will show what type of drug it is.

Before diving into these murky waters where causes are largely unknown, let us first look back at the well-mapped terrain we are leaving behind. That terrain has a large enclosure on it with a sign saying ALLERGIC RHINITIS. You will have been excluded from that enclosure if you had no positive skin-prick tests and no positive blood tests for IgE (see chapter 6). These tests are generally good, but unfortunately they do exclude a few people who rightly should be in the allergic enclosure. This problem is discussed at the end of this chapter.

There are several other enclosures available that have already been described. These include infection or its consequences, exposure to irritants at work or at home, rhinitis medicamentosa, and hormonal effects.

When all these possibilities have been excluded, then you will be consigned to the murky waters, where causes cannot be identified but treatment is still possible.

At this point, the ear, nose, and throat specialist will generally take a tiny sample from the lining of the nose and send it to a laboratory for examination. If the laboratory finds that there are a large number of immune cells known as **eosinophils** present, then the diagnosis will be **nonallergic rhinitis with eosinophilia,** sometimes abbreviated as **NARES.** If there are few eosinophils, the diagnosis will probably be **vasomotor rhinitis,** although some doctors prefer a different term for reasons that will be explained later. A third possibility, but one that occurs only rarely, is that the nose will be rich in mast cells. The diagnosis in this case is **nasal mastocytosis.** We will look at each of these three conditions in turn.

NARES

Nonallergic rhinitis with eosinophilia or NARES (also called eosinophilic nonallergic perennial rhinitis) is a disease that has been identified properly only in the last few years. In the past, people with this problem were usually diagnosed as having vasomotor rhinitis.

NARES is the diagnosis given when large numbers of eosinophils are found in the nose but the patient has not given any positive test reactions for allergy. As well as a congested and runny nose with bouts of sneezing, patients with NARES often lose their sense of smell.

The fact that eosinophils have converged on the nose in the thousands shows that some kind of immune reaction is going on there. Exactly why is at present unknown. Mast cells are also releasing some mediators in the nose of a patient with NARES.

Hand-in-hand with this immune reaction, there is an imbalance in the autonomic nervous system producing hyperreactivity in the nose (see the box "Nerves in the Nose" later in this chapter). Recent research shows that there are many subtle interactions between the autonomic nervous system and the immune system, and it is difficult to say which is the fundamental problem in NARES—the inflammation or the malfunctioning nervous controls. Either of these could be the underlying problem that has sparked the other disorder.

You may remember that eosinophils also flock to the nose during the late phase of an allergic reaction (see chapter 3). But with an allergic reaction there are also many basophils (another type of immune cell) as well, so the lab finding will be a little different for someone with allergic rhinitis. It is possible, however, that a few patients diagnosed as having NARES are actually suffering from allergic rhinitis, which has somehow been overlooked by conventional allergy tests (see "Rhinitis Due to Undetected Airborne Allergens" later in this chapter).

With the realization that NARES is distinct from vasomotor rhinitis (see

"Vasomotor Rhinitis" later in this chapter) and involves inflammation, an effective treatment has been found. Nose drops containing corticosteroids reduce the inflammation and produce very good results in most patients, but must not be overused (see "Corticosteroids" in chapter 7). Cod-liver oil may also be valuable (see page 228).

ASPIRIN SENSITIVITY, ASTHMA, RHINITIS, AND NASAL POLYPS

For many years, allergists have been noticing a set of patients with a rather odd combination of problems: they usually have asthma and perennial rhinitis, they are very prone to nasal polyps (see the box "Nasal Polyps" later in this chapter), and they are extremely sensitive to aspirin, so that a couple of ordinary aspirin tablets will produce an unpleasant reaction. The most severe reactions to aspirin are similar to anaphylactic shock (see page 135). However, the patient does not produce any IgE molecules to aspirin, so this is no ordinary allergic reaction. Some of these patients also have urticaria (hives). This condition became known as the **triad** because of the three typical symptoms: asthma, polyps, and aspirin sensitivity.

Recently it has been realized that there is a link between NARES and this triad syndrome. People diagnosed as having NARES *sometimes* go on to become triad patients. And triad patients show an influx of eosinophils into the nose very like that in NARES, although there may be other immune cells as well.

This link may point the way to explaining both NARES and triad. Aspirin affects the production of substances called **prostaglandins.** (This action by aspirin is largely beneficial in the normal person, helping to reduce inflammation in the joints, for example.) Prostaglandins can be produced by almost any cell in the body, although they are also among the mediators released from mast cells (see chapter 3). There are at least 20 different types of prostaglandins and they are involved in the regulation of inflammation, but in a very complex way: the actions of different prostaglandins often oppose one another. They interact with each other, and with other parts of the immune system, through a complicated network of checks and balances.

Researchers in this area now believe that both NARES and triad may be disorders in the production or regulation of the prostaglandins. Prostaglandins are known to affect the autonomic nervous system and vice versa, which might explain why inflammation and autonomic imbalance (see page 226) go together in NARES. The arrival of eosinophils in the nose could just be a response to the initial inflammation, but a response that would aggravate the inflammation.

NERVES IN THE NOSE

The brain helps to control what is going on in the nose by means of the **autonomic nervous system.** The autonomic nervous system is the equivalent of "autopilot" in an airplane—a system that can run things by itself, without any conscious thought on our part. The autonomic system regulates the heart, ensures that we breathe in and out, and organizes the breakdown of food without our even being aware of these activities.

The autonomic system has two separate networks of nerves. One is called the **parasympathetic system** and its basic message to the body is, "Don't panic, everything is fine." The other is called the **sympathetic system** and its basic message is, "Action needed." Having these two opposing systems allows the body to adapt to different situations. When danger threatens, or when we simply have to run upstairs, the heart must beat faster, the lungs work harder, and the airways let in more air. The sympathetic system gears up the body for these more energetic moments of the day. The parasympathetic is involved in calming things down again afterward and making sure that important maintenance tasks are carried out—tasks such as digestion and the clearing of dust from the airways.

The parasympathetic promotes secretion of many important substances in the body, including mucus in the nose and bronchi. The mucus helps to pick up dust and microbes, so that they can be swept out of the nasal passages and down the throat. When something irritates the nose, a message goes to the brain and stimulates the parasympathetic system, which in turn steps up the production of mucus.

When it comes to the control of the blood vessels in the nose, both the sympathetic and the parasympathetic are involved. There are many small blood vessels in the lining of the nose, and if they enlarge, the lining itself grows thicker as a result, which makes the air passages narrower. The parasympathetic has this effect. The sympathetic system makes the blood vessels smaller, which widens the nasal passages so more air can get through.

In the healthy nose, the sympathetic system opens up the airways when more air is needed, while the parasympathetic restores the status quo afterward.

The **hyperreactive** nose is one where the parasympathetic system has become much too busy and the sympathetic a little lazy. Instead of restoring the blood vessels in the nose to their normal width, the parasympathetic can make them expand and expand until the nasal passages are uncomfortably narrow. The sympathetic, meanwhile, does not do enough to compensate. Instead of producing a useful amount of mucus to clear out the nose, the parasympathetic produces an excessive amount, so that the nose runs constantly. And rather than reacting to irritants such as smoke when they reach potentially damaging levels, the parasympathetic reacts to them in mere traces.

This process (also called **autonomic imbalance**) plays some part in almost all the diseases described in this book. Any nose that is inflamed is also hyperreactive—the nervous controls are disturbed by the inflammation process in the membranes. That is why people with hay fever can find strong scents, tobacco smoke, or paint fumes unusually troublesome to the nose during the pollen season.

Autonomic imbalance can be an important feature in asthma, too, with an overzealous parasympathetic system narrowing the bronchi and stimulating too much mucus production.

In triad patients, the prostaglandin disorder has become serious enough to make the interplay of prostaglandin reactions fundamentally different from that in normal people. This in itself causes symptoms such as asthma, rhinitis, and nasal polyps, but it also makes the prostaglandin balance fragile and susceptible to interference from outside—so that the action of two aspirin tablets is highly disruptive and damaging.

The treatment of triad involves several different measures aimed at the different symptoms. Corticosteroid nose drops (see "Corticosteroids" in chapter 7) are often effective in treating the rhinitis seen in triad patients, but must be used carefully. Corticosteroid inhalers are valuable for controlling the asthma. Polyps are often treated surgically or with corticosteroids. The new antileukotrine drugs (see pages 104–106) can be valuable as well.

Anyone who has ever reacted badly to aspirin should be careful about taking painkillers in the future. Many contain, if not aspirin itself, an aspirin-like drug that can have much the same effect. Several drugs used to treat rheumatoid arthritis also belong in this family. A guide to avoiding these medicines is given on page 71.

Several doctors have tried out diets that are low in salicylates for their triad patients, salicylates being the natural counterparts of aspirin. They are

NASAL POLYPS

Nasal polyps are small, soft, bulbous outgrowths from the lining of the nose. Except in a few, very rare cases, they have nothing to do with cancerous tumors. These polyps are entirely harmless, and cause concern only when they block the nasal passages. This can make nose-breathing difficult or reduce the sense of smell.

Many healthy people have nasal polyps, but they are far more frequent in those suffering from rhinitis. At the end of a long hot summer, people with severe hay fever may develop nasal polyps, although they are far more common in year-round rhinitis. The group with the greatest tendency to polyps is triad patients, closely followed by those with NARES.

Polyps that develop during the hay fever season will probably go away again of their own accord. For those with year-round rhinitis, polyps are usually treated by removing them surgically, but they tend to reappear. Unfortunately, surgery on the nose can sometimes make asthma much worse or cause it to recur in someone who had apparently outgrown it. Thus, it is wise to explore other treatment options before resorting to surgery.

Sometimes small nasal polyps can be persuaded to shrink by the use of corticosteroid drops alone. It is important to allow the drops to penetrate as far as possible into the nasal passages, and the "head down" position shown on page 228 is the best way to achieve this.

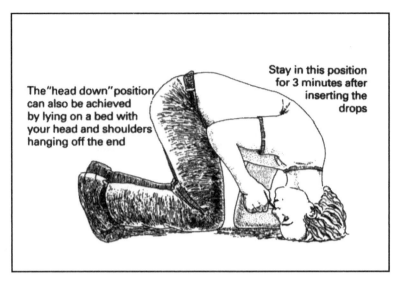

The"head down"position can also be achieved by lying on a bed with your head and shoulders hanging off the end

Stay in this position for 3 minutes after inserting the drops

Treating nasal polyps with nose drops

found in a variety of fruits, vegetables, herbs, and spices. The diet is quite difficult to stick to and rarely produces any major benefits, so this treatment is probably not worth trying.

With the growing understanding of NARES and triad, it is likely that new forms of treatment may become available in the future, such as drugs that address the basic problem of the prostaglandin disorder. One intriguing discovery is that some triad patients show an improvement in their asthma and polyps if they take a tiny amount of aspirin every day. However, you should *definitely* not try this for yourself without the agreement of your doctor, because the reaction to aspirin is potentially dangerous.

One treatment that you can try for yourself is to take cod-liver oil. Some substances found in this oil influence the production of prostaglandins by the body, tending to reduce their pro-inflammatory action. They may therefore be particularly useful to NARES and triad patients. Only two teaspoons a day should be taken—too much can be toxic. Eating oily fish such as herring or mackerel at least twice a week will have a similar effect.

VASOMOTOR RHINITIS

This is a term that can mean a variety of different things and tends to create considerable confusion as well as controversy. To begin with, we will explain what vasomotor rhinitis *should* mean.

As already explained, nerves in the nose play a crucial part in narrowing or widening the air passages and in producing mucus. A **hyperreactive nose** is one where the parasympathetic system is overactive, making the nose blocked and runny most of the time or making it respond too readily to irritants, or both. This hyperreactivity occurs in any inflamed nose, adding to the misery of allergy sufferers.

For some patients, hyperreactivity in the nose, due to autonomic imbalance (see the box "Nerves in the Nose" earlier in this chapter), is thought to be their primary problem. This hyperreactivity may even be the sole problem, or it may be accompanied by some inflammation as well. If hyperreactivity is the fundamental problem, then a diagnosis of vasomotor rhinitis is entirely appropriate: "vasomotor" implies that the blockage of the nose is largely due to the action of the autonomic nerves on veins in the lining of the nose. Where the fault arises is unknown. It could originate in the part of the brain that controls the autonomic system.

With true vasomotor rhinitis, a runny and congested nose is usually the main symptom, with little sneezing or itchiness in the nose. Sometimes the blockage shifts from one nostril to another. Unlike allergic problems in the nose, vasomotor rhinitis usually comes on in adulthood, often in the elderly.

Unfortunately, the term "vasomotor rhinitis" has been much abused in the past. If no infection or allergy could be identified in someone with rhinitis, and no other explanation could be found, it was assumed that the symptoms must be due to autonomic imbalance. This led to many people being wrongly diagnosed as having vasomotor rhinitis. Some had what we would now call NARES. Others were allergic to something, but this had not been picked up by allergy tests for various reasons (see "Rhinitis Due to Undetected Airborne Allergens" later in this chapter). Some had food intolerance (discussed later in this chapter).

Techniques of diagnosis have improved greatly in the past 20 years, and this mislabeling is far less common now. Even so, it can still occur: There is no way to show that a disorder is truly vasomotor rhinitis; a foolproof test cannot be devised because there is some degree of hyperreactivity in most forms of rhinitis. The doctor simply assumes that the patient has vasomotor rhinitis because all the other possibilities have been ruled out. For this reason, some specialists prefer to use the term **nonallergic rhinitis without eosinophilia**. It may be a mouthful, but at least it is an honest way of saying, "We don't know what you've got, actually."

Anyone diagnosed as having vasomotor rhinitis some years ago should ask to see a specialist again, especially if the treatment is not helping a great deal or if new problems have developed, such as asthma. If you have never had a sample taken from the nose, then the possibility of NARES has not been ruled out.

For true vasomotor rhinitis, the most logical treatment is an **anticholinergic drug,** one that largely blocks the action of the parasympathetic nervous system. The main drugs used are *atropine* and *ipratropium,* both given as nasal drops. Unfortunately, this type of treatment is not available in the United States or Canada. The standard drug treatment is with corticosteroid drops or spray, or antihistamines. Corticosteroids are generally more useful, especially if the nose is blocked. Antihistamines can help to dry up nasal mucus. In severe cases that do not respond to drug treatment, parasympathetic and sympathetic nerves leading to the nose can be cut, which gives complete and prompt relief. Sadly, the nerves grow back again within a year or two, so the operation has to be repeated.

A simple form of self-help is to take some strenuous exercise. Any vigorous activity requires the sympathetic nervous system to come into play, and this has a beneficial side effect in unblocking the nose. Obviously, you should take your exercise in clean air, away from potential irritants such as smoke.

These are the irritants that can provoke a reaction when there is hyperreactivity in the nose:

- Cigarette smoke and other pollutants

- Cold air, hot air, or changes in temperature

- A change from damp to dry air, or vice versa

- Some foods, particularly hot spicy ones

- Alcoholic drinks

- Bright lights

- Strong smells such as those of perfume, flowers, wet paint, and smoke

- Emotional upsets

Although these are important in vasomotor rhinitis, remember that such overreaction to airborne irritants can also occur in any form of nasal disease.

There are certain specific diseases that seem to be forms of vasomotor rhinitis. One of these is **skier's nose,** a response to the cold dry air of the mountains. Although there are some inflammatory mediators released, the main reaction is probably hyperreactivity by the parasympathetic system. A somewhat more embarrassing problem is **postcoital rhinitis,** which may be accompanied by postcoital asthma.

At one time, doctors thought that this was a rare condition, but a paper in the scientific journal *Allergy* in 2001 suggests otherwise. Doctors in Seville, Spain, found 23 individuals with this problem among those attending an allergy clinic. All had allergies to either grass pollen, olive pollen, or dust mites.

None developed allergy-type symptoms in the nose following exercise, so that did not explain the sneezing and runny nose that came on immediately after intercourse; nor were they allergic to latex (so condoms were not the cause) or to semen (a source of allergic reactions in some women). Yet the problem did seem to be an allergic reaction—as evidenced by the fact that symptoms recurred five to eight hours later, something known as the "late-phase reaction," which frequently follows an allergic attack.

The Spanish scientists who carried out this research suggest that postcoital rhinitis is caused by the intense emotional arousal of intercourse producing a temporary autonomic imbalance (see the box "Nerves in the Nose" in chapter 13) and so generating rhinitis symptoms. Orgasm, as they point out, is accompanied by a surge of parasympathetic nervous system activity.

According to these doctors, overactivity of the parasympathetic nervous system can actually trigger mast cells into action, which would account for the allergy-style late-phase reaction that followed.

This down-to-earth physiological account of postcoital rhinitis is in contrast to the traditional explanation that links it with anxieties and inhibitions about sex. This theory held that emotional disturbances were responsible for the symptoms, and that counseling on sexual relationships was the best treatment. While that might be true for some people (and emotional difficulties are undoubtedly the cause of postcoital asthma in certain cases), the new findings imply that most people with postcoital rhinitis have a medical, rather than a psychological, problem and should be treated with drugs, not therapy.

It would make sense to take some treatment before intercourse begins. If your existing allergy treatments don't help, then try adding anticholinergic drops (see page 230).

NASAL MASTOCYTOSIS

This problem is thought to be very rare. It occurs in people with no sign of allergy whatsoever, yet they have very high numbers of mast cells in the nose. The problem may come on suddenly, and then seem like a cold that never goes away. For other people it begins gradually.

The rhinitis suffered by people with nasal mastocytosis is often made worse by drinking alcohol or by exposure to smells such as turpentine and perfume. All these seem to act by triggering the many mast cells in the nose, but again this is not an allergic reaction.

Antihistamines do not seem to work well for this disease, but *sodium cromoglycate* (see "Mast-cell Stabilizers" in chapter 7) may help.

RHINITIS CAUSED BY FOOD INTOLERANCE

Some people who have been told that they are suffering from "perennial non-allergic rhinitis" or "vasomotor rhinitis" are actually being affected by the food they eat. Because this relationship between food and the nose is not widely recognized by most conventional doctors, few patients with this problem get satisfac-

MARY

Mary's allergic disposition showed up as a small child, when she suffered from eczema. The cause was never discovered, but she grew out of the eczema within a few years. In her teens Mary developed hay fever and sinusitis, with the sinusitis persisting and becoming very painful, particularly in winter. In her early 30s, the sinusitis became much worse and reached a crisis on her return from a vacation abroad. An X-ray showed a buildup of fluid in the sinuses, which was causing the intense pain, and an operation was performed to drain away the fluid.

Despite this improvement Mary was now suffering symptoms similar to hay fever all year round. There were occasions when the symptoms changed, or got worse, and Mary began to notice a certain pattern to these. Drinking wine, for example, was always followed by a badly blocked nose the next morning. A course of vitamin B tablets seemed to make her nose far more blocked and uncomfortable than usual. As an experiment, she tried stopping the vitamins and then restarting them a few days later—the severe symptoms in her nose followed suit. Her doctor could not make sense of these observations and referred her to a specialist. The specialist realized that vitamin B tablets are often made from dried yeast, and wine is also rich in yeast. He suggested that Mary try a yeast-free diet for a while, cutting out bread, yeast extract, mushrooms, beer, wine, cider, and certain other foods (see table 1 on page 237 for a complete list). The effect pleased Mary greatly: her nose was no longer blocked or runny, and she found that she also felt far more energetic than before.

By accident she ate some gravy in a restaurant not realizing that it would contain yeast extract. Within a few hours, she had developed severe symptoms in the nose, which lasted until the following day. Clearly, her year-round rhinitis was due to yeast sensitivity, and on the yeast-free diet Mary remained well. Later, she was able to return to a more normal diet by using neutralization therapy (see chapter 9) for yeast. During the pollen season, her hay fever returned, but was not as severe as before.

tory treatment. And because the symptoms do not come on as soon as they eat the food, the patients themselves are generally unaware of the connection. However, they can diagnose themselves and get rid of the symptoms pretty easily.

The term that covers this reaction, and a number of other reactions to food (including food-induced asthma, migraine, irritable bowel syndrome, and joint pains), is **food intolerance.** It should not be referred to as "food allergy," although it often is, particularly by alternative practitioners. Skin-prick tests (see chapter 6) for the foods are almost always negative, which sets it apart from true allergic reactions. Calling the reaction "food allergy" only perpetuates the problem of nonacceptance by mainstream medicine, since food allergy (see page 161) is a clearly defined disease whose symptoms come on immediately and are largely different from food intolerance.

Food intolerance, as an explanation for your perennial rhinitis, is worth considering if:

- You have no positive skin-prick tests to airbone allergens

- You have positive skin-prick tests to pollen, but not to other allergens, yet your rhinitis continues to some extent all year long

First, make sure that:

- You are definitely not suffering from a prolonged infection (see page 221)

- There is no possibility of rhinitis medicamentosa (see page 222) or any hormonal effect (see page 222)

- You have ruled out the possibility of irritants or allergens in the workplace causing your rhinitis (see page 215)

- You are not suffering from the "triad" of asthma, nasal polyps, and aspirin sensitivity (see page 225)

You can test for food intolerance quite simply with an elimination diet. The diet suggested here is not a particularly restrictive one, and there is no need to consult your doctor before starting it unless you are already undernourished or seriously unwell. If you have ever suffered from *anorexia nervosa,* you should have medical supervision when on the diet. Children can safely be put on this diet for a few weeks, as long as they are healthy and well fed at the outset, but if you identify problem foods and decide to keep the child off them permanently, check with your doctor that the diet being eaten is adequate. It is all too easy for children to suffer nutritional deficiencies.

There are several other forms of elimination diet used, some of which permit very few foods at the outset with the aim of identifying every possible food sensitivity, even the most unusual ones. (One of the best known is the lamb-and-pears diet.) While a diet of this type has its uses, we feel that a less restrictive diet will help almost everyone with food-induced rhinitis. Should the diet outlined here not help you, or if it leaves you with some symptoms, and you wish to try a more thorough diagnostic diet, one is given in *Food Allergies and Food Intolerance,* by Jonathan Brostoff, M.D., and Linda Gamlin (Healing Arts Press, 2000).

Exclusion Phase

This is the first phase of the diet. For a week or so you cut out many of the foods you commonly eat—it is the everyday foods that are the usual offenders in food intolerance. The important point here is that you must stick to the diet absolutely. It is not like a weight-loss diet where the odd lapse is allowed. Not a molecule of the excluded foods must cross your lips.

The foods you must eliminate are:

Yeast and all yeast-containing foods (see the table 1 on page 237)
Mushrooms and any other fungi
Wheat (which means anything made from flour, unless rice flour)
Rye and oats
Corn
Milk
Cheese, butter, yogurt, and all milk products
Eggs
Fish
Citrus fruits (oranges, tangerines, lemons, grapefruit, etc.)
Peanuts
Tea
Coffee
Chocolate
Anything containing preservatives or colorings
Anything containing sulfur dioxide (see appendix 7)
Sugar and honey, and any food containing them
Alcoholic drinks

You should add to this list any food that you are really "addicted to," something you eat every day and cannot imagine going without. This may be the hardest part, but it could make all the difference: for some strange reason, those with food intolerance are often "hooked" on their problem food.

These are the allowed foods:

Any kind of meat
Most fruit if peeled (but not citrus fruits, dried fruits, or anything overripe
      because of yeast contamination)
Freshly squeezed fruit juice
All vegetables
Beans and lentils
Soy milk
Potatoes
Rice
Rice cakes (good as a temporary substitute for bread)
Rice noodles (try Chinese stores)
Buckwheat and buckwheat spaghetti (try health food stores)
Yams
Sweet potatoes
Eddoes (taro) and Jerusalem artichokes
Milk-free margarine (available in health food stores; ordinary brands
      contain some milk)
Cooking oil, olive oil, nut oils
Almond butter, cashew butter
Nuts, other than peanuts
Sunflower seeds and pumpkin seeds
Herb teas, other than red bush (rooibos) and maté

There is plenty here for a good healthy diet, and you are unlikely to be hungry if you approach the matter intelligently. Don't be in a rush to start—you need to plan for the diet in advance and stock up on suitable foods; otherwise you can suddenly find yourself hungry and with nothing on hand that you are allowed to eat. Bananas, nuts, and seeds make good snacks to replace cookies and cakes. Make sure that no great social event, such as Thanksgiving or a wedding, is going to occur within the next ten weeks.

The best way to avoid mistakes is to cook your own food and keep meals plain and simple, using pure ingredients that are exactly what they seem. When eating out, have something simple like steak, fries, and a salad. Anything "instant" can be a source of forbidden food. Bouillon cubes and packaged soups contain yeast, for example, sauces contain flour or corn starch, while eggs and milk turn up in a variety of ways and are often not named as such on the label. Certain packaged foods, such as rice cakes, are acceptable because they contain just one ingredient. Avoid gluten-free breads and similar products at this stage.

For lunches at work, take food in a plastic container (e.g., a mixture of potatoes and stir-fried vegetables with beans or meat). Breakfast can seem problematic, especially if you dislike soy milk. One good substitute for conventional breakfast foods is precooked rice, heated gently in a mixture of almond butter and cooking oil, with apple, banana, or other fruit added.

Pay special attention to avoiding yeast because this is often the guilty party in rhinitis caused by food. Look at table 1 on the next page and scrupulously avoid everything on it during the exclusion phase.

Be careful not to eat huge amounts of any one food, and try to keep meals varied. If you have a large appetite normally, overdoing one of the starchy foods is a risk. Try out some of the exotic substitutes, such as sweet potatoes, yams, and millet. They are best if boiled first and then fried. Boiled millet can be mixed with a nut butter while still warm, then shaped into cakes and fried— another good breakfast food.

Possible Outcome of the Exclusion Phase

Feeling much worse

This can happen, particularly in the first few days. Keep going: it is usually a sign that food intolerance is indeed your problem.

If you still feel terrible after ten days, try reintroducing all the foods, but not tea, coffee, alcohol, or sugar. Stay on this diet for several weeks and you will probably improve.

Feeling about the same

Keep going for two weeks. If at the end of that time your symptoms are unchanged, then it is unlikely that food has anything to do with them. (However, you could try a more stringent elimination diet to check other foods— see page 236.)

Feeling partially better

Keep going for two weeks. If at the end of that time there is still only a partial improvement, try cutting out potatoes and any other food that you normally eat every day. Stay on the exclusion phase for another week. If there is no

TABLE 1: FOODS CONTAINING YEAST

Main sources of yeast

Bread, including some pita bread and pizza, but excluding soda bread, matzo, and chapatis

Buns and cakes made with yeast—e.g., doughnuts

Yeast extract (Marmite, Vegemite, etc.)

Bouillon cubes and most other stock cubes

Anything labeled "hydrolyzed vegetable protein"

Beer, wine, and cider

Vinegar and pickles

Sauerkraut

Vitamins with B complex, unless labeled "yeast-free"

Secondary sources of yeast

Dried fruit

Overripe fruit

Any unpeeled fruit

Commercial fruit juices

Anything labeled "malt"

Yogurt, buttermilk, and sour cream

Synthetic cream

Soy sauce

Tofu

Any leftover food, unless eaten within 24 hours, or 48 hours if in a refrigerator

Whiskey, vodka, gin, brandy, and other spirits

Other sources of fungi that may affect some people

Mushrooms, puffballs, truffles, and other edible fungi

Quorn, mycoprotein (meat substitutes derived from fungi)

Cheese, especially Brie and Camembert

Yeasts and molds in the air

Stay away from damp houses, greenhouses (unless very dry and clean), compost heaps, and rotting leaves. After you have been on the diet for a while, you can test whether such exposure makes you ill.

further improvement, you could try testing some foods (see below, under "Re-introduction Phase"). If your improvement is only slight, return to your ordinary diet and assume that food is not involved.

Feeling a lot better

This is a pretty clear sign that food is at fault, unless your symptoms tend to come and go a great deal anyway. When you have been feeling fine for four days, go on to the reintroduction phase. Do not delay for too long, or you may not get clear results.

Reintroduction Phase

Continue with the same diet as during the exclusion phase, but reintroduce the following foods, recording those tested and any reappearance of symptoms in a notebook.

First test

Take two yeast tablets or a spoonful of yeast extract. If you get no reaction, repeat every day for three days, stopping if a reaction occurs. Then leave a day without testing any food.

If nothing happens, you can relax the restrictions on yeast to some extent—you can eat unpeeled fruits, drink commercial fruit juices, and not worry about overripe fruit or leftovers (see table 1, page 237). But do not reintroduce any major yeast-containing foods or alcoholic drinks.

Do not begin the second test if you still have any symptoms from the first. Allow at least one symptom-free day in between tests. This applies to all subsequent tests as well.

Second test

Drink a glass of milk or eat some plain cottage cheese or cow's milk yogurt. If you get no reaction, repeat every day for three days, stopping if a reaction occurs.

Leave a day without testing any food. Even if nothing happens, cut out milk again for now.

If you experience a very strong reaction to either yeast or milk, then you may prefer to cut short the testing program. Among foods, these two are the most common causes of rhinitis, and often the sole offenders. If yeast provoked a reaction, consult table 1 again to see which foods contain yeast and omit all those for the moment. (You can experiment later with the ones that are only secondary sources of yeast, or affect only some people.) If milk brings on symptoms, consult table 2 (see page 241) for synonyms of milk used on package labels and avoid these too. Apart from these restrictions, you can go back to a normal diet. In the unlikely event that your symptoms recur, you will need to cut out everything again, wait for the symptoms to die down, and then resume testing.

Third test

Eat four pieces of rye crispbread (it should be pure rye). If you get no reaction, repeat every day for three days, stopping if a reaction occurs.

Leave a day without testing any food. Even if nothing happens, cut out rye again for now.

Fourth test

Eat something that is pure wheat, such as pasta (check the label for other ingredients), puffed wheat, or shredded wheat (moisten with fruit juice, if necessary). Bulgur wheat could also be used for this test. If you get no reaction, repeat every day for three days, stopping if a reaction occurs.

Leave a day without testing any food. Even if nothing happens, cut out wheat again for now.

Fifth test

Eat some fish. If you get no reaction, repeat every day for three days, using a different type of fish each time, but stopping if a reaction occurs.

Leave a day without testing any food. Even if nothing happens, cut out fish again for now.

Sixth test

Eat two or more eggs, cooked in any way you like. If you get no reaction, repeat every day for three days, stopping if a reaction occurs. Leave a day without testing any fodod.

At this point you have tested most of the likely culprits and you can reintroduce any food that caused no problem when tested, to give yourself a more normal diet. (If you proved sensitive to yeast but not to wheat, you can eat soda bread, matzo, and chapatis. Consult table 1 again to see which foods are a source of yeast and should therefore be avoided. At a later date you can experiment with the secondary sources of yeast, to see if you are able to tolerate these.)

Eat this new and more relaxed diet for a week. You should remain well, in which case you can continue testing foods. (If you relapse, which is most unlikely, then you need to cut out all the foods, wait for the symptoms to clear again, and then start retesting. This time, test each food for a week before going on to the next.)

During this week you should, at some point, test out sulfur dioxide. This is a mild irritant given off by several foods and can provoke rhinitis in sensitive people. Assuming you are not sensitive to yeast, try chewing some uncooked dried apricots or golden raisins (not if they are labeled "unsulfured" or "no preservatives," nor if they are very dark in color, which is a sign that sulfur dioxide has not been used). If you are sensitive to yeast, then buy Campden tablets (sold to home wine-makers), dissolve in warm water, and sniff the fumes coming off. Should either of these tests produce your symptoms, you are almost certainly sensitive to sulfur dioxide; refer to appendix 7 for the foods that can produce this gas.

Assuming you have stayed well while eating your expanded diet for a week, continue testing the remaining foods, with three days for each. Once they have been tested, cut out the foods again, even if they caused no reaction.

Seventh test

If you did not react to rye or wheat, you can reintroduce oats without testing them. If you *did* react to rye or wheat, test oats either using oatmeal or oatcakes (make sure they contain no forbidden ingredients). If you never normally eat oats, don't bother to test them, unless you are keen to have them as a substitute for wheat.

Eighth test

Test oranges, satsumas, tangerines, and clementines. If you have discovered that you are yeast-sensitive, use fresh fruit only. Should you prove tolerant of oranges and their kin, introduce lemons and grapefruit the next day. If there is no reaction, then leave one test-free day and continue.

Ninth test

Test peanuts using plain salted peanuts (not dry-roasted) or plain peanut butter as sold in health food stores. Eat a good handful of nuts or a thick spread of peanut butter.

Tenth test

If you were not affected by milk, yogurt, or cottage cheese, then test ordinary cheeses (but not Brie or Camembert if you have proved to be yeast-sensitive; you can experiment with these later).

Eleventh test

Test corn by eating a large portion of frozen sweet corn.

Table 2: Avoiding Milk in Food

The following words, seen on food labels, denote items derived from milk:

Casein

Caseinate

Lactalbumin

Whey

You should avoid all these initially if you are sensitive to milk. You may later be able to tolerate them, as they are usually present only in very small amounts.

Dairy-free

Many people who are sensitive to cow's milk also react to goat's milk and, less frequently, to sheep's milk. Should you see the term "dairy-free" on standard packaged foods, this means that the contents are free from goat's and sheep's milk as well as cow's milk. But be more cautious about homemade or locally produced foods labeled "dairy-free"—some small producers think that "dairy" refers only to cow's milk.

No milk fat

The words "no milk fat" sometimes mislead people if they just glance quickly at labels. The fact that a product contains no milk fat does not, of course, mean that it is entirely milk-free—remember to look for all the synonyms for milk listed above.

Twelfth test

Whether or not you were sensitive to yeast, test mushrooms, trying different kinds (button, field, etc.).

Any of this second batch of foods that proved harmless can now be reintroduced. This means that (with the exception of foods that produced symptoms) you are on a normal diet apart from alcohol, sugar, tea, coffee, chocolate, and certain additives (preservatives and colors). Add each of these back into the diet at the rate of one a week.

With alcohol, try a small tot of pure spirit such as vodka or white rum on the first day, whiskey on the second, sherry on the third, wine on the fourth, beer on the fifth, and so on. Obviously, if you are yeast-sensitive, beer, wine, and cider are unlikely to be tolerated, but you may wish to test spirits. If you proved sensitive to sulfur dioxide, you may also have problems with these drinks (see appendix 7).

At the end of the reintroduction phase, you should know what foods bring on your nasal problems (and you may have found that some other ailments were also related to food). Avoid those foods for at least six months, using table 2, page 241 to spot hidden ingredients in packaged foods. After about six months, you can retest each of the incriminated foods to see if you still react to them. If you do react, then try again six months later. If not, you can begin eating them once every four days or so. Continue in this way for a year, then increase the frequency a little if you like. Some people can go back to eating the food normally, but most find that they can never eat the food every day again, or in large amounts. If symptoms recur, cut out the culprit foods entirely for a couple of months.

If you find it very difficult to avoid your problem foods, you could try neutralization therapy (see chapter 9). This can work well with food intolerance. Nose drops containing *sodium cromoglycate* (see "Mast-cell Stabilizers" in chapter 7) may also help.

The reintroduction phase for foods should take about eight weeks. If it takes any longer than this (because you get flu in the middle, for example), then there is a risk of lost sensitivity—the food-intolerant person becomes less reactive after avoiding the culprit food for a time. If you are still testing foods after eight weeks, you should eat each test food every day for a week, rather than for three days.

RHINITIS DUE TO UNDETECTED AIRBORNE ALLERGENS

This is possible with both perennial rhinitis and seasonal rhinitis (see below).

There are two ways in which allergies can go undetected. First, if patients are allergic to something that no one tests for, their sensitivity will not be detected (see "Limitations of Skin Testing" in chapter 6). Rare pollen allergens (see pages 4–7) or insect allergens (see pages 81–82 and 211) are the most likely candidates here, and both could cause either perennial or seasonal symptoms. Second, some people with genuine allergic reactions to common allergens fail to react to the usual tests. It seems that they have the allergy antibody IgE in the nose and nowhere else, causing both skin tests and blood tests to be negative. For these patients, the allergy will be revealed only by nasal provocation testing—something that an allergist can carry out.

One good (but not foolproof) sign is violent sneezing on waking up. This rarely occurs with nonallergic rhinitis but is often seen with allergy to dust mites.

In a situation where your opinion differs from that of the doctor treating you, there is a case for being persistent and seeking a second or even a third opinion. Occasionally, patients with genuine allergies have gotten the treatment they needed only by such persistence. However, you should also keep an open mind about the possible cause of your illness, and be prepared to accept that it may, after all, be nonallergic.

SEASONAL NONALLERGIC RHINITIS

This is a disease that does not appear in the medical textbooks, since in theory it does not exist! All seasonal rhinitis is assumed to be allergic. However, researchers in Sweden have found people with all the symptoms of spring hay fever but no allergic response to pollen or other likely allergens. There are occasional reports from other parts of the world as well. The possible explanations for this problem (apart from undetected allergy—see above) are as follows:

- The nose is hyperreactive (see page 226), particularly to volatile chemicals (see page 115) given off from plants—e.g., from birch twigs, tree buds, or perfumed flowers.

- There is no allergy to pollen, but the grains are acting as an irritant; this has been demonstrated with pine pollen, which has big grains and is very abundant in the air, allowing large amounts to be inhaled.

- Pollen grains are carrying pollutants that irritate the nose.

- There is food intolerance (see page 232) to something eaten only in summer (such as fresh strawberries) or to something consumed in larger quantities (such as additives or coloring in orange soft drinks).

- There is a reaction to an irritant that is more common in the air in summer, such as ozone (see appendix 6). This explanation is just speculative at present.

Chapter 14
AVOIDING ALLERGIES IN YOUR CHILD

Most people want a better life for their children, and those with severe hay fever will surely hope that their children can be spared the same fate. Unfortunately, you cannot take any measures that will guarantee a hay fever–free future for your child, but you can reduce the chances that he or she will develop the same disease.

To try and prevent hay fever alone is not a logical approach, however. What is passed on from parent to child is a general tendency to allergy, called **atopy** (see page 38). Your children will not necessarily inherit this allergic predisposition, but if they do, it could appear in a variety of ways—as eczema, for example, or perennial rhinitis, asthma, or food allergy. If you have hay fever, there is a *slightly* greater chance that your children (if atopic) will have hay fever rather than one of these other allergic diseases, but it would make no sense to take precautions against hay fever alone. For this reason, the measures outlined here are those that will minimize the chance of allergic reactions in general, not just reactions to pollen.

What is the chance of your child inheriting the allergic tendency? It is impossible to say exactly, but where one parent has allergies, the child has roughly a 20 to 40 percent chance of developing them. The chance is higher if it is the mother who is allergic. Where both parents have allergies, the figure is 40 to 60 percent, but higher if it is the same *type* of allergic reaction in both—that is, both have asthma or both have hay fever. For these children the risk is 60 to 80 percent. Where neither parent has allergies but one of their children does, then a new baby has a 25 to 35 percent risk. Should there be a large number of other close relatives with allergies, you can assume that the risk is higher.

A difficult birth may make allergy more likely, while low birth weight with a slow increase in weight just after birth can be a sign of greater susceptibility to allergy.

You need to make a rough assessment of the risk to your baby, bearing all these factors in mind, and then decide just how careful you should be in protecting the child from allergens. Few people will feel able to take all the precautions described here, but do what you can.

There is a test that can be done at birth. Some blood is taken from the umbilical cord and the amount of IgE is measured. IgE is the antibody that plays a key role in allergy (see page 29), and a high level indicates that the child is definitely at risk. This test is not done routinely, but if you ask the hospital, it may be possible to arrange. Blood tests for IgE can also be carried out on the baby after birth. A high level of IgE would indicate that it was worth taking the more difficult measures described here.

Some advance planning is helpful in allergy avoidance, and it is valuable to start thinking about the matter well before you get pregnant. (However, there is still a great deal you can do if you are pregnant as you read this, or even if the baby has already been born.) The most crucial period for allergy prevention is from birth to about one year of age. Reducing exposure to allergens during this time can drastically reduce the risk of allergies. One recent study, which employed only some of the measures described here, saved two out of three susceptible children from developing allergies in their first year of life.

MEASURES TO TAKE BEFORE BECOMING PREGNANT

First, you can try to plan the timing of your child's birth. There is some evidence that being born during or just before the pollen season increases the risk of hay fever. The effect is strongest for tree pollens, notably birch, but it may also be a factor in allergy to grasses and ragweed. Low-risk months are those just after the pollen season. High-risk months are the season itself and two to three months beforehand. It seems that babies are most vulnerable to sensitization by pollen in the first three to six months of life. Use appendix 1 to check when the main pollen seasons occur.

As the effect of birth timing is not that great, you should not worry too much if you fail to get it right. Should your plans not work out at all and the baby is born at the worst time of year, then you could consider using an air cleaner or other measures (see "Avoiding Pollen at Home" in chapter 8), which would at least reduce the pollen levels indoors.

Another aspect of planning is to make sure you do not move or undertake major structural work just before the birth. A remarkable number of parents do fall into this trap by realizing that they will need more living space only after the baby is conceived. The hazards of renovation include the stirring up of house dust, which contains a rich variety of allergens, and the release of many mold spores into the air. There are ways of partially combating these hazards, by using air cleaners and cleaning up carefully (see pages 187–188), but it is much better not to create the problem in the first place. Plastering or laying concrete floors will establish a reservoir of water in the house that continues to ooze moisture into the air for up to a year afterward (see page 198). This affects both new and renovated houses. If you have already gotten into this situation and the baby is due during the autumn or winter, a dehumidifier may be the only option to keep down the humidity. Moisture promotes the growth of both molds and dust mites (see chapter 12).

Should your house be suffering from damp penetration or condensation, sort out such problems as soon as you can (see page 198). Bringing a baby home to a severely damp house is taking an unnecessary risk with its health.

Mothers who smoke should stop before becoming pregnant. Smoking has a variety of bad effects on an unborn child, but one of them is to increase the risk of allergies. Since there must be no tobacco smoke in the house once the baby is born, it is as well for the father to give up at the same time.

Finally, mothers with allergies should also bear in mind other risks to the baby. If you suffer from asthma, it is important that you get the best possible treatment for it during pregnancy (see "Coping with Hay Fever or Asthma When Pregnant" in chapter 7).

MEASURES TO TAKE DURING PREGNANCY

There is no need for the expectant mother to avoid any allergens while pregnant—various studies have looked at this and shown that it has few benefits. Some babies do become sensitized while in the womb to foods eaten by the mother, but this occurs so rarely that it is not considered worth putting pregnant mothers on a special diet. The important thing to do at this stage is to prepare the house for its new inhabitant, reducing the allergens to levels that will not sensitize the baby.

With airborne allergens, the levels needed to sensitize someone (that is, to start up an allergic reaction) are much higher than the levels needed to produce symptoms in someone who is already sensitized. Thus, the actions you need to take against dust mites, for example, are not as drastic as those needed by someone with a severe allergy to mites.

Reducing Dampness in the House

Minimizing dampness is an important part of the battle against both dust mites and molds. Once the baby is born, there will be a lot of laundry to dry, which can increase the amount of moisture in the house at the very moment when you most want to keep it down. Before the baby arrives, organize a good method of drying clothes, particularly if the baby is due in the autumn or winter, or if you have nowhere to dry clothes outside. A tumble-dryer is a good investment. Make sure it is vented to the outside. A cheaper alternative is to dry clothes on a porch or in a utility room, but it must have good ventilation so that the moisture goes outside rather than coming in. If this is not possible, dry clothes in a room that has some heating and a partially open window, keeping the door closed to prevent the moist air from traveling into other rooms.

If your house is well insulated and draft-free, get into the habit of increasing the ventilation so that the air inside is drier (see chapter 12, especially page 189). The sooner you begin to do this, the better.

Specific Action against Dust Mites

For a baby, dust mites are a major source of allergic problems. Reducing mite allergens to a minimum will be one of the most worthwhile measures you can take in lowering the risk of allergy.

Making sure that the newborn's mattress and bedding are free from mite allergens is a simple matter (see pages176–177 and 189), and if you can manage no other changes around the house, at least take this step.

It is also valuable to reduce mite allergens in carpets, since the child will start to play on them when a few months old. Simply increasing the ventilation in the house and taking other measures against damp will do quite a lot to combat mites. If you have begun this early on in pregnancy, the mite levels will have been declining for many months before the baby arrives. Thorough vacuuming must also be carried out to remove the existing reservoir of mite allergens. Buy a good-quality HEPA vacuum cleaner (see appendix 3) to ensure that the allergens are not dispersed into the air. Spraying the carpet and furniture a few times with tannic acid (see appendix 3) to denature the allergens may also be worthwhile, but this is not recommended as a long-term measure if you have small children in the house. It is worth doing only if you are also increasing the ventilation and reducing dampness so that mite numbers are reduced.

Assuming you can afford it, a more drastic mite-eradication program for your floors and furniture would certainly be very valuable. There are various approaches to this. You might decide, for example, to recarpet the house, replace your upholstered furniture with something less congenial to mites, and purchase a dehumidifier to guard against reinfestation. Chapter 12 provides more details.

Cats, Dogs, and Other Pets

Once upon a time, the standard advice to atopic (allergy-prone) parents was "Get rid of your dog or cat before the baby is born." Atopic children did (and still do) develop allergic reactions to pets in the house. These reactions can be severe and a real nuisance—they make it very difficult for the child to visit other people who have a dog or cat, and the allergy may be lifelong.

But research data gathered in the 1990s have turned our ideas about animals and allergy upside down. As explained at the end of chapter 4, close contact with animals early in life can *reduce* the risk of allergies developing—not just allergies to animals, but all other kinds of allergies as well. In other words, having a pet cat or dog means your child has less chance of allergies *overall,* but if allergies do develop, cat or dog allergy is likely to be among the child's problems.

For a first child, with no older brothers or sisters, dogs and cats are especially useful in protecting against allergy. This is probably because the pet makes the environment less hygienic for the child, exposing him or her to minor infections (probably symptom-free infections that none of you notices) that nudge the immune system away from allergy and toward healthier disease-fighting reactions. In this case the pet is fulfilling the same antiallergy role as siblings would in the early life of a child.

If you can give your child the kind of grubby childhood that seems to protect against allergy—lots of rolling about in the garden, with a minimum of hand-washing—the additional protection provided by a pet may well be superfluous.

On the other hand, you probably love your pet and want very much to keep it—so you could regard it as having both pros and cons in the battle against allergy and decide to let it stay, although minimizing its potential for causing allergies. That means reducing the allergen load from the animal as much as possible: ensure that the house is well ventilated so pet allergens don't build up to very high levels indoors, and keep the animal out of the child's bedroom so that he or she is not breathing huge amounts of the allergen while asleep. Let the child have close contact with the animal during the day, having made sure it is treated by a vet for more dangerous infections, such as parasites, that can harm a child.

Smaller caged pets, such as guinea pigs, hamsters, and mice, are probably best avoided. They pump a lot of allergen into the air of the house, and it seems unlikely that they would provide the same kind of bacterial challenge that a cat or dog provides, although this has not been investigated.

Reducing Pollutants in the Home

Any decorating that needs doing should be completed some months before the baby is due. All too often fathers decorate the nursery while the mother is in the hospital, and the baby comes home to a room smelling of fresh paint. If the decorating has to be done less than eight weeks before the baby is due, use a low-odor paint—these are now widely available.

Tobacco smoke is one of the worst pollutants that a baby can be exposed to, making asthma far more likely. Even if both parents have stopped smoking, there may be problems with guests. The best way to deal with this is to designate a "smoking room" well away from the baby. An ionizer or air cleaner (see appendix 3) in this room will clear the smoke from the air and prevent it from seeping into the rest of the house.

A gas stove in a poorly ventilated kitchen can be a source of nitrogen dioxide. This gas, if it becomes sufficiently concentrated, may increase the chance of a child developing an allergic reaction to an allergen in the air (see page 57). Consider installing an extractor fan.

Formaldehyde acts as an irritant to the airways, and you should consider whether there may be high levels in your home (see page 214). Unpainted particleboard and plywood could be painted to reduce the amount of formaldehyde being given off. Simply increasing ventilation will reduce the level of this pollutant.

There are other potential sources of irritants to the nose and airways, such as air fresheners, polish, mineral spirits, and cleaning fluids. Eradicate these whenever possible (see appendix 6).

Preparing Yourself for Breast-feeding

Breast-feeding is thought to help in preventing allergies in babies, particularly a bad reaction to cow's milk. There is a great deal of controversy about how much difference breast-feeding makes, so the advice given here is based on the best evidence available at present.

On one point there is no doubt: the practice of giving "supplementary" or bottle feeds to newborn babies while in the hospital carries a risk of sensitizing them to cow's milk. Unfortunately, this practice is still routine in some hospitals, and the mother is usually unaware that the bottle feed has been given. Sometimes cow's milk is the first food a newborn baby receives.

As early as possible in your pregnancy, find out about the policy on supplementary feeds in the hospital where you will give birth. Make it very clear to your doctor or midwife that you do not wish your baby to have anything but breast milk—no glucose water, formula, or pacifier. Ask whether you will be able to have your baby with you and feed him or her on demand—that way you will be able to ensure that your baby is not given a bottle or pacifier. Feeding on demand is also far more conducive to establishing successful breast-feeding than is a system that is ruled by the clock. Putting the baby to the breast soon after birth, within four hours at most, is also important in establishing successful breast-feeding, and you should ask about hospital policy on this.

If the hospital does not allow rooming-in, then you should ask that a notice be put on the baby's crib stating that bottle feeds or pacifiers must not be given. Ask that your baby be brought to you often. Newborns need to nurse frequently—every two to three hours during the day and night. Many hospitals offer new mothers gift packs that contain formula samples or coupons. Lactation consultants recommend that breast-feeding mothers turn down these offers and trust that their body's own milk is their baby's best food.

Where there is a hospital policy of not putting babies to the breast during the night, breast milk can be "expressed" and stored, to be given from a bottle by a nurse. However, this is a somewhat unsatisfactory solution for the newborn baby, because it is easier to suck milk from a bottle than from a breast, so the baby learns to suck less hard. Since the intensity of sucking influences the amount of milk produced, a mother may begin to produce less milk under this system, and the baby may refuse the breast.

If your inquiries about feeding policy at the hospital are not being treated sympathetically, ask to speak to the head of the maternity unit. Be prepared to stick your neck out a little, if necessary, and insist on your rights.

As well as finding out about the hospital, you should learn as much as you can about breast-feeding before you give birth. Since breast-feeding is a natural process, it is often assumed that it "comes naturally." Unfortunately, this is not always the case, and many mothers give up because they have not been shown how to breast-feed properly, or because they have sore nipples, or as a result of other problems. These problems can be overcome, but nursing staff generally find it more convenient to fall back on bottle feeds. The idea that some mothers "don't have enough milk" is a prevalent one, but the truth is that the supply is established by the demand—that is, by the frequency and intensity of feedings. If the breast-feeding relationship between mother and baby has been established properly, there is unlikely to be any problem with the amount of milk produced.

Sore nipples frequently occur because of incorrect positioning. If the baby is positioned properly, soreness is generally temporary and minor—lasting only 5 to 15 seconds after the baby latches on. Other tips for preventing soreness include using only water to wash the breasts, before and after the birth, because soap and cleansers dry the skin. Allow air circulation around the nipples for as much time as possible: try going braless for a few hours a day and wear loose T-shirts. Let your nipples air-dry after feedings.

If you tend to have dry skin, you could also apply modified lanolin (available as Lansinoh) twice a day during the last month of pregnancy, and after every feeding once the baby arrives, to prevent soreness before it starts.

The best preparation for breast-feeding is to contact your local La Leche League leader during pregnancy and attend a few meetings (see appendix 5). She can provide essential information on the best positions for nursing your baby, as well as moral support during those first challenging weeks.

A final word on maternity hospitals: One study from Britain found that babies who spent the first night after birth with their mother (rather than in the hospital's communal nursery) were significantly less likely to suffer from hay fever as young adults. The exact cause of this effect is a mystery—careful analysis of the data showed that it was not explained simply by differences in breast-feeding. Perhaps it is due to the exposure to microbes that a newborn baby has when sleeping with its mother. Whatever the explanation, the moral is clear: Try to find a hospital that will let you keep your baby with you day and night, right from the start. This has great benefits in establishing a good breast-feeding relationship as well.

MEASURES TO TAKE AFTER THE BIRTH

If breast-feeding is not possible, for whatever reason, you should not feel guilty about the situation. Fortunately, there are alternatives that carry less risk of allergy than standard infant formulas. These are formula mixtures known as **hydrolysates** and are available with a prescription. They are made from either cow's milk or soy protein that has been treated to break up the allergens. When broken up into smaller pieces, the proteins are far less allergenic. Consequently, these hydrolysates are far safer than ordinary cow's milk formulas, although a tiny minority of children do react to them. Note that soy hydrolysates are *not* the same as standard soy formulas, where the soy allergens have not been broken up: children can become sensitized to these intact soy allergens in time.

If you have established successful breast-feeding, continue it for as long as you can, preferably for six months, although continuing for four or five months is also valuable. Do not give any solids until the baby is at least four months old. Should the baby seem to need extra food, a hydrolysate formula can be used. Learning to express and store breast milk will give you some much needed freedom during this time; breast-feeding advice groups can help with this.

When you do introduce solid foods, do so gradually, so that breast milk still supplies most of the child's needs. If some breast-feeding can be continued until the child is a year old, so much the better.

When it comes to introducing new foods, those with low allergenic potential should be given at first, and the foods that most often produce allergic reactions withheld for a time. The main problem foods are eggs, milk (including all milk products such as butter, yogurt, cheese, and cottage cheese), fish, peanuts, wheat, rye, barley, nuts, soy (including all soy products such as tofu and soy milk), citrus fruits, and chocolate. Delay the introduction of eggs until the child is close to one year, and do not offer foods that contain peanut until age three. Delay introducing the baby to the rest of these foods until at least nine months old, and then introduce them slowly, one per week. If there are any reactions to the foods, or if the child shows an intense dislike for them, take them off the menu again.

Another measure that can have some benefit in reducing allergies is for a breast-feeding mother to avoid certain foods herself, especially those containing the most powerful allergens. Small amounts of food allergen do pass unchanged from the mother's stomach into her breast milk, and these can sensitize some children who are prone to allergy. The foods to avoid are milk and all milk products, eggs, fish, and peanuts.

Restricting your diet in this way while breast-feeding and caring for a baby can prove too much of a burden, but try it for a while and see if you can cope. To get the maximum benefit, you should continue avoiding these foods until the child is eating them as solids. If you cannot manage this, simply avoiding the foods for a month or two may be helpful. Always check packaged food to see that it does not contain milk or eggs (and see the synonyms for these foods, given in table 2, page 241). Calcium tablets can be prescribed to make up for the lack of calcium in a milk-free diet.

A breast-fed baby who develops colic may be reacting to traces of food allergens in his or her mother's milk. If you are breast-feeding but not restricting your diet and the baby becomes colicky, try cutting out milk, eggs, fish, and peanuts for a week. This will often cure the colic. If there is no improvement, eliminate soy, chocolate, all nuts, wheat, and citrus fruits as well.

The measures for reducing dampness and combating dust mites, already described in chapter 12, should continue for the first year of the baby's life, and longer if possible. When soft toys are bought, make sure that they are ones that can be laundered easily.

For as long as possible, keep the baby away from areas of high traffic pollution when outdoors.

Finally, and perhaps most important, ease up on hygiene. Encourage your child to play outdoors, and give him or her plenty of contact with other children and animals from an early age. Don't worry too much about unwashed hands. It is difficult, and goes against the grain for most of us, but the overwhelming evidence from scientific studies now (see page 63) is that a bit of dirt is just what the young immune system needs. There may be the occasional tummy ache as a result, but that is a small price to pay for an allergy-free life.

Appendix 1
POLLEN SEASONS
AROUND THE WORLD

The authors would like to acknowledge the help of Dr. Jean Emberlin, of the Pollen Research Unit at the University of North London, in compiling these lists, and to thank Professor Eugenio Dominguez-Vilches of the University of Cordoba for supplying information on behalf of REA (Spanish Aerobiology Network). Special mention should also be made of Professor Walter H. Lewis and Dr. Prathiba Vinay of Washington University, whose excellent publications on allergenic pollen, both in the U.S. and around the world, have been immensely useful as a source of reference.

THE REGIONAL LISTINGS

The regions of the world are dealt with in the following order:

USING THIS APPENDIX

The information given here can be useful in several different ways, as follows. For most people, planning hay fever–free vacations will probably be the most important consideration.

Diagnosis

By comparing the time when you suffer symptoms with the pollen seasons given for the area where you live, you may be able to identify the particular pollen or pollens responsible for your hay fever. This can help in everyday pollen avoidance (see chapter 8), although it is not essential.

Identification of the pollen allergen is essential before any type of desensitization treatment (see chapter 9), but in this case a skin-prick test or other diagnostic test must be used beforehand for precise diagnosis.

In trying to pinpoint the source of your problems, bear in mind that you may be sensitive to more than one type of pollen. Sensitivity to mold spores (see page 192) can also confuse the picture, as these sometimes produce seasonal symptoms. You could be sensitive to mold spores alone, or to both mold spores and pollen.

Allergies to other airborne allergens, such as dust mites or animal proteins and skin particles (see chapter 12), can produce year-round symptoms. These are frequently milder than hay fever. If your "hay fever" drags on for much of the year but is worst in one of the pollen seasons identified below, this may be the explanation.

The information given here is fairly generalized, and local features (such as mountain ranges and forestry plantations) can make enormous differences to the pollen in the air. A local doctor or allergist may have more specialized knowledge of potentially allergenic pollens in your immediate area. See your doctor if you feel you need more guidance or a skin-prick test to confirm the diagnosis.

The dates given here may not hold true in every year. Changes in the seasonal weather can affect the timing of pollination; in temperate climates, for example, a warm spring will advance the grass pollen season by as much as three weeks.

Bear in mind that there are also "minority interest" pollens, which cause problems for a few people only. These are not included here. However, you are very unlikely to react to a pollen of this type unless you are also sensitive to another pollen that is a major allergen (that is, if you are already disposed to react allergically to pollens). The exception to this rule arises when people are breathing in huge amounts of a minority pollen, either at home or at work. This can happen when people work with plants or cut flowers, or live close to fields or orchards where a single crop is grown (see pages 5–7). It can occasionally affect gardeners who are keen growers of one type of plant.

Getting Away from Your Problem Pollen

The lists in this appendix can also be used to show where you will find lower concentrations of your problem pollen if you need to escape during the pollen season. Again, keep in mind that this information is generalized and does not cover local variations.

Also remember that an unusual variation in the weather can change the timing of the pollen season in your "retreat" area. These changes should not be more than a week or two, however. Allow a margin of error of two weeks for any of the dates given below.

People with very severe hay fever are sometimes driven to moving from their houses, or even emigrating. The list following can help you choose a new home area, but more specific advice is definitely advisable in this case. If you are already very allergic to one pollen, the chance of developing a new sensitivity to a different pollen is fairly high. Such sensitivities generally appear within two to three years of arriving in a new area. The more potently allergenic the pollen, the more likely a new sensitivity, so areas with high pollen counts for particularly notorious allergens (e.g., ragweed, birch, and grasses) should be avoided.

Planning Vacations

Before making any travel arrangements, always check the regional lists. Choosing the right time of the year can make all the difference to your vacation.

Local variations are again important here, and are not covered in the lists below. For example, one side of a holiday island may have much higher pollen counts than the other, while mountain areas may be lower (or higher) in certain pollens.

Using the Lists

For a variety of reasons, the plants are not arranged alphabetically, but in groups. These are the groups, in the order that they appear within each region:

Grasses
Trees and tree crops
Shrubs and hedging plants (only in those regions/countries where relevant)
Crops (only in those regions/countries where relevant)
Weeds (i.e., wild plants other than grasses)

These groupings are useful for diagnosis because, in seasonal climates, each major group pollinates in a particular season. The trees tend to pollinate in the spring, the grasses in early summer, and the weeds in late summer and autumn.

If you have symptoms in the spring, for example, and you are trying to identify your problem pollen, your strategy should be to read through all the entries for trees and look for clues as to the likely culprits. These are some questions to ask yourself as you read: Which of the trees mentioned are common in my area? How closely do their pollinating seasons compare with the timing of my symptoms? Did my hay fever get worse (or vanish) when I lived in a different place?

You may be able to refer to the lists for other areas where you have lived or visited on vacation to check out your hunches about the culprit pollen.

If you live in a region with year-round warmth, especially California or Florida, the pollination seasons of the major plant groups are less well-defined and the potential culprits are far more diverse because so many different plants have been introduced. Identifying your culprit pollen is more difficult for these areas, and you may need to read every plant entry for your region in your diagnostic quest.

Within each major plant group in each region/country, the most potent allergens—those that cause the most cases of hay fever in that region—are dealt with first and covered in more detail. For example, ragweed heads the list of Weeds in all areas of the United States (but not in Europe, where it is still a rare plant and not yet a major cause of allergies), while birch heads the list of Trees in any region where it is common.

These very potent allergens tend to be involved in cross-reactions (see page 159) with other pollens. Suppose you are allergic to ragweed, for example; you might also react to various related plants, such as goldenrod, dandelions, marsh elder, or groundsel bush. These cross-reactions can make your symptoms last longer than the pollen season for ragweed—or you may mysteriously develop symptoms while living in or visiting countries where ragweed doesn't grow.

Plants that are likely to be involved in cross-reactions generally appear immediately after the entry for the primary allergen (such as ragweed or birch). So when you are planning vacations, read the next few entries down the list to find out about other potential problem plants—but do remember that cross-reactions are not inevitable.

The grasses, including grass crops, are dealt with first in each area because they are the most common cause of hay fever worldwide. Although there are many different species of grass, they all flower at about the same time within a given area, and can therefore be dealt with as a single group. Grasses do not provoke cross-reactions with other plants, so if you are sensitive to grass and no other pollen you need to read only the entry for grasses.

Finally, remember always to check the scientific name (shown in parentheses) as well as the common name. This is especially important when traveling because common names differ around the world. For example, sagebrush is a cause of hay fever in parts of the U.S. It belongs to the same genus *(Artemisia)* as European plants known as mugworts and wormwoods and almost certainly shares their allergens. By looking down the list for *Artemisia,* you would be able to locate plants that could cause trouble for someone sensitized to sagebrush. Where possible, alternative common names have been included.

Travelers who are already sensitized to a plant in their home country may react to small amounts of that pollen abroad, whereas the levels are too low to sensitize local people. To help travelers, plants that are common allergens worldwide have generally been included in the lists, even if they cause little or no hay fever in the region where they are listed. While every effort has been made to give complete coverage in this respect, there may be a few omissions due to lack of information, because pollens that are locally unimportant as allergens may not be recorded. Additionally, pollens that are known as allergens in certain countries but do not cause much hay fever worldwide—e.g., those of willows, poplars, elms, maples, limes (lindens and basswoods), chestnut trees, horse chestnut trees, plane trees, walnut trees, elder, privet, heather, goldenrod, cocklebur, and dandelion—appear only in those areas where they are significant allergens.

AFRICA

EAST AFRICA

There is little information available, but the pollen season for grasses can be given. The peak seasons occur in the months following the rains. Some areas have one rainy season per year, others have two. Kenya's grasses flower from September through October and again from December through January. In the savannas of Tanzania, the savanna grass pollinates from June through December with a peak in September and October. In Zimbabwe pollen is present in the air year round, but peak grass pollen counts occur from July through August and again from October through November. In Malawi the peak is from October through February. There are reports of hay fever–like symptoms at the time of the corn harvest in Malawi, which could be due to mold spores.

NORTH AFRICA

Along the northern coast of Morocco, Algeria, and Tunisia, the vegetation is very similar to that of the Mediterranean region but the pollination seasons may be earlier. The grass season, for example, runs from March through May. Olives (*Olea*) pollinate mainly in May. Lamb's-quarters or goosefoot (*Chenopodiaceae*) and mugwort or sagebrush (*Artemisia*) pollen can reach high levels in some areas.

Egypt has a desert climate over large areas, with low pollen counts, but many of the most visited regions are in the Nile Delta, where pollen seasons are very long. Around Alexandria, for example, grass and other pollens are abundant from mid-February through early December. The nettle (*Urtica*) season lasts from late February or early March through to November, with peak counts in April. Goosefoot, (*Chenopodiaceae*) flowers from late February through November. Cairo has much lower counts owing to the very dry climate.

SOUTHERN AFRICA

Botswana has peak grass pollen counts from November through April. In South Africa, there may be some grass pollen in the air in most months of the year. Around Cape Town the peak for grass pollen counts is from November through January. The area around Johannesburg and Pretoria has a shorter peak season, from December through January. The grass pollen counts are generally very high, as are counts for mold spores.

Mesquite (*Prosopis*), a cause of hay fever in the southern regions of North America, also grows here and may cause problems for visitors sensitized to its pollen.

WEST AFRICA

Little information is available for this area, but the flowering season for grasses in the savanna regions can be given. These stretch from the edge of the rain forests north to the Sahel and include much of Nigeria and northern Ghana. Most of the grasses pollinate from April through July, with a peak in May. There will be some grass pollen in the air through to November.

AUSTRALIA

NEW SOUTH WALES

Grasses (Gramineae or Poaceae)
August through May
There will be some grass pollen in the air all year round. The peak season is from September through March.

White cypress pine or Murray pine (Callitris columellaris)
August through November
A conifer but not a true pine. Pollen counts are lower after the end of October. An important allergenic tree. Less common in northern areas.

She-oak or "Australian pine" (Casuarina)
July through April

Neither an oak nor a pine, so cross-reactions with these trees are unlikely. An important allergen in the central and southern areas; often planted for shelter. The season varies from one part of the state to another.

Silver birch (Betula pendula)
September through October

A tree introduced from Europe; grows mainly in cooler areas.

Wattles (Acacia)
June through December

High pollen counts in wattle scrub and woodland; also grown in gardens.

Olive trees (Olea)
October through November

The peak is in November, when pollen counts can be high near olive-growing areas in the south of the state.

Gum trees (Eucalyptus)
All year

A rare cause of hay fever but visitors from California or Hawaii may be sensitized.

Privet (Ligustrum)
September through November

The pollen count can be high in October and November. Can cross-react with olive pollen and people may become allergic to it in this way.

Cypresses (Cupressaceae)
August through November

Not a particularly important allergen locally but may affect those sensitized elsewhere. Planted for shelter in the south.

Paterson's curse or Salvation Jane (Echium plantagineum)
September through December

A weed that commonly causes hay fever. Found only in the south and in inland areas.

Plantains (Plantago)
June through February

The season varies from one part of the state to another. A very common weed and an important source of hay fever.

Docks and sorrels (Rumex)
September through February

The pollen peak is from September through November.

Lamb's-quarters or goosefoot (Chenopodiaceae)
December through February

The pollen is in the air all year long but peaks in late summer. Common throughout the state.

Pellitory-of-the-wall (Parietaria judaica)
June through April

In the Sydney area, it is mainly found on the lower North Shore, but is colonizing the inner city. The weed has also been found growing in Melbourne, Adelaide, and Freemantle, but not yet in sufficient numbers to cause hay fever.

Capeweed (Arctotheca calendula)
September through November

High pollen counts except in the north.

Wormwoord or sagebrush (Artemisia)
December through January

Mainly in inland areas.

NORTHERN TERRITORY

Very little information available. In the north, grass pollen is likely in summer (October through March).

QUEENSLAND

Grasses (Gramineae or Poaceae)
September through May

There is likely to be some grass pollen in the air all year round in many areas. Pollen counts are much higher in the south of the state, lower on the northeast coast.

White cypress pine or Murray pine (Callitris columellaris)
September through November
A conifer but not a true pine. Peak pollination occurs in October. Only grows in the south of the state (below the Tropic of Capricorn).

She-oak or "Australian pine" (Casuarina)
September through February
Confined to the central and southern part of the state. Neither an oak nor a pine, so cross-reactions are unlikely.

Wattles (Acacia)
May through October
Some pollen in the air all year round. Pollen counts higher inland, in areas of wattle scrub and woodland. Also grown in gardens.

Gum trees (Eucalyptus)
All year
A rare cause of hay fever but visitors from California or Hawaii may be sensitized.

Privet (Ligustrum)
September through November
Not considered a particularly important allergen in this area, but may affect those sensitized elsewhere. Only in the south of the state; planted for hedging.

Sunflower (Helianthus)
December through May
A frequent cause of hay fever where it is cultivated. Can cross-react with ragweed.

Plantains (Plantago)
August through March
An important type of allergenic pollen in the south of this region.

Docks and sorrels (Rumex)
September through February
The pollen count is lower after the end of November. Mainly in the south of the state.

Lamb's-quarters or goosefoot (Chenopodiaceae)
September through April
The peak is from December onward. Considered an important allergen in the south.

Capeweed (Arctotheca calendula)
September through December
Not particularly common except in the south of this state.

SOUTH AUSTRALIA

Grasses (Gramineae or Poaceae)
July through March
Plentiful pollen in the air for much of the year; airborne in lesser amounts even in May and June.

White cypress pine or Murray pine (Callitris columellaris)
August through October
A conifer but not a true pine. Planted for shelter; also grows wild.

She-oak or "Australian pine" (Casuarina)
August through September, March through July
Pollination season very variable. Grown for shelter and found in the wild. Neither an oak nor a pine, so cross-reactions are unlikely.

Silver birch (Betula pendula)
September through November
Planted for shelter in some cooler areas.

Wattles (Acacia)
July through November
Very common in the wild and planted in gardens.

Olive trees (Oleo)
September through November
Peak is in November. Pollen counts are high only where olive groves are found.

Gum trees (Eucalyptus)
August through March
A rare cause of hay fever but visitors from California or Hawaii may be sensitized.

Privet (Ligustrum)
September through November
Cross-reactions with olive may produce sensitivity.

Cypresses (Cupressaceae)
August through October
These conifers can be a source of hay fever where planted for shelter.

Paterson's curse or Salvation Jane (Echium plantagineum)
July through December
The peak is in October and November. A common cause of hay fever when found in abundance.

Plantains (Plantago)
August through March
The peak is from September to January. A widespread weed that often causes hay fever.

Docks and sorrels (Rumex)
September through December
A common weed throughout the area.

Lamb's-quarters or goosefoot (Chenopodiaceae)
December through April
The peak is at the end of the season in March and April. Native species are known as salt bushes.

Capeweed (Arctotheca calendula)
August through November
The peak is in September and October. A very common weed throughout the state and an important allergen.

TASMANIA

Grasses (Gramineae or Poaceae)
September through April
The peak is in December. Pollen counts can be high.

She-oak or "Australian pine" (Casuarina)
June through December
Neither an oak nor a pine, so cross-reactions are unlikely. Grows wild; also planted in some areas.

Silver birch (Betula pendula)
September through November
Widely planted.

Wattles (Acacia)
August through February
Pollen counts higher in the north.

Cypresses and pines (Cupressaceae and Pinaceae)
July through November
Planted for shelter. Cypresses are likely to cause hay fever only in hot dry areas. Pines are more likely to act as irritants than as allergens.

Gum trees (Eucalyptus)
August through February
A rare cause of hay fever but visitors from California or Hawaii may be sensitized.

Plantains (Plantago)
October through March
A common weed in most parts of the island and an important allergen.

Docks and sorrels (Rumex)
September through May
The peak is in November and December.

Capeweed (Arctotheca calendula)
September through January
Pollen counts are lower after October. Considered an important allergen.

VICTORIA

Grasses (Gramineae or Poaceae)
September through May
There is some pollen in the air all year long.

White cypress pine or Murray pine (Callitris columellaris)
June through October
A conifer but not a true pine. The season varies from one part of the state to another. Found mainly in the north and not particularly common.

She-oak or "Australian pine" (Casuarina)
March through April, July through August
Pollination season may vary. Confined to the north of the state and not common except where planted for shelter. Neither an oak nor a pine, so cross-reactions are unlikely.

Silver birch (Betula pendula)
September through October
Planted for shelter in southern areas.

Wattles (Acacia)
July through January
The peak of the season is in August and September. Common throughout the area; also grown in gardens.

Olive trees (Olea)
October through November
Grown mainly in the north of the state.

Cypresses (Cupressaceae)
April through September
Widely planted for shelter in the south.

Pines (Pinaceae)
August through September
Commonly planted for shelter in the south.

Gum trees (Eucalyptus)
All year
A rare cause of hay fever.

Privet (Ligustrum)
October through December
Commonly used for hedging and considered a likely cause of hay fever.

Clovers (Trifolium)
September through February
Peak is in October and November. May cause some hay fever where common.

Paterson's curse or Salvation Jane (Echium plantagineum)
August through December
The peak is in October. Not common except in the northeast.

Plantains (Plantago)
October through March
Peak pollen counts are from November to January. A very common weed throughout the state.

Docks and sorrels (Rumex)
August through February
The peak is in October and November. Common throughout the state.

Lamb's-quarters or goosefoot (Chenopodiaceae)
December through April
Common only in the north.

Capeweed (Arctotheca calendula)
August through December
Common throughout, and an important allergen.

WESTERN AUSTRALIA

Grasses (Gramineae or Poaceae)
September through March
The peak is from September to November. However there can be some grass pollen in the air at any time of the year. While the pollen count is generally lower from March to September, there is a small peak in June.

White cypress pine (Callitris columellaris)
August through October

A conifer but not a true pine. Commonly a cause of hay fever in this area. Planted for shelter and found growing wild.

She-oak or "Australian pine" (Casuarina)
July through November

Neither an oak nor a pine, so cross-reactions are unlikely. Pollination shows a peak during July and August, then a lull, followed by a second peak in November. Planted for shelter, and found growing wild.

Wattles (Acacia)
May through February

The highest pollen counts are from July to October. Note that cross-reactions are likely with cultivated mimosas.

Olive trees (Olea)
November through December

Not a particularly common source of hay fever here, but may affect those sensitized elsewhere.

Cypresses (Cupressaceae)
August through October

Widely planted for shelter.

Pines (Pinaceae)
July through November

Planted for shelter in some areas. Pollen may produce allergic reactions or simply act as an irritant.

Gum trees (Eucalyptus)
October through March

A rare cause of hay fever, but some visitors from California or Hawaii may be sensitized.

Privet (Ligustrum)
August through November

Planted for hedging in some areas and may cause some hay fever. Cross-reactions with olive are possible.

Sunflower (Helianthus)
October through February

May cause local problems where cultivated. Can cross-react with ragweed.

Paterson's curse or Salvation Jane (Echium plantagineum)
October through November

A shorter season than in some other parts of Australia.

Plantains (Plantago)
August through February

The most allergenic species pollinates in October.

Docks and sorrels (Rumex)
September through January

Common weeds but not a major cause of hay fever in this area.

Lamb's-quarters or goosefoot (Chenopodiaceae)
September through February

The native species are known as salt bushes. Common in dry and windy places.

Capeweed (Arctotheca calendula)
July through November

The pollination peak is during September and October. A common allergenic weed.

BRITAIN AND IRELAND

Grasses (Gramineae or Poaceae)
May through July

Grasses are the prime cause of hay fever in the British Isles. About 12 major species seem to be responsible, and most patients react to several of these.

The grass pollen season usually begins first along the warm coasts of Cornwall, west Cork, west Kerry, and southwest Clare, sometimes at the beginning of May. A week later, southern Britain, the Midlands, Wales, East Anglia, and the southwestern counties of Ireland follow suit. Much of the north of England and all the rest of Ireland begin a week later. Another week passes before pollination begins in Durham, Northumberland, and much of Scotland. The highlands of Scotland follow a week later, but the extreme north, beyond Loch Shin, waits another week. In all, there may be a five-week difference between the southwest tip of Cornwall and Ireland and the extreme north of Scotland. However, the pollen season ends in the north only a week or two later than in the south, so the season in the extreme north is substantially shorter. In southern Britain the pollen peak is usually in the second week of June, and this is when most people suffer symptoms. A warm spring with temperatures above average in March, April, and the first half of May will bring on the pollen season earlier.

There are some variations from one region to another. Cities surrounded by countryside, such as Cardiff and Glasgow, show higher pollen counts than extensive conurbations such as London. Pollen counts are usually lower at the tops of mountains and on breezy coasts.

Birches (Betula)
April through May

Some people show cross-reactions (see page 156) with alder and hazel, which belong to the same plant family (see above).

Alder, hornbeam, and hazel (Alnus, Carpinus, and Corylus)
February through April

Birch-sensitive people who also react to alder and/or hazel may experience symptoms before the birch season begins. For hazel, pollination is usually in March, but it can be as early as the beginning of February, or even January in a mild winter. (In a few sheltered gardens, it can begin in December.) Alder pollen comes out later than hazel, in March or April. Hornbeam pollen is very scarce in some years, abundant in others.

Oaks and beeches (Quercus and Fagus)
April through May

The allergens in the pollen can cross-react with those of birch (see page 156).

Ashes (Fraxinus)
April through May

Not a particularly strong allergen, but those already sensitive to olive pollen may become allergic to it through a cross-reaction (see page 157).

Poplars and willows (Populus and Salix)
March through May

Pollen counts are generally moderate. May affect North American visitors already sensitized to the pollen.

Plane trees (Platanus)
April through May

Particularly common in London and some other cities, where it may cause a certain amount of hay fever. In general, however, pollen counts are low and they affect relatively few people.

Maples and sycamores (Acer)
April through May

Pollen counts are low, but may affect a few North American travelers who are already allergic to maple pollen. The most allergenic of the maples, the wind-pollinated box elder or ash-leaved maple *(Acer ne-gundo)*, is grown in parks and gardens, especially in London. It flowers in early March.

Lindens and basswoods *(Tilia)*
June through July

Known as lime in Britain. Pollination is by insects and the pollen does not generally travel very far on the wind. Pollen counts are low to moderate, but may be high near the trees.

Horse chestnuts *(Aesculus)*
April through May

Not considered a source of hay fever in the British Isles, but gives some positive skin-prick tests among birch-sensitive patients in Scandinavia, and is reported as an allergen in Turkey. Pollen counts are moderate and may be high in the vicinity of the trees.

Elms *(Ulmus)*
February through March

Pollen counts are low to moderate.

Walnuts *(Juglans)*
May through June

Walnut trees seem to have less allergenic pollen than their close relatives the hickories and pecans. Most people reacting to walnut have probably been sensitized by these more allergenic pollens. Very few hickories and pecans are found in Britain—just the occasional specimen in a botanic garden or large park. Walnuts are much more common, though not native. You may find them in parks and large gardens, and sometimes naturalized in the countryside. The pollen count for walnuts is generally low, and they are not known to cause hay fever among Britons, but North American visitors already sensitized to hickories may suffer symptoms when near the trees.

Chestnuts *(Castanea)*
June through July

Pollination does not begin until late June. Chestnuts are not believed to cause hay fever in Britain, though they do in other parts of Europe, owing largely to cross-reactions with birch. Cross-reactions with oak and beech are also likely. Chestnuts are fairly widespread in southern England, less common elsewhere. Pollen counts are low.

Pines (Pinaceae)
April through May

Not a cause of hay fever in Britain, but there is ample pollen in the air, which might affect visitors from other countries who are already sensitized.

Cypresses (Cupressaceae)
April, June

Although these are grown widely in Britain, there is very little pollen in the air. Not a cause of hay fever locally and unlikely to affect those sensitized elsewhere.

Japanese red cedar
  (Cryptomeria japonica)
February

Grown as an ornamental tree and also tried as a timber tree (a few small plantations remain in parts of Devon, for example). It is uncommon except in the west of Britain. Pollen counts are negligible except in the immediate vicinity of the trees.

Privet *(Ligustrum)*
May through June

One species grows wild and another is used very widely for hedging (although regularly clipped hedges do not flower). Pollen counts are very low. Due to cross-reaction, it may provoke symptoms in people who have been sensitized to olive pollen abroad (see page 157).

Elders (Sambucus)
May through July

A very common shrub in Britain, and some pollen becomes airborne, but pollen counts are low.

Heathers (Erica and Calluna)
July through September

Not reported as a cause of hay fever in Britain, but heathers seem to affect some people who are sensitive to birch. Heathers grow mainly in moorland areas. Pollen counts are significant only in areas such as Scotland, where heather is abundant.

Sweet gale (Myrica gale)
April through May

Not considered a source of hay fever in Britain (where it is known as bog myrtle). Pollen counts are very low or nonexistent. The plant is scarce throughout most of the country, but boggy moorland country in northern Scotland and the west of Ireland often has extensive colonies, and pollen counts could be higher in such areas. Travelers from Canada already sensitized to sweet gale (or to birch—they cross-react) might be affected in these regions.

Nettles (Urtica)
June through July, August through September

Common weeds with two separate spurts of pollination. Not particularly allergenic, but they do cause some summer hay fever.

Plantains (Plantago)
July through September

Do not usually begin pollinating until late July. Only small amounts of pollen are produced, but the pollen is very allergenic.

Mugwort and wormwoods (Artemisia)
July through September

Do not usually begin pollinating until late July. The pollen could affect U.S. visitors sensitized to sagebrush.

Docks and sorrels (Rumex)
May through July

Do not usually begin pollinating until mid-May, and there is relatively little pollen in the air after the end of June. Pollen counts are generally low.

Goosefoot and amaranths (Chenopodiaceae and Amaranthaceae)
May through October

Various species grow widely, but there is relatively little pollen in the air. Rural areas can have slightly higher pollen counts. Whether these would affect North American visitors already sensitized to goosefoot, lamb's-quarters, pigweed, and related species is unknown.

Ragweeds (Ambrosia)
June through September

Pollen counts are very low and do not seem to cause any symptoms in either residents or visitors. There may, however, be localized areas with higher levels of pollen, especially near seaports and on wasteland with ragweed colonies (e.g., around London and in East Anglia).

Goldenrod and dandelion (Compositae or Asteraceae)
April through September

These and other plants belonging to the Asteraceae, may cause problems through cross-reactions for visitors who are highly sensitive to ragweed (see page 159).

CANADA

BRITISH COLUMBIA

Grasses (Gramineae or Poaceae)
May through September
The peak is in June and July, but there are variations with altitude. The season starts two weeks earlier in the south than in the north and is longest in the coastal areas. Pollen counts are not particularly high since grassland areas, except in some coastal regions, are mostly restricted to small areas.

Birches *(Betula)*
May and June
Pollen counts are highest near the tree line on mountain slopes, but birches are found throughout the area.

Alders *(Alnus)*
April through May
Can cross-react with birch. West of the Rockies, it is a more potent allergen than birch.

Poplars and willows *(Populus and Salix)*
April through May
The willow season is later, from May to early June, in the north and at high altitudes.

Maples *(Acer)*
May through June
The most common cause of hay fever among the maples, box elder *(Acer negundo)*, does not grow in this area. Local species are not particularly allergenic.

Cypresses, junipers, and "cedars" (Cupressaceae)
February through June
The peak is in April. Rarely a cause of hay fever in this area, but the pollen may affect those sensitized in warmer climates.

Sweet gale *(Myrica gale)*
April through June
The same species grows in Scandinavia where it is known to cross-react with birch. May also cause symptoms in birch-sensitive patients in Canada. Cross-reaction with bayberry or wax myrtle of the U.S. is likely.

Ragweeds *(Ambrosia)*
August through September
The season begins earlier here than in eastern Canada. Pollen counts are highest in the south and close to settlements.

GREAT PLAINS OF CANADA

This region comprises Alberta, Saskatchewan, and Manitoba.

Grasses (Gramineae and Poaceae)
May through August
The peak is in June and July, when grass pollen can be very abundant in parts of the southern prairies. Pollen counts are generally moderate in the north because areas of grassland are limited, but they can be high locally, such as in the Peace River valley in the northwest, where there is more pastureland.

Birches *(Betula)*
April through May
Birches are scattered throughout this region and are more widespread in southern Manitoba. There can be unexpected cross-reactions to sweet gale, a low-growing shrub (see below).

Poplars and quaking aspen *(Populus)*
April through May
Balsam poplar and quaking aspen *(P. balsamifera* and *P. tremuloides)* are believed to be prime offenders in hay fever and are found throughout this area. Aspens are most common in southern Manitoba.

Maples *(Acer)*
May through June
The highly allergenic box elder or ash-leaved maple *(Acer negundo)* is found in the south of this area, notably in southern Manitoba.

Oaks *(Quercus)*
May
Found in southern Manitoba only.

Elms *(Ulmus)*
May through June
Found in the southern prairies only.

Cypresses, junipers, and "cedars" (Cupressaceae)
March through June
The peak is in April. These trees, mainly found in the Rocky Mountains, rarely cause hay fever locally, but the pollen may affect those sensitized in warmer climates.

Sweet gale *(Myrica gale)*
April through June
Not found in the far south of this region. The same species grows in Scandinavia, where it is known to cross-react with birch. May also cause symptoms in birch-sensitive patients in Canada. Cross-reactions with bayberry or wax myrtle of the U.S. is likely.

Ragweeds *(Ambrosia)*
August through September
Found only in the far south of this region, mainly within 125 miles (200 km) of the U.S. border.

Lamb's-quarters or goosefoot and plantains (Chenopodiaceae and Plantago)
August through September
The season may end earlier in the north. These weeds grow only where there are settlements and are therefore more scattered in the north.

Sagebrush, mugwort, and wormwoods (Artemisia)
August through September
These weeds grow mainly around settlements and are therefore more common in the south.

NORTHEAST CANADA

This area comprises northern Ontario, northern Quebec, Labrador, and Newfoundland.

Grasses (Gramineae or Poaceae)
July
Pollen sparse in northern Ontario. May be prolific in the northeast, but the season is very short. May cross-react with sedges.

Birches *(Betula)*
May through June
The season is short, usually from late May through early June only. There can be unexpected cross-reactions to sweet gale, a low-growing shrub (see below).

Spruces, firs, and larches (Pinaceae)
July through August
Prolific pollen producers, but very rarely produce allergic reactions. Might cause some irritation.

Sweet gale *(Myrica gale)*
April through June
The same species grows in Scandinavia, where it is known to cross-react with birch. May also cause symptoms in birch-sensitive patients in Canada. Cross-reaction with bayberry or wax myrtle of the U.S. are likely.

NORTHERN CANADA

Grasses (Gramineae and Poaceae)
May through September
The season is shorter in the very north from July to August and is shorter at high

altitudes. There can be high concentrations of pollen in some areas.

Pollen counts are low in forest areas, higher on the tundra (where sedges also contribute to symptoms), and in transitional vegetation zones.

Birches (Betula)
May through June

The peak is in April. The season is later in the north and at high altitudes. Pollen counts can be very high. There can be unexpected cross-reactions to sweet gale, a low-growing shrub (see below).

Alders (Alnus)
April through May

Can cross-react with birch, lengthening the season for those with birch sensitivity. Most abundant in western mountain areas.

Poplars and willows (Populus and salix)
April through May

Found throughout the forest zones. Balsam poplar *(P. balsamifera)* and quaking aspen *(P. tremuloides)* are a the most likely to cause hay fever.

Sweet gale (Myrica gale)
April through June

The same species grows in Scandinavia, where it is known to cross-react with birch. May also cause symptoms in birch-sensitive patients in Canada. Cross-reaction with bayberry or wax myrtle of the eastern seaboard in the U.S. or southern U.S. is likely.

SOUTHEAST CANADA

This area comprises Southern Ontario and Quebec, New Brunswick, Nova Scotia, and Prince Edward Island.

Grasses (Gramineae or Poaceae)
May through August

The peak is in June and July. In Ontario the season is shorter, from the end of June to the end of July, starting later in the north. There is extensive grassland in some areas around the St. Lawrence seaway.

Birches (Betula)
May through June

The season does not begin until late May in most parts, but south of the St. Lawrence and around Montreal it may start in early May. Pollen production can vary from year to year, with very high counts in some years. There can be unexpected cross-reactions to sweet gale, a low-growing shrub (see below).

Alders (Alnus)
April

Can produce cross-reactions in those sensitized by birch.

Oaks and beeches (Quercus and Fagus)
May through June

Not abundant pollen producers except in Ontario and along the St. Lawrence seaway. Can pollinate as early as April in the south of this area. Cross-reactions are possible with birch.

Hickories (Carya)
May through June

Found only in the most southern parts of Ontario and Quebec. A highly allergenic pollen, but the grains are large, so it does not disperse widely.

Mulberry (Morus)
April through June

Found in the air in the Toronto region. A highly allergenic pollen.

Willows and poplars (Salix and Populus)
April through May

The season is later in the north, from May to June. Can produce high pollen counts in some parts of the region.

Maples *(Acer)*
May through June
Can be as early as April in the south. Maples growing in this area are all insect-pollinated and probably of low allergenicity. Box elder *(Acer negundo)*, the most allergenic species of maple, is not found here.

Lindens and basswoods *(Tilia)*
July
Only a moderately potent allergen.

Pines and spruces (Pinaceae)
June through August
The season is earlier in the south. Not considered to be a common cause of true allergy but can act as an irritant.

Elms and hackberries *(Ulmus* and *Celtis)*
May through June
The season is later in the north.

Ashes *(Fraxinus)*
April through May
Not a potent allergen; may affect those sensitized by olive pollen.

Privet *(Ligustrum)*
May through June
Only in the southern part of this region, and the number of people affected is small. Those affected have often been sensitized by olive pollen, which cross-reacts with privet.

Sweet gale *(Myrica gale)*
April through June
The same species grows in Scandinavia, where it is known to cross-react with birch. May also cause symptoms in birch-sensitive patients in Canada. Cross-reactions with bayberry or wax myrtle of the U.S. is likely.

Ragweeds *(Ambrosia)*
August through September
Mainly found around settlements and on disturbed ground. Pollen counts can be very high in the south. They decline sharply with the first frosts.

Sagebrush, mugwort, and wormwoods (Artemisia)
August through September
Very high counts in some areas, such as around Montreal. Mainly on disturbed sites and near settlements.

Lamb's-quarters or goosefoot, pigweeds, and Russian thistle (Chenopodiaceae)
July through September
May cause some hay fever in the Great Lakes region.

Plantains *(Plantago)*
July through October
Only in the Great Lakes region and along the St. Lawrence seaway.

THE CANARY ISLANDS

There is very little grass on some islands (e.g., Gomera) except in the small fields beside streams. Other islands may have more grass, but it flowers early, in April. The islands have a specialized native flora and are home to very few of the more troublesome hay fever plants. Along the coasts of the islands, particularly in the north, pollen counts are very low because of the strong onshore winds.

Tree heather *(Erica arborea)* grows on some islands and has been implicated in hay fever elsewhere (e.g., Turkey). Olives *(Olea)* may be grown on some islands. Palm trees are common and might affect some visitors from California or Florida if sensitized already.

THE CARIBBEAN

The list below may omit some important local allergens, as the allergenic properties of the native trees have been very little studied.

Pollen is in the air during all seasons because the tropical climate allows plants to grow and flower all year round. Overall, the highest counts occur from October through January, and the lowest during the dry season, from August through late September. If you are a traveler visiting the islands, concentrate on avoiding pollens to which you are already sensitive. If you are highly sensitive to several pollens, stick to the dry season and stay in a coastal resort.

Grasses (Gramineae or Poaceae)
October through March, June through July
There are hundreds of different grasses and sedges, with a great range of flowering times. There will be some grass pollen in the air all year round, but the main season is from October through March. There is another burst of flowering in June and July but the pollen count is much lower then.

There are variations between lowlands and mountains, with the greatest differences on large islands, such as Jamaica. The lowest pollen counts are found on coasts with onshore winds.

She-oak or "Australian pine" *(Casuarina)*
February through April
Introduced trees often planted in sandy coastal areas and at up to about 1,320 feet (400 meters) altitude. Irregular pollen producers—very high in some years, very low in others. Neither oaks nor pines, so they are unlikely to produce cross-reactions with these trees.

Paper mulberry
(Broussonetia papyrifera)
April through May
Planted in some areas for rearing silkworms. Note that silkworms themselves can produce airborne allergens (see page 211).

Sugarberries or hackberries *(Celtis)*
June through October
Produces particularly strong allergens. Occurs in woodland, especially on limestone, as in parts of Jamaica. Belongs to the elm family, so may cross-react with elm pollen.

Pellitory-of-the-wall
(Parietaria judaica)
December through August
A weed of open habitats that also grows in crevices in banks and walls. Found at altitudes up to 4000 feet (1,200 meters). A problem only in some localities.

Nettles *(Urtica)*
March through June
Some pollen is in the air at other times of year as well. A common weed on waste ground in lowland areas, especially around centers of population.

EUROPE

THE BALKANS AND TURKEY
Turkey, Bulgaria, Romania, and the countries of the former Yugoslavia. No data available for Albania.

Grasses (Gramineae and Poaceae)
May through September
Counts are highest in May and June for much of this region, falls sharply at the end of June, and is fairly low by mid-July. Rye is grown in Croatia, adding to the pollen count. In southern Bulgaria the

season may start at the end of April, but for northern Bulgaria the peak pollen season is in July.

Sedges and reeds, pollinating in April and May, may cross-react with grass pollen. Counts may be high near large lakes.

Birches *(Betula)*
April through May
Common only in Romania, Bulgaria, and other parts of the Balkans, but the species found in Turkey produces highly allergenic pollen.

Alder, hornbeam, hop-hornbeam, and hazel (*Alnus, Carpinus, Ostrya,* and *Corylus*)
February through May
The pollen counts for hazel can be fairly high in some areas. The hazel season in Turkey is largely over by April.

Olive trees *(Olea)*
May through June
Significant only in Turkey, mainly in coastal regions.

Poplars *(Populus)*
March through April
Considered an important allergen in the countries of the former Yugoslavia.

Ashes *(Fraxinus)*
March through April
Pollen counts can be high in parts of Turkey and on the Adriatic coast.

Cypresses (Cupressaceae)
March through May
Pollen counts can be high in Turkey, but the season ends in April.

Pines (Pinaceae)
April through July
The season is shorter in Turkey, from May to June, but counts are very high.

Oaks, beeches, and plane trees (*Quercus, Fagus* and *Platanus*)
April through May
Planes produce very high counts for a brief period in parts of Turkey.

Box elder or ash-leaved maple (*Acer negundo*)
March through May
A tree introduced from the U.S. that is found in parts of Turkey and produces highly allergenic pollen.

Horse chestnuts *(Aesculus)*
April through May
Gives some positive skin-prick tests among birch-sensitive patients in Scandinavia, and is reported as an allergen in Turkey. Pollen counts are moderate and may be high in the vicinity of the trees.

Tree heather *(Erica arborea)*
April through May, September through October
Produces highly allergenic pollen.

Plantains *(Plantago)*
May through August
Season does not start until June in Turkey. The pollen can be highly allergenic.

Lamb's-quarters or goosefoot and pigweeds (Chenopodiaceae and Amaranthaceae)
June through October
Peak pollen production is in August and September. An important source of allergenic pollen along the Bulgarian coast.

Pellitories *(Parietaria)*
May through August
Pollen counts are not particularly high except on the Romanian plains, along the Adriatic coast, and in parts of Croatia.

Mugwort and wormwoods *(Artemisia)*
July through September

Close relatives of the U.S. sagebrush species. Common allergens in Romania and Bulgaria, not particularly important elsewhere.

Docks and sorrels *(Rumex)*
April through June

Pollen counts are generally low.

Nettles *(Urtica)*
March through August

Not a particularly important allergen. Counts can be high in Bulgaria.

Ragweeds *(Ambrosia)*
August through September

Recorded in Bulgaria, along the Adriatic coast, and in much of Croatia, where the pollen count is steadily rising.

NORTHERN AND EASTERN EUROPE

This includes northern France, Belgium, Luxembourg, the Netherlands, Germany, Switzerland, Austria, Hungary, Slovakia, the Czech Republic, and Poland.

Grasses (Gramineae or Poaceae)
April through September

The most important allergenic pollen throughout this region. As well as wild and cultivated grasses, fields of rye contribute to the pollen count in Germany, Austria, and eastern Europe.

The season is much shorter in the west and north of this region, ending in July. The Rouen area, for example, has very high grass pollen counts from April through June. In Belgium and the Netherlands the grass pollen season is later, from mid-May through mid-July. In the west of Germany it runs from May through July. In central France, central Germany, Austria, and eastern Europe the grass season

is long, from May through to September, although counts are fairly low after mid-August. Hungary has a relatively short season, from May through mid-July. At high altitudes, the pollen season generally runs from June through July.

Counts are lower on the west coast of France and near the Brittany coast; in forest areas, notably the Black Forest, and in the high Alps. They are high in the upper Loire valley in June and on the north German plain from June through early July. Reeds and sedges can provoke cross-reactions in those sensitive to grass pollen, and areas with many reeds, such as Lakes Balaton and Velencei in Hungary, can provoke severe symptoms; the reed pollination season is from April through early July.

Birches *(Betula)*
April through May

The season can begin earlier, during March, in eastern Europe. In western Germany it runs from mid-March through June, with the peak in late April and early May. Mountainous areas generally begin one to three weeks later than nearby lowlands.

High counts occur in Belgium, Luxembourg, Austria, and parts of northern Germany, but not in France, except around Paris and to the east of Paris.

Alder, hornbeam, and hazel
(*Alnus, Carpinus,* and *Corylus*)
February through May

Peak pollen production is in March and April. Hazel can begin pollinating in January.

Oaks and beeches (*Quercus* and *Fagus*)
April through June

The pollen count peaks in May. Beech pollen is highest in eastern France. Oak pollen can be high in central Germany and the eastern lowlands of Austria.

Chestnuts (Castanea)
June through July
Those sensitive to this pollen usually react to birch pollen as well. Chestnuts are common in France, particularly around Paris, but counts are relatively low. They can be high in the south and east of Austria.

Plane trees (Platanus)
March through May
Widely planted on city streets. There is a high count for planes in Paris, usually from late March and ending in early May; similarly in some Swiss and Austrian cities, from April through May. Not a particularly common cause of hay fever.

Ashes (Fraxinus)
April through May
Not a particularly strong allergen, but those already allergic to olive pollen may be sensitive to it through cross-reaction.

Cypresses (Cupressaceae)
February through May
Peak is in March and April. Not considered a cause of hay fever in this region, but might affect visitors sensitized elsewhere. Pollen counts are low in the north, higher in the south.

Yew (Taxus)
March through April
Causes some hay fever in northern Switzerland and northern Austria, but not elsewhere in this region nor in most other parts of the world.

Pines (Pinaceae)
April through July
The season is shorter in the north and in central and eastern Europe: from May through June. In Switzerland it is longer, continuing into August. Pollen counts are especially high in the Black Forest. Not considered a cause of hay fever anywhere in this region, but might affect visitors sensitized elsewhere.

Mugwort and wormwoods (Artemisia)
July through September
The main pollen season is in August. Could affect U.S. visitors sensitized to sagebrush because they are closely related.

Plantains (Plantago)
May through September
A long flowering season, but pollen counts are never particularly high. The maximum levels occur in July. Fairly common as a cause of hay fever in Belgium and parts of Austria.

Pellitories (Parietaria)
May through September
The season starts later in the north, usually in June. Widespread in France, Slovakia, the Czech Republic, Austria, and Hungary, but found only in certain localities in the other countries making up this area. Abundant along the banks of the Danube.

Docks and sorrels (Rumex)
May through August
Counts are generally low after the end of June, so sensitivity to docks and sorrels may be mistaken for grass-pollen hay fever. There is less pollen in the air in the north of the region. Docks are considered an important allergen in Poland.

Nettles (Urtica)
June through September
Very high pollen counts have been recorded in some areas (e.g., Belgium), yet this is not a common cause of hay fever. The season is earlier in central Germany and Austria, from mid-May through to the end of August.

Ragweeds (Ambrosia)
August through September

Grows significantly only in Switzerland, around the lakes of northern Italy, and in the east of Austria, from Vienna to the Hungarian border. May be spreading into the upper Rhône valley from the Lyon area. In eastern Europe, ragweeds are an increasing problem (see page 130).

Lamb's-quarters or goosefoot and pigweeds (Chenopodiaceae and Amaranthaceae)
May through October

The main pollen season is from June through September. Various species grow widely. There is relatively little airborne pollen in most areas, though significant amounts have been found in northeastern France and eastern Europe. Not considered a common cause of hay fever in this region, but could well affect North American visitors who are already sensitized to it.

SCANDINAVIA

This area comprises Finland, Sweden, Norway, and Denmark.

Grasses (Gramineae or Poaceae)
May through August

A more common cause of hay fever than birch in some parts of Scandinavia, but grasses rank second in the northern and central areas, where the grass season is shorter (mid-June through mid-August) and pollen counts are low.

Birches (Betula)
April through June

The main season, for most of Scandinavia, is during May and early June. The season begins earlier in Denmark (mid-April through early June). South and central Finland experience birch pollen from April through May. In the far north the season begins in late May and continues into July. Counts are lower here than elsewhere. The highest counts are in central Norway and Sweden, and central and southern Finland.

Birch is one of the trees that produces varied amounts of pollen year to year.

Alder and hazel (Alnus and Corylus)
April through May

In the past, the hazel pollen season in Norway, Sweden, and Finland has been short, beginning in late April. With milder winters in recent years, hazel has begun to release pollen in January and February around Oslo and in the south. This has had a noticeable priming effect (see pages 38–39) on those with birch pollen sensitivity.

In Denmark, hazel pollinates from January or February. Northern Scandinavia has very low pollen counts for hazel.

The alder season has also been getting longer, due to warmer weather. It begins earlier in Denmark, from mid-February or early March. Pollen counts are moderate in most areas, very low in the far north.

Horse chestnuts (Aesculus)
May through June

Gives some positive skin-prick tests among birch-sensitive patients in Scandinavia, and is reported as an allergen in Turkey. Pollen counts are moderate and may be high in the vicinity of the trees.

Oaks (Quercus)
May through June

Significant pollen counts are found in southeastern Sweden and Denmark only.

Ashes (Fraxinus)
May

Only in the south of the region.

Elms *(Ulmus)*
March through May
Cross-reactions with birch may occur.

Pines *(Pinaceae)*
May through July
Only Denmark is likely to have appreciable amounts of pollen in the air before mid-May.

Cypresses (Cupressaceae)
May through July
Low pollen counts in most areas, peaking in June. Not observed in Denmark, but junipers (which cross-react with cypresses) pollinate from March through June.

Sweet gale or bog myrtle (Myrica gale)
April through May
Cross-reacts with birch pollen.

Mugwort and wormwoods *(Artemisia)*
July through September
Rarely begin pollination before mid-July and peak in August. Pollen counts are highest in Denmark and around the Oslo fjord region, but low in central and northern Scandinavia. Could affect U.S. visitors sensitized to sagebrush because they are closely related.

Nettles *(Urtica)*
June through August
The season begins earlier in Denmark and continues into September. Pollen counts are very low in central and northern Scandinavia.

Docks and plantains (Rumex and Plantago)
June through August
Pollen counts are low in most areas, but dock pollen reaches moderate levels in central Scandinavia.

Grasses (Gramineae or Poaceae)
April through June
Although the highest counts are in the spring and early summer, there can be some airborne pollen all year round in the warmest areas. Portugal has significant counts from late March through to early September.

On the Costa del Sol, the main season begins at the end of April. The rest of Andalusia and the Madrid area follow in May. There are a great many variations due to weather. Dry winters delay the season; wet ones hasten it.

In general, pollen counts inland are higher than those near the coast.

Olive trees *(Olea)*
May through June
There is considerable variation in the pollen count from one year to another.

The season begins much earlier in Portugal—in March. It is early on the Costa del Sol and in the southwest, later in the northeast. In the warmest areas, pollen is the heaviest in the last week of May.

Few olives are grown in the north; main growing regions are Portugal, Andalusia, Catalonia, and central Spain.

Cypresses (Cupressaceae)
January through March
Although pollen peaks in early spring, there is some in the air almost all year. In the south, peak season starts in February.

Birches *(Betula)*
April
Common only in the mountainous areas of northern Spain. Where it does occur, birch is an important allergen.

Alders *(Alnus)*
February through March
Common only alongside rivers and in the mountains. The pollen counts are usually low.

She-oak or "Australian pine" *(Casuarina)*
October through November
Pollen counts can be quite high wherever this tree has been planted. It could affect sensitized visitors from California or Florida. The season is two or three weeks earlier on the Costa del Sol.

Plane trees *(Platanus)*
March, April, or May
The season is short, only about a week. It occurs in March in the south, as late as June in the far northwest or the high mountains. A very common street tree, so pollen counts can be high.

Oaks *(Quercus)*
March through June
There are large areas of oak that produce high pollen counts. Not a particularly allergenic pollen.

Ashes *(Fraxinus)*
February through May
Common alongside rivers, mainly in Castille, around Madrid, and in the north. Cross-reacts with olive pollen, so it may cause symptoms in those sensitized to olive.

Pines *(Pinaceae)*
March through July
A rare cause of hay fever in Spain, but could affect North American visitors already sensitized.

Eucalyptus or gum tree *(Eucalyptus)*
May through June
Some pollen in the air year round. Not a powerful allergen; no cases of hay fever have so far been recorded in Spain, but it could affect visitors from California or Hawaii who are already sensitized.

Sunflower *(Helianthus)*
June through August
Although sunflowers pollinate from June to July, many people experience symptoms during the harvest period in August. The reason for this is unknown. Mainly grown in southern Spain. People living near sunflower fields may be sensitized. Can cross-react with ragweed.

Lamb's-quarters or goosefoot and pigweeds (Chenopodiaceae and Amaranthaceae)
May through September
Among the most important allergenic weeds in this region, mainly in the driest areas. There may be some pollen in the air year round, but the peak is in summer. In southern Spain, the peak comes in May and June; in central and northern Spain, in July and August. The season is generally shorter in Portugal, running only from July through August.

Pellitories *(Parietaria)*
March through May or May through July
The season varies, depending on which species grow locally. Pellitories are not a common cause of hay fever here, but are in other Mediterranean countries. It seems that the local species produce less pollen that is less allergenic. Pellitory hay fever is common only in Catalonia. May affect U.S. visitors already sensitized.

Nettles *(Urtica)*
May through July
Common weeds throughout the region, causing some hay fever.

Mugwort and wormwoods *(Artemisia)*
August through September
Close relatives of the U.S. sagebrush spe-

cies. Very common in drier areas and in the mountains of the south, southeast, east, and center of the Iberian peninsula.

Plantains *(Plantago)*
March through June
The season begins first on the Costa del Sol, later in Catalonia, and not until May in the center and south.

INDIA AND PAKISTAN

During the monsoon rains, the air is practically free of pollen. The period immediately afterward sees very high pollen counts for most plants, including grasses. This continues for about two months, then the grass pollen count declines for about two months, followed by a period with low or moderate pollen counts. This is a very generalized picture. The monsoon seasons vary from north to south and within particular regions, so the grass pollen season will also be variable. Try to find out the timing of the rainy season in the area you plan to visit, and avoid the months immediately after this. For most of the subcontinent, excluding the far south, the period from February through April will have the lowest pollen counts.

There are many other plants that cause hay fever in India, such as mesquite *(Prosopis)* and American feverfew *(Parthenium)*. The latter cross-reacts with ragweed but, curiously, is not thought to be a significant cause of hay fever in its own right in the U.S.

JAPAN

Grasses (Gramineae or Poaceae)
April through June
Many hay fever sufferers reacting to grasses are also sensitive to Japanese red cedar.

Although grass pollen can continue into September, the pollen counts are low after June. The season begins later in the north and at higher altitudes.

Highest pollen counts are in the central areas such as Matsukawa where there are extensive apple orchards.

Japanese red cedar or "sugi" *(Cryptomeria japonica)*
February through April
More than 90 percent of patients with hay fever in Japan are allergic to Japanese red cedar. This tree is also grown in parts of California, so some U.S. visitors may already be sensitized. Visitors may also be affected if they are already allergic to cypress (Cupressaceae) pollen due to cross-reaction between these pollens. Reactions to Japanese red cedar seem to be considerably worse in towns and along roads with serious air pollution.

The main pollination period for Tokyo and surrounding areas is in February and March. The season begins later farther north and at higher altitudes.

The tree is native to the northern part of Honshu, the main island. It grows in forests between 730 and 1320 feet (220 and 400 meters) above sea level, sometimes alone, sometimes mixed with cypresses. Elsewhere it is grown in plantations for timber. A very beautiful conifer with glossy green foliage, it is also widely grown in gardens, palaces, and sanctuaries, providing a source of pollen within towns.

The amount of pollen produced varies enormously from year to year. Patients who are not particularly sensitive may be free from symptoms in low-pollen years.

Cypresses (Cupressaceae)
March through April
Cypresses grow wild, particularly in the mountains. They are also cultivated

widely in gardens, and are grown as bonsai, or miniature trees. Since bonsai trees are brought indoors for special occasions, cypress pollen can be liberated in the home itself.

Those sensitive to cypress may be allergic to Japanese red cedar as well.

The season usually ends in early April but sometimes continues to late April. The amount of pollen produced varies greatly from one year to another.

Birches (Betula)
February through May
The season does not usually begin until late February. Pollen production is prolific and the pollen spreads widely, but a relatively small proportion of hay fever sufferers are affected.

Birches grow mostly in mountain valleys in light woodland. They also border coniferous forests along the tree line at high altitudes.

Alders (Alnus)
March through April
Alders have recently been identified as a cause of hay fever in Japan. A large number of cases of alder hay fever are found close to alder plantations. Cross-reactions between birches and alders are known to occur.

Ragweeds (Ambrosia)
July through August
The season does not usually begin until late July. Introduced from America about a hundred years ago and now widespread in open habitats.

Mugwort (Artemisia)
July through September
This pollen does not spread widely, so it causes only localized problems in areas where mugwort grows. Could affect U.S.

visitors sensitized to sagebrush because they are closely related.

Hops (Humulus)
July through August
Localized in lowland areas, so a relatively rare cause of hay fever. Hops and hemp (cannabis) belong to the same plant family, and there are occasional reports, from various parts of the world, of hay fever reactions to their pollen.

Lamb's-quarters or goosefoot, plantains, and nettles (Chenopodiaceae, Plantago, and Urtica)
August through September
Widespread weeds of open habitats, but pollen does not spread far. Reactions to them are relatively rare in Japan, but they could cause problems for visitors from abroad.

THE MEDITERRANEAN

Southern France, Italy, Greece, and the Mediterranean islands. For northeastern Greece, the information for Turkey and the Balkans may be more relevant.

Grasses (Gramineae or Poaceae)
April through September
The season is much shorter in Greece, from mid-April to June. Throughout the region, grass pollen counts are much lower than in northern Europe, particularly in hot dry areas, where they may be insufficient to provoke hay fever. Sicily and the Greek islands have low counts, as do the Bordeaux region, Calabria, and the Adriatic coast of Italy.

A few species of grass flower in winter in Greece and might cause problems in some areas.

Olive trees (Olea)
March through July
Peak pollination is in May and June. In southern France and southern Italy, the season starts in late April or early May.

Cypresses (Cupressaceae)
December through June
The season is earlier in Italy and Greece and along the Mediterranean coast of France (December or January to May). It is later (February to June) in inland areas of southern France. Cypress hay fever is rising rapidly in southern France, where many cypresses have been planted to protect crops and fruit trees from the wind.

Birches (Betula)
April through May
Pollen counts are generally low. Significant only in mountainous areas of France and northern Italy.

Alder and hazel (*Alnus* and *Corylus*)
January through May
The season begins in January only on the Mediterranean coast. Pollen counts can be quite high in northern and central Italy; elsewhere they are very low.

Pines (Pinaceae)
March through July
Pollen counts are not particularly high, yet there are isolated cases of pine allergy reported. Could affect North American visitors sensitized to pine.

Oaks (Quercus)
April through June
Not a major source of hay fever.

Chestnuts (Castanea)
June through July
Common only in southern France and northern and central Italy, where they may cause some hay fever.

Mimosas (Acacia)
February through May
Important only in the area around Nice.

Poplars (Populus)
March through April
Grown for shade in some parts of Greece and may cause hay fever.

Paper mulberry (Broussonetia papyrifera)
April through May
Grown only in southeastern France.

Pellitories (Parietaria)
March through July, September through November
This very long season, with a lull in midsummer, is typical of southern Italy only. In Sicily, there may be some pollen in the air year round. In Greece, the hot dry climate keeps the season shorter, from April to June, with low levels continuing until September. In central and northern Italy and in southern France, the season is from April to October, beginning later in the north.

Nettles (Urtica)
April through June
Some pollen in the air all year round.

Docks and sorrels (Rumex)
April through September
Moderate amounts are found in the air in southern France and northern Italy, but not elsewhere in this region.

Plantains (Plantago)
May through September
Pollen counts are negligible in Greece.

Mugwort and wormwoods (Artemisia)
August through October
Close relatives of the U.S. sagebrush species. Pollen counts are fairly low everywhere, especially in the far south.

Lamb's-quarters or goosefoot, pigweeds, and Russian Thistle (Chenopodiaceae and Amaranthaceae)
May through October
Russian thistle is a common cause of hay fever in some areas.

Ragweeds *(Ambrosia)*
August through September
The season may start in mid-July in northern Italy. It continues into October in parts of Italy. Ragweed pollen is particularly abundant in the Rhône valley, around Lyon, and around the lakes of northern Italy.

THE MIDDLE EAST

In most of the area, desert conditions prevail and pollen counts are very low, especially from July through January. What pollen there is becomes airborne in April. Where there are extensive tree plantations, as in Saudi Arabia, the pollen may cause hay fever. Grass pollen is found in Israel, Lebanon, and the western regions of Jordan and Syria. The season runs from March through May, continuing into June in parts of Israel. The same regions have olive *(Olea)* pollen in May and June and some mugwort-sagebrush *(Artemisia)* from August through October. Goosefoot (Chenopodiaceae) is widespread on dry soils, particularly Russian thistle *(Salsol kali)*, which is a common source of symptoms in parts of Iran. Cypress (Cupressaceae) pollinates in winter, continuing into February, and is an increasing cause of hay fever. Rural areas in Israel growing irrigated crops produce very high pollen counts (see page 52) and hay fever is a serious problem. Australian she-oak *(Casuarina)* and wattle *(Acacia)* are planted for shelter and have been impli-

cated in hay fever. Both have been planted in California and Florida too, and some U.S. visitors may be sensitized.

NEW ZEALAND

Grasses (Gramineae or Poaceae)
October through February
Grasses are the largest pollen producers and the major cause of springtime hay fever.

The grass pollen season starts earlier in the north than in the south, with a four-week difference between the northern end of North Island and the southern end of South Island. The season ends earlier in the far south, so it is two months shorter there.

There is a lot of variation in concentration from place to place. Cities and large towns are often surrounded by grazing lands, and therefore experience higher concentrations of grass pollen. The pollen counts are highest in inland pastoral areas, where seasons can be severe. Concentrations are lower in coastal areas.

Wattles and mimosas *(Acacia* and *Albizia)*
August through November
These are potent allergens, but the pollen concentration is high only in the immediate vicinity of the trees.

Birches *(Betula)*
August through October
Introduced from Europe, and therefore found only in a few areas. Produces pollen abundantly, so these localized pockets can cause problems for sensitized people.

Cypresses (Cupressaceae)
July through November
Only a small percentage of New Zealanders react to this pollen, but some North American visitors may be sensitized already and suffer symptoms. Prob-

lems occur mainly in drier areas if people live near dense banks of cypresses.

Oaks *(Quercus)*
August through October
Introduced from Europe, and therefore found only in a few areas. These localized pockets can cause problems for a few sensitized people.

Pines (Pinaceae)
July through October
Huge amounts of pine pollen come from forestry plantations of *Pinus radiata*. The pollen is not highly allergenic, and only a small proportion of patients with hay fever and asthma are genuinely allergic to it. However, by virtue of its size, quantity, and certain chemicals carried on the pollen wall, this particular pine pollen may cause some irritation in the nose if a very large amount is inhaled. The reaction is not an allergic one.

Visitors from New England who are genuinely allergic to *Pinus strobus* (see page 292) might suffer symptoms from irritation, allergy, or both.

Privet *(Ligustrum)*
October through March
Produces plenty of pollen, but most of it does not travel far. Can cross-react with olive pollen, a much more strongly allergeric pollen.

Docks *(Rumex)*
January through March
Not a very heavy pollen producer. Dock is a common weed, and while relatively few people react to it, those who do tend to react vigorously.

Plantains *(Plantago)*
October through February
Only small amounts of pollen are produced, but the pollen is very allergenic.

SOUTH AMERICA

Pollen information for South America is very limited, but some educated guesses can be made on the basis of the seasonal weather patterns and type of vegetation.

In countries north of the Equator there will be a grass pollen season from April through July, peaking in May. The coastal plain of Venezuela may have some grass pollen in the air year round.

In northern Brazil there are reports of an increase in the amount of grass pollen in some areas due to the replacement of the rain forest by pastureland, causing hay fever from October through December. Around Rio de Janeiro there may be grass pollen in the air year round, with the highest concentrations likely to occur from December through March, the lowest from June through October.

Ecuador has sufficient warmth and moisture to encourage grass pollen year round. For Peru, the peak counts for grass occur from October through January, with low counts from February through June.

Buenos Aires has the right conditions for grass growth year round, with peak production likely to occur from October through February. It is reported from Argentina that reaction to hackberry *(Celtis)* is very common; this pollen may cross-react with that of elm.

UNITED STATES

ALASKA

Grasses and sedges (Gramineae and Poaceae; *Carex*)
May through early September
Peak pollen counts occur early on and pass quickly. The humidity and high rainfall on the tundra take most of the pollen out of the air rapidly. There will

be higher counts in the temperate agricultural and urban regions. Counts are generally low in forested areas, although there may be grasses and sedges along streams and where forests have been felled and are regenerating.

Birches *(Betula)*
May through June
The peak is in April. The most important source of tree-pollen hay fever. Pollen counts can be very high due to extensive areas of birch/spruce forest.

Alders *(Alnus)*
April through May
Can cross-react with birch. Common in mountain regions alongside streams.

Poplars, aspens, and willows (*Populus* and *Salix*)
April through May
Found throughout the forest regions, especially alongside streams and in areas of regenerating forest.

Lamb's-quarters or goosefoot (*Chenopodium*)
August through September
Only in the south, and pollen counts are generally low. Can cross-react with several other plants (see page 160) and may affect visitors sensitized elsewhere.

Sagebrush or wormwoods *(Artemisia)*
August through September
Mainly in the temperate agricultural regions. Will affect visitors from farther south sensitized to other *Artemisia* species. Can also cross-react with ragweed (see page 160).

Bulrush *(Scirpus)*
August through September
Around lakes and streams. Pollen counts can be high locally.

Plantains *(Plantago)*
August through September
Mainly in the temperate agricultural regions.

Docks and sorrels *(Rumex)*
August through September
Only in the south, and pollen counts are generally low.

Nettles *(Urtica)*
August through September
Only around settlements, and pollen counts are generally low.

Spearscale *(Atriplex)*
August through September
Mainly in the temperate agricultural regions. Will probably affect those sensitized to other *Atriplex* species and related plants (see page 159).

ARIZONA AND NEW MEXICO

Irrigation in Arizona, particularly in gardens, has allowed a greater variety of plants to be grown. As in Israel, irrigated plants in a dry area can produce very high pollen counts. The number of allergenic pollens in the air has increased considerably in the past sixty years.

Grasses (Gramineae or Poaceae)
February through November
In New Mexico the season is a little shorter, from April through September.

Cypresses, junipers, and "cedars" (Cupressaceae)
September through March
Pinchot junipers produce pollen from September through November, other species from December through March.

Olive trees *(Olea)*
May through June
Introduced from the Mediterranean re-

gion. Can cause problems where grown as a crop.

Ashes *(Fraxinus)*
February through March
An important cause of hay fever in Arizona. Olive pollen can cross-react with that of ash, making sensitivity to ash more likely in areas where olives are grown.

Mesquite *(Prosopis)*
May through July
Could provoke cross-reactions in anyone allergic to wattle *(Acacia).*

Sagebrush *(Artemisia)*
July through September
A common cause of hay fever. Cross-reacts with mugwort and wormwood.

Ragweeds and bur ragweed *(Ambrosia* and *Franseria)*
August through September
Cross-reactions can occur between these two closely related groups. Certain species of ragweed flower during the winter in parts of Arizona.

Lamb's-quarters or goosefoot and pigweeds (Chenopodiaceae and Amaranthaceae)
April through October
Several species are known locally as pigweeds and saltbushes. Most are moderate allergens, but Mexican tea *(Chenopodium ambrosioides)* and Russian thistle *(Salsola kali)* are both potent allergens, and cross-reactions with other species are common. Russian thistle flowers from July through October.

Docks and sorrels *(Rumex)*
March through September
Pollination coincides with the peak period for grass, so hay fever caused by these plants is easily mistaken for grass-pollen hay fever.

CALIFORNIA

Grasses (Gramineae or Poaceae)
April through October
The season peaks in May and June in the south and during June and July in the north, where it ends by the end of September. Parts of southern California have some grass pollen in the air all year round.

The highest pollen counts occur inland and up to the middle slopes of the mountains.

Cypresses, junipers, and "cedars" (Cupressaceae)
September through March
The peak is from January through March. One species pollinates later, in April and May. A moderately common cause of hay fever, as in other warm dry climates.

Poplars *(Populus)*
April through May
Balsam poplar and quaking aspen *(Populus balsamifera* and *P. tremuloides)* both grow in this region and are more allergenic than other poplars.

Alders and birches *(Alnus* and *Betula)*
December through May
Alders are found at higher altitudes in the north of the state. They pollinate first, from December through February, with lower counts continuing into April. Birches pollinate from April through May. Cross-reactions between the two are common.

Oaks *(Quercus)*
February through April
In the south, flowering ends in March; in the north it does not begin until March and continues into April. Local species of oak are considered highly allergenic.

She-oak or "Australian pine" (Casuarina)
February through May, September through November

Seasons are variable. An Australian tree planted as a windbreak and for erosion control, and a cause of some hay fever as the pollen is highly allergenic. Neither an oak nor a pine, so cross-reactions with these trees are unlikely.

Walnuts, pecans, and hickories (Juglans and Carya)
March through May

Where cultivated, these produce high pollen counts causing many cases of hay fever, but the pollen does not travel far.

Olive trees (Olea)
May through June

Can cause problems where grown as a crop.

Ashes (Fraxinus)
February through April

The season ends in March in the south, just as the season in the north is beginning. May affect those already sensitized by olive pollen due to a cross-reaction.

Elms (Ulmus)
February through April, August through October

In southern California, the species of elm that flower in autumn (*Ulmus crassifolia, U. serotina,* and *U. parvifolia*) are important allergens. The season for these trees can sometimes continue to November. Cross-reactions with hackberry *(Celtis)* are likely.

Japanese red cedar (Cryptomeria)
March through April

Planted for landscaping and windbreaks and a potential source of hay fever locally. May cross-react with cypress; see page 284.

Paper mulberry and mulberries (Broussonetia and Morus)
March through May

Paper mulberry produces highly allergenic pollen that tends to strongly affect the eyes. Cases of hay fever from these have been reported in southern California. The two groups are related and will cross-react.

Maples (Acer)
March through May

Considered a fairly common cause of hay fever. The most allergenic maple, box elder or ash-leaved maple *(Acer negundo),* grows in parts of California.

Palms (Arecaceae)
June through December

Those affected are mainly people pollinating the palms or living on streets where palms are planted.

Gum trees (Eucalyptus)
December through March

Introduced from Australia. A rare cause of hay fever there but does affect some from California. Those sensitized will be affected by *Eucalyptus* if visiting Australia or southern Europe, where the trees are also planted widely.

Wattles and acacia (Acacia)
January through October

Widely planted as ornamental shrubs and trees. Pollen counts are high only close to where the plants are growing. May cause cross-reactions with mesquite, which belongs to the same family.

Mesquite (Prosopis)
May through July

Found in the southeast and thought to cause some hay fever.

Privet (Ligustrum)
March through June

Produces plenty of pollen, but most of it does not travel far. Only a modest allergen, and the number of people affected is small. Those affected have often been sensitized by olive pollen, which cross-reacts with privet.

Bayberry or wax myrtle (Myrica)
February through May

The south sees flowering during February and March, the north from April through May. A moderately strong allergen affecting a few hay fever patients. Note that this is the same genus as the sweet gale of Canada, Scandinavia, and parts of Britain (where it is called bog myrtle). Cross-reactions may occur.

Ragweeds (Ambrosia)
April through December

There may be some pollen in the air year round from ragweed (see page 159) or from closely related plants that cross-react with it. However, pollen counts are generally low.

Poverty weeds and marsh elders (Iva)
August through November

These cross-react with ragweed pollen and are common in some areas.

Lamb's-quarters or goosefoot, pig-weeds, and careless weed (Chenopodiaceae and Amaranthaceae)
April through December

The pollen levels are fairly high from June onward in southern California and remain so until late November.

Plantains (Plantago)
May through November

The pollen peak coincides with the grass pollen season in many areas.

Docks and sorrels (Rumex)
All year

The peak pollen season is from March through August.

Sagebrush (Artemisia)
July through September

A powerful allergen. Will cross-react with mugwort.

Nettles (Urtica)
January through September

The cause of some hay fever in southern California.

Pellitories (Parietaria)
February through July

Found in some parts and may affect visitors sensitized elsewhere.

HAWAII

It may be small in terms of total land area, but Hawaii has a staggering array of different habitats, so the vegetation is very diverse and can change markedly in a short distance. Introduced plants from all over the world add to the diversity, and hay fever sufferers visiting these islands stand a good chance of being ambushed by their culprit pollen. However, pollen counts vary greatly from one island to another, and within the islands.

Hay fever seasons are not clear-cut because there is an almost continuous growing season in most areas. Grasses and weeds may be flowering all year round, though there tend to be peak periods. All the pollen seasons given should be regarded as a very general guide only.

Grasses (Gramineae and Poaceae)
All year

There is generally less pollen in the air in late December. In addition to native grasses, there are about 500 species of grasses introduced from elsewhere in the world.

Japanese red cedar *(Cryptomeria)*
January through April

A potent allergen. Planted (most unwisely) for landscaping and windbreaks. Will affect sensitized visitors from Japan and a few from California and Florida, where it has also been introduced.

Gum trees *(Eucalyptus)*
January through April

Not a common source of hay fever in Australia, where it originates but, curiously, it seems to sensitize quite a few Hawaiians. Visitors from California who are already sensitized will also be affected.

She-oak, "Australian pine," or beefwood *(Casuarina)*
January through April

A powerfully allergenic tree that should not be planted, but is frequently used as a windbreak. Visitors from California and Florida may already be sensitized.

Wattles *(Acacia)*
January through April

Cross-reacts with cultivated mimosa, an occupational allergen for some flower pickers. Also grown as an ornamental in warmer areas of North America; a few visitors from California and Florida may already be sensitized.

Cypresses and junipers (Cupressaceae)
No defined pollen season

Visitors from some western parts of the United States and Canada may already be sensitized.

Date palms *(Phoenix dactylifera)*
Pollen season unknown

There might be cross-reactions with other species of palm.

Mesquite *(Prosopis)*
Pollen season unknown

Some visitors from the southern United States may already be sensitized.

Paper mulberry *(Broussonetia papyrifera)*
January through April

A particularly potent allergen. Visitors from warmer areas of the United States may be sensitized already.

Olive trees *(Olea)*
March through July

Quite a powerful allergen. Those sensitized may also react to privet *(Ligustrum)*.

Ragweeds *(Ambrosia)*
Mid-May through December

An unfortunate introduction from the mainland United States. Found chiefly on disturbed ground.

Saltbush/Scale *(Atriplex)*
Mid-May through December

Will affect North American visitors already sensitized.

Sagebrush, pigweeds, and plantains *(Artemisia, Amaranthus,* and *Plantago)*
Mid-May through December

Pollen counts are generally low but could be higher in some areas.

KENTUCKY AND TENNESSEE

Grasses (Gramineae and Poaceae)
May through August

The season is longer in Tennessee, continuing until early December in the south.

"Cedars" and junipers (Cupressaceae)
January through March

These cross-react with cypress pollen.

Maples *(Acer)*
February through March
Box elder or ash-leaved maple *(Acer negundo)*, the most powerfully allergenic of the maples, is plentiful in this region.

Willows *(Salix)*
March through April
Moderate allergen. Can cross-react with poplar.

Oaks *(Quercus)*
April through May
Moderate allergen. Can cross-react with birch.

Ragweeds *(Ambrosia)*
August through October
The most important allergenic pollen in this region.

Wormwoods *(Artemisia)*
August through October
Will cross-react with mugwort and sagebrush. Particularly common in Tennessee.

Docks and sorrels *(Rumex)*
April through September
The peak season is from May to August.

Plantains *(Plantago)*
May through November
Only small amounts of pollen are produced, but the pollen is very allergenic.

THE MIDWEST
This area comprises Iowa, Indiana, Minnesota, Michigan, North and South Dakota, Nebraska, and Wisconsin.

Grasses *(Gramineae or Poaceae)*
May through July
Begins in early May in the south, late May in the north. The season ends earlier in the east.

Maples *(Acer)*
April through May
The main allergen is the pollen of the box elder or ash-leaved maple *(Acer negundo)*.

Birches *(Betula)*
April through May
Powerful allergens that cross-react with several other trees, notably alder, hazel, hornbeam, and oak. More common in the north of this region.

Hazel, ironwood, hornbeam, and alders *(Corylus, Carpinus, Ostrya,* and *Alnus)*
February through April
Can provoke cross-reactions in those sensitive to birch.

Elms *(Ulmus)*
March through April
Can cross-react with hackberry and sugarberry *(Celtis)*, which belong to the same family (Ulmaceae).

Oaks *(Quercus)*
April through May
Can cross-react with birch.

Willows and poplars *(Salix* and *Populus)*
March through April
Moderate allergens. Most common in the Great Lakes region and northern Minnesota. Balsam poplar and quaking aspen *(Populus balsamifera* and *P. tremuloides)*, both noted allergens, are found in this area.

Ashes *(Fraxinus)*
April or May
The season is during April in the south of the region, during May in the north. Moderate allergens, most likely to provoke reactions in those already sensitized to olive pollen.

Privet *(Ligustrum)*
May through June
Produces plenty of pollen, but most of it does not travel far. Only a modest allergen, and the number of people affected is small. Those

affected have often been sensitized by olive pollen, which cross-reacts with privet.

Ragweeds (Ambrosia)
July through October
The most important allergen in the region. There are many related plants that can cross-react with ragweed allergens, including bur ragweed (Franseria) and marsh elders (Iva), both of which flower at about the same time.

Nettles and clearweed (Urtica and Pilea)
July through September
The season continues into October in the west of the region. Only moderately allergenic.

Pellitories (Parietaria)
July through September
Not reported as a common source of hay fever in this area, but may affect visitors sensitized elsewhere.

Docks and sorrels (Rumex)
May through September
The peak season usually coincides with that of grass. Mainly found in the east of the region.

Plantains (Plantago)
May through November
Very little is found in the west of this region but counts can be high in the east, particularly in July.

Hemp or cannabis (Cannabis sativa)
June through September
A fairly common cause of hay fever in Nebraska and the Dakotas.

Lamb's-quarters or goosefoot and pigweeds (Chenopodiaceae and Amaranthaceae)
June through October
Local names for these plants include sowbane.

MONTANA, IDAHO, AND WYOMING

Grasses (Gramineae and Poaceae)
May through September
The season is much shorter in Wyoming (ends in late July) and Montana (ends in June).

Birches (Betula)
April through May
An important allergenic pollen.

Willows and poplars (Salix and Populus)
March through May
Most species finish pollinating by the end of April. Two of the more allergenic poplars, quaking aspen and balsam poplar (Populus tremuloides and P. balsamifera), grow here; both flower from April through May.

Oaks (Quercus)
April through May
Can cross-react with birch and related trees.

Cypresses (Cupressaceae)
January through February
May cause some hay fever locally and could affect those sensitized elsewhere.

Ragweeds (Ambrosia)
August through September
The most important allergenic pollen.

Docks, sorrels, and plantains (Rumex and Plantago)
May through November
Docks and sorrels stop pollinating earlier, by the end of September.

Lamb's-quarters or goosefoot and pigweeds (Chenopodiaceae and Amaranthaceae)
June through October
Pigweeds are generally of the family Amaranthaceae but the name "pigweed" may also be applied to some species of goosefoot. Burning bush (Kochia scoparia),

which grows in dry places, also belongs to this group; its pollen is a potent allergen. "Russian thistle" *(Salsola kali)* is common in Idaho and is likewise a powerful allergen. Smotherweed *(Bassia)* and greasewood *(Sarcobatus)*, found growing locally, are also members of this group. Cross-reactions are common among plants of this group (see page 159).

Sagebrush *(Artemisia)*
August through September
Considered an important allergen in Idaho.

Alders, ironwoods, hornbeams, and hazels *(Alnus, Ostrya, Carpinus, and Corylus)*
February through April
Can cross-react with birch, producing symptoms before birch begins to pollinate. Hazel pollen declines in March, and alder pollen in April. Hornbeam and ironwood flower from April to May.

NEVADA, UTAH, AND COLORADO

Grasses (Gramineae or Poaceae)
March through October
This very long season is seen only in the west of the zone. The season in Utah runs from May to July, while in much of Colorado it lasts from May to September. Pollen counts are low in dry areas, but irrigation greatly increases the amount produced. At high altitudes, where there is more rainfall, counts can be high.

Cypresses, junipers, and "cedars" (Cupressaceae)
January through March
The most important allergenic trees in the mountains.

Poplars *(Populus)*
April through May
Balsam poplar and quaking aspen *(Pop-*

ulus balsamifera and *P. tremuloides)*, two of the more allergenic poplars, both grow here. At high altitudes the season may start and end later.

Lamb's-quarters or goosefoot and pigweeds (Chenopodiaceae and Amaranthaceae)
June through October
These include various species known as pigweeds *(Chenopodium* and *Amaranthus)*, saltbush or orach *(Atriplex)*, smotherweed *(Bassia)*, greasewood *(Sarcobatus)* and "Russian thistle" *(Salsola kali)*. The last is a particularly potent sensitizer. Extensive cross-reactions occur among the plants of this group (see page 159), making them a widespread source of hay fever.

Ragweeds *(Ambrosia)*
August through September
Only Colorado has high pollen counts.

Pellitories *(Parietaria)*
July through September
The pollen of these plants is a potent sensitizer. Found growing on disturbed ground.

Docks and sorrels *(Rumex)*
May through September
Pollination coincides with the peak period for grass, so hay fever caused by these plants is easily mistaken for grass-pollen hay fever.

THE NORTHEAST AND NEW ENGLAND

This area comprises Connecticut, Delaware, Maine, Maryland, Massachusetts, New Hampshire, New Jersey, New York, Pennsylvania, Rhode Island, Vermont, Virginia, Washington D.C. and West Virginia.

Grasses (Gramineae and Poaceae)
May through July

Counts can be very high in June and July. The season continues until early August or even September in the Virginias and Delaware. Throughout the region, some pollen may remain in the air until October.

Birches *(Betula)*
April through May

Some pollen may still be airborne in June. A strongly allergenic pollen. Birches are more common in New England and the Appalachian Mountains than in any other part of the U.S.

Alders, ironwoods, hornbeams, and hazels *(Alnus, Carpinus, Ostrya,* and *Corylus)*
April through May

Some alders may begin pollinating in March or even February, particularly in the south of this region. All these pollens can cross-react with birch.

Oaks and beeches *(Quercus)*
April through May

Oaks are the main allergen, but in some areas, such as New Jersey, beeches seem to cause hay fever. The two groups cross-react with each other and with birches.

Elms *(Ulmus)*
February through April

Pollen counts can be very high. The season is later in Delaware and the Virginias, from April to May. Cross-reactions with hackberry *(Celtis)* pollen are likely.

Maples *(Acer)*
February through May

The most allergenic species is box elder or ash-leaved maple *(Acer negundo).*

Willows and poplars *(Salix* and *Populus)*
March through April

Cross-reactions between these two groups are common. The season may begin earlier and end later in the south of the region. Willows are particularly common in the north of this region (e.g., in Maine).

Lindens or basswoods *(Tilia)*
June through July

Considered an important cause of hay fever in Virginia.

"Cedars" and junipers (Cupressaceae)
March through May

Can cross-react with cypress.

Pines (Pinaceae)
April through May

New England has the highest recorded rate of genuine allergy to pine pollen in the world. The species concerned is *Pinus strobus,* which grows in other countries as well. Why it should prove so allergenic here is a mystery.

Ashes *(Fraxinus)*
May

The season can begin in April in the south of this region. Only a moderate allergen, but may affect those sensitized by olive pollen. Grows mainly on moist lowland soils.

Privet *(Ligustrum)*
May through June

Produces plenty of pollen, but most of it does not travel far. Only a modest allergen, and the number of people affected is small. Those affected have often been sensitized by olive pollen, which cross-reacts with privet.

Bayberry or wax myrtle *(Myrica)*
April through July

Found only on the coastal plain. A fairly strong allergen. Cross-reactions are likely with sweet gale *(Myrica gale)*, which grows throughout Canada and Scandinavia and in parts of the British Isles (where it is known as bog myrtle).

Sweet fern *(Comptonia peregrina)*
April through June

Not a true fern, but a shrub with fernlike leaves. This invasive plant is a fairly strong allergen and is spreading rapidly. A member of the same family as bayberry (Myricaceae), so cross-reactions might occur, but this possibility has not been investigated.

Ragweeds *(Ambrosia)*
July through October

Ragweeds are the major cause of hay fever in this region. The peak season is from August to September but can continue into early November in the Virginias. Several other members of the same family (Compositae or Asteraceae) can provoke cross-reactions in those sensitive to ragweed pollen, and some flower at other times, thus prolonging the season.

Marsh elders or poverty weeds *(Iva)*
August to October

These are the most common of the plants that cross-react with ragweed.

Nettles and clearweed *(Urtica* and *Pilea)*
May through October

The main season is from August to September. Moderately allergenic. Found mainly on disturbed ground and around abandoned buildings.

Pellitories *(Parietaria)*
June through October

The peak is in August and September. May cause some hay fever. A highly potent allergen but pollen counts are fairly low.

Lamb's-quarters or goosefoot and pigweeds (Chenopodiaceae and Amaranthaceae)
June through October

Pollen counts are never as high as in the western U.S. and cases of hay fever to these plants are correspondingly fewer. Some patients who have symptoms in the ragweed season may actually be reacting to these plants, not to ragweed.

Docks and sorrels *(Rumex)*
May through September

The peak season coincides with that for grass. Counts are lower after the end of August.

Plantains *(Plantago)*
June through August

Where English plantain *(Plantago lanceolata)* grows, there may be some pollen in the air until October. In the south of the region (Delaware, Maryland, Virginia, and West Virginia), the season continues until November. Plantains are considered a minor cause of hay fever.

THE SOUTH

This area comprises Texas, Louisiana, Mississippi, and Alabama.

Grasses (Gramineae and Poaceae)
March through December

The season runs from March through October in Texas, with west Texas having a slightly longer season than east Texas. Some areas of southern Texas have grass pollen in the air all year round. In Louisiana the grass pollen season runs from April through November or December. In much of Mississippi, the season begins in April but ends earlier, in October. Alabama's season is from May through November.

Junipers and "cedars" (Cupressaceae)
September through March
The main season is from January through March. Only one species, the pinchot juniper, flowers from September through November. Mountain cedar *(Juniperus ashei)* grows on neglected grassland and has become a particular problem.

Maples *(Acer)*
February through May
The main allergen is box elder or ash-leaved maple *(Acer negundo)*.

Elms, hackberries, and sugarberries (*Ulmus* and *Celtis*)
January through April, August through October
The peak season is from January through March, with very high counts in February, particularly in Texas.

Hickories and pecans *(Carya)*
March through May
Where cultivated or planted as street trees, these are often the second most important cause of hay fever, after ragweed. Pecans and hickories are widely cultivated in Texas.

Mulberries and paper mulberry (*Morus* and *Broussonetia*)
March through May
Paper mulberry, in particular, is highly allergenic and can cause severe symptoms, especially in the eyes. It is widely planted in this area.

Osage orange or hedgeplant *(Maclura)*
April through June
Used for hedging and moderately allergenic. Can cross-react with paper mulberry and mulberry, which belong to the same family (Moraceae).

Privet *(Ligustrum)*
March through June
May produce a few cases of hay fever in some parts of this region. Those affected have often been sensitized by olive pollen, which cross-reacts with privet.

Southern bayberry or wax myrtle (*Myrica cerifera*)
March through April
Pollination may begin in February in the southeastern part of this region, toward Florida. A moderately allergenic pollen sometimes producing severe symptoms in those affected. May cross-react with sweet gale *(Myrica gale)*, found in Canada and Scandinavia and in parts of Britain (where it is known as bog myrtle).

Ragweeds *(Ambrosia)*
July through November
The pollen of some species may appear from May onward, but early counts are low. Peak season is from mid-August through October. Ragweeds are the main cause of hay fever in this region.

Marsh elders, poverty weeds, and dune elders *(Iva)*
August through November
Related to the ragweeds, so cross-reactions are common. Some species may begin pollinating as early as June. Found mainly in coastal areas and the lower Mississippi valley.

Groundsel bush or tree (*Baccharis halmilifolia*)
August through November
Can begin pollinating much earlier in parts of Texas. May cross-react with ragweed. Many other plants belonging to the same family (Compositae or Asteraceae) grow throughout this area and can provoke cross-reactions in those with rag-

weed hay fever (see page 159). There may be some pollen in the air for most of the year, with the lowest pollen counts in January and February and the highest from August through December.

Lamb's-quarters or goosefoot and pigweeds (Chenopodiaceae and Amaranthaceae)
June through December
Many different species can provoke cross-reactions with other plants in these two related families (see page 160). Local names include southern water hemp and tumbleweed.

THE SOUTH-CENTRAL STATES

This area comprises Kansas, Oklahoma, Missouri, and Arkansas.

Grasses (Gramineae or Poaceae)
April through November
The season lasts for eight months in Arkansas but is shorter elsewhere in the region, usually from May through August.

Maples (Acer)
February through May
The most allergenic of the maples, box elder or ash-leaved maple *(Acer negundo)*, grows in this region and is a major cause of hay fever.

Birches (Betula)
March through May
A fairly common source of hay fever. The most common species grows on the banks of rivers and streams; pollen counts will therefore be highest in these areas.

Oaks (Quercus)
April through May
Can cross-react with birch pollen.

Hackberries and sugarberries (Celtis)
February through March
Particularly common in Oklahoma.

Ashes (Fraxinus)
February through March
Only a moderate allergen. Found growing in wet lowland areas.

Paper mulberry (Broussonetia papyrifera)
March through May
Grown in Oklahoma and a powerful allergen. Tends to provoke severe symptoms and affects the eyes in particular.

Osage orange or hedgeplant (Maclura)
April through May
Widely planted for hedging. Can cross-react with paper mulberry and mulberries.

Southern bayberry or wax myrtle (Myrica cerifera)
March through April
A moderately allergenic pollen sometimes producing severe symptoms in those affected. May cross-react with sweet gale *(Myrica gale)*, found in Canada and Scandinavia and in parts of Britain (where it is known as bog myrtle).

Ragweeds (Ambrosia)
August through September
The season can continue into mid-October in Oklahoma. The major allergenic pollen in this region. Other members of the same family (Compositae or Asteraceae) also grow in this region and may cross-react, prolonging the hay fever season until November or December.

Lamb's-quarters or goosefoot and pigweeds (Chenopodiaceae and Amaranthaceae)
April through October
Local names for these plants include redroot.

Docks and sorrels (Rumex)
May through September

The peak season coincides with that of grass, so allergy to docks and sorrels is often wrongly attributed to grass pollen.

Plantains (Plantago)
May through November

Peak pollination is from May through July.

Sagebrush (Artemisia)
July through September

Mainly found in the dry western areas. Cross-reacts with mugwort and wormwoods.

THE SOUTHEAST

This area comprises Georgia, Florida, North Carolina, and South Carolina. The range of plants found growing in Florida is much wider than that of the other states, and growing seasons are longer. This is particularly true of southern Florida, and some of the plants listed below are relevant only for this region.

Grasses (Gramineae or Poaceae)
March through October

In southern Florida the season is much longer, and there is sufficient grass pollen in the air throughout the year to produce year-round symptoms in many people. The peak in Florida is from April through October.

"Cedars," cypresses, and junipers (Cupressaceae)
December through March

Peak levels begin in January and last until March. Visitors sensitized to cypresses elsewhere will probably show cross-reactions to these conifers.

Oaks (Quercus)
February through May

In southern Florida the season starts in December. The highest counts are during March and April in all areas and can be very high in southern Florida. Oak pollen can cross-react with that of birch.

Elms (Ulmus)
March through May

The season is much longer in southern Florida, with one species, Chinese elm *(U. parvifolia)*, pollinating from September to December and other species beginning in January and continuing through to March.

Birches (Betula)
February through April

Pollen counts are not high, except in the Appalachian Mountains of North Carolina and northern Georgia.

Bald "cypress" or swamp "cypress" and pond "cypress" (Taxodium)
December through March

The peak is from January through March. These are not true cypresses but relatives of the redwoods. Found in the swamp forests of southern Florida. A moderate allergen.

She-oak or "Australian pine" (Casuarina)
February through April, October through December

The season is quite variable; they may pollinate intermittently throughout the year in the Tampa Bay area of southern Florida. Unwisely planted in parts of Florida for windbreaks. A strongly allergenic pollen. Neither a pine nor an oak, so cross-reactions with these trees are unlikely.

Hickories and walnuts (Carya and Juglans)
April through May

In southern Florida, hickory pollen can be airborne in February.

Willows and poplars (Salix and Populus)
March through May

Willows are generally less common in Florida, but the southern willow, which does grow in southern Florida, can begin pollinating in January or February.

Maples (Acer)
March through May

The box elder or ash-leaved maple *(Acer negundo)* may be a problem in some areas, notably in Florida.

Everglades palms
(Acoelorrhaphe wrightii)
April through June

Seems to cause some hay fever in the small area of southern Florida where it grows.

Paper mulberry
(Broussonetia papyrifera)
March through June

The peak is in April and May. Not found in the northern part of this area, but widely planted in the south. It has become naturalized in parts of southern Florida. A powerful allergen that can cause very severe symptoms, particularly in the eyes. Cross-reactions with mulberry *(Morus)* are likely.

Mimosas or silk trees (Albizia)
April through June

Affects some in southern Florida.

Pines (Pinaceae)
December through June

Peak is from February to March. There are very high pollen counts in some areas, notably southern Florida. These may affect visitors who are already sensitive to pine, either as an allergen or as an irritant.

Gum trees (Eucalyptus)
December through March

A rare cause of hay fever in Florida.

Osage orange or hedgeplant (Maclura)
April through May

Widely planted for hedging. Can cross-react with mulberry and paper mulberry.

Privet (Ligustrum)
May through June

Produces plenty of pollen, but most of it does not travel far. Only a modest allergen, and the number of people affected is small. Those affected have often been sensitized by olive pollen, which cross-reacts with privet.

Bayberry or wax myrtle (Myrica)
February through April

A potential allergen in southern Florida. May cross-react with sweet gale *(Myrica gale)* of Canada, Scandinavia, and parts of Britain (where it is known as bog myrtle).

Ragweeds (Ambrosia)
July through November

There is some ragweed pollen in the air throughout the year, but the counts are generally low from January through March. They may be fairly high near the Florida coast, even in these months, where one species of ragweed flowers at this time.

By way of compensation, ragweed pollen counts at the height of the season (August through October) are not as high as in the northeastern U.S. or the states of the Midwest.

Other plants in the same family (Asteraceae or Compositae) can provoke cross-reactions. Among those growing here is dog fennel or boneset *(Eupatorium),* which flowers from October through November and produces large amounts of airborne pollen. Groundsel bush or tree *(Baccharis halmilifolia)* and feverfew *(Parthenium)* also contribute to the pollen load.

Marsh elders and dune elders *(Iva)*
August through September

Found in the coastal areas, notably the salt marshes of Florida. Allergens are likely to cross-react with those of ragweed.

Lamb's-quarters or goosefoot and pigweeds (*Chenopodiaceae* and *Amaranthaceae*)
April through October

Pollen counts are never as high as in the western U.S., and cases of hay fever to these plants are correspondingly fewer. However, some patients who have symptoms in the ragweed season may actually be responding to these plants, not to ragweed. In southern Florida, there may be some pollen in the air all year round, but levels are low from January through March.

Docks and sorrels *(Rumex)*
April through June

May continue producing some pollen until September.

Plantains *(Plantago)*
May through November

English plantain *(Plantago lanceolata)*, the most allergenic species, is widespread.

Pellitories *(Parietaria)*
January through June

Pollen counts are low, but this is a powerful allergen and may affect those sensitized elsewhere.

Nettles and clearweed (*Urtica* and *Pilea*)
August through October

Nettles are not found in southern Florida.

WASHINGTON AND OREGON

The seasons tend to be later to the east of the Cascade Mountains. All seasons are about two weeks longer in the south than in the north.

Grasses (Gramineae or Poaceae)
April through September

The peak is in June and July. Pollen counts are moderate in most regions.

Alders *(Alnus)*
February through April

A common cause of hay fever due to very high pollen counts, particularly in March. Allergenically more important than birch in this area.

Birches *(Betula)*
April through May

Can cross-react with alder and thus prolong the season.

Poplars and willows (*Populus* and *Salix*)
March through May

Two of the more allergenic poplars, balsam poplar and quaking aspen (*Populus balsamifera* and *P. tremuloides*), both grow here.

Oaks *(Quercus)*
April through May

Has the potential for cross-reactions with birch and alder.

Maples *(Acer)*
April through May

Considered a fairly common source of hay fever.

Coast redwood *(Sequoia)*
March through May

Moderately allergenic pollen.

Cypresses, junipers, and "cedars" (Cupressaceae)
March through May

May cause some hay fever, but not to the same extent as in California owing to the cooler climate.

Ragweeds *(Ambrosia)*
July through October
Pollen counts are not as high as in other states and are generally lower to the west of the Cascade Mountains.

Docks and sorrels *(Rumex)*
May through September
The peak is in early summer, coinciding with the grass pollen season, so allergies to docks and sorrels can easily be misdiagnosed.

Plantains *(Plantago)*
May through November
High pollen counts in July and August, which lessen in September. Considered moderately significant as a cause of hay fever.

Lamb's-quarters or goosefoot and pigweeds (Chenopodiaceae and Amaranthaceae)
June through October
The amaranths are known locally as redroot pigweed and spiny pigweed. Widespread weeds in this area.

THE FORMER USSR

In Russia (west of the Urals), Belarus, the Ukraine, and the Caucasus region, the pollen seasons are similar to those of eastern Europe. Ragweeds *(Ambrosia)*, introduced from the U.S., is a major allergen in large parts of this area, often the most common cause of hay fever. Rye *(Secale)*, grown as a crop, boosts the grass pollen count in early summer. Birches *(Betula)*, alders *(Alnus)*, hazels *(Corylus)*, wormwoods-sagebrush *(Artemisia)*, plantains *(Plantago)*, and goosefoot (Chenopodiaceae) are other notable allergens. Sunflowers *(Helianthus)* cause hay fever in some localities and can cross-react with ragweeds.

Information is sparse for other countries in this region. Ragweeds *(Ambrosia)* grows in Georgia, and probably in several other states.

Appendix 2

PARTICLES, DROPLETS, AND DUST: THE RANGE OF SIZES

(A micron is a thousandth of a millimeter.)

Type of particle	Size (diameter) of particle
Absidia spores	2–4 microns
Alder pollen	22–34 microns
Alternaria spores	4–10 microns, some larger
Amaranth pollen	20–40 microns
Arthrinium spores	4–10 microns
Ash pollen	18–27 microns
Aspergillus spores	2–4 microns, some smaller than 2 microns
Aspergillus tereus	less than 2 microns
Aureobasidium spores	2–10 microns
Australian white cypress pine	20–24 microns
Bacteria	0.1 micron–5 microns
Bald "cypress" pollen	28–36 microns
Birch pollen	18–28 microns
Bird allergens	see "Feather allergens"
Cat allergen	less than 2.5 microns (perhaps as low as 0.05 micron) up to 20 microns or more
Cladosporium spores	4–10 microns
Coal dust	1–100 microns
Coniophora cerebella spores	14 microns x 9 microns
Cryptostroma spores	2–4 microns
Cypress pollen	19–38 microns
Diesel exhaust particulates	1–10 microns; most are 2.5 microns or less
Dock pollen	21–27 microns
Dog allergen	no figures available
Dry rot spores	4–10 microns

Dust mites	200–300 microns
Dust-mite droppings	4–20 microns
Epicoccum spores	over 10 microns
Feather allergens	most are 1 micron
Flour	1–90 microns
Fog and mist	2–100 microns
Goosefoot pollen	20–30 microns
Graphium spores	2–10 microns
Grass pollen	25–37 microns
Greasy particles found in domestic air	0.01 micron–5 microns
Hazel pollen	18–23 microns
Horsetail *(Equisetum)* spores	38–56 microns
Japanese red cedar pollen	24–32 microns
Micropolyspora faeni spores	less than 2 microns
Mold spores	less than 2 microns to over 10 microns (see individual entries if you know which mold is your allergen)
Mucor spores	2–10 microns
Nocardia asteroides spores	less than 2 microns
Mugwort pollen	18–24 microns
Olive pollen	17–28 microns
Paxillus panuoides spores	4–5 microns
Pellitory pollen	14–19 microns,
Penicillium spores	mostly 2–4 microns, some larger
Pine pollen	60–85 microns, but air bladders keep it airborne despite its large size
Plane pollen	18–25 microns
Plantain pollen	16–36 microns
Pollen (general)	5–200 microns, although the main allergenic pollens fall in the range 10–40 microns, with the majority between 20 and 35 microns (see individual entries if you know which pollen is your allergen)
Pollen fragments*	0.5 micron upwards
Privet pollen	28–38 microns
Puccinia spores	over 10 microns
Ragweed pollen	19–20 microns

Rat urinary proteins	associated with particles of 5–10 microns
Redwood pollen	22–25 microns
Smog	0.01 micron–2 microns
Smoke from cigarettes	see "Tobacco smoke particles"
Smoke from coal fires and boilers	0.01 micron–4 microns
Smoke from oil-burning boilers, etc.	0.04 micron–1 micron
Sporobolomyces spores	2–10 microns
Thermoactinomyces spores	less than 2 microns
Tobacco smoke particles	0.01 micron–1 micron
Ustilago spores	4–10 microns
Viruses	0.02–0.3 micron
Wet rot spores	see *Coniophora cerebella* spores and *Paxillus panuoides* spores

* Covers all smaller-than-pollen-grain particles carrying pollen allergens. This includes both fragmented pollen grains and very small particles containing pollen-type allergens that are released by the plant at the same time as the pollen. These are known to exist for ragweed, some grasses, Japanese red cedar, and Australian white cypress pine. They may exist for other plants, but this has not been widely investigated.

APPENDIX 3

USEFUL PRODUCTS AND SUPPLIERS

One of the problems facing allergy sufferers is that the trade in protective goods is not well regulated. To quote just one example, there is a small aerosol spray containing herbal extracts that claims to "safely clear the air of smoke and pollen." The claim is absurd, but there is apparently nothing to prevent this spray from being sold. Most manufacturers' claims are not as misleading as this, but one still needs to be wary of believing everything that is claimed about certain air cleaners, for example, or some of the laundry additives or antipollution masks. The details given here are primarily intended to make potential buyers more informed about the goods available and better able to choose the right product. They will also help you assess whether the customer- service people at an allergy supply company actually know what they are talking about. Not all do, and the level of knowledge (or ignorance) you encounter during your inquiries can give you some indication of whether a company is dedicated to selling goods that work or just selling anything that will make a profit.

The names of suppliers are given here. For their addresses and Web sites, please turn to the end of this appendix. The inclusion of a supply company here does not indicate that we think everything it sells is wonderful—there are many companies, unfortunately, that sell some very dubious products alongside reputable and useful items.

Similarly, the fact that a company is not included here doesn't necessarily mean that we think it is without merit—it is just that there are a lot of different organizations now selling allergy products and we don't have space to list them all. If you want to find others, go to www.allergy-intolerance.com or, for an exhaustive list, www.allallergy.com.

While we have made every effort to ensure that the details given here are correct, we cannot take any responsibility for errors or omissions. Nor have we carried out any independent testing of the products, although we have relied, wherever possible, on independent and objective studies carried out by others. Purchasers should check all details carefully before buying any product.

THE ALLERGY-INTOLERANCE WEB SITE

For more information on allergy products along with regular updates, please go to www.allergyintolerance.com, the Web site that accompanies this book.

STEAM INHALERS

These can be useful for relieving the symptoms of hay fever and perennial allergic rhinitis (see page 142) and may help in chronic sinusitis too.

Suppliers include: Allergy Control Products, The Allergy Store, National Allergy Supply

HUMIDIFIERS/VAPORIZERS

Note that room humidifiers are also marketed for treatment of sinus pain and are featured on the Web sites of several allergy supply companies. These really are a bad idea—if you need moisture to relieve sinus symptoms, go for a steam inhaler, which directs the steam to your nose. Anything that makes the air in a room generally more moist will be promoting the growth of dust mites and molds and could make your problems worse. Indeed, molds growing in the sinus cavities may be contributing to the inflammation of the sinuses, and some studies have found that people with chronic sinusitis have the same mold species growing in the house and within their sinuses. Damp houses, then, are very bad news in chronic sinusitis, so a humidifier could actually make matters worse. Even if you live in a desert region, you are unlikely to benefit from a humidifier—it is probably indoor pollution rather than dry air that irritates your nose (see page 200). Chronic sinusitis needs dedicated expert treatment that tackles the source of the problem—for further details see *Asthma: The Complete Guide to Integrative Therapies* (Healing Arts Press, 2000), by Jonathan Brostoff, M.D., and Linda Gamlin.

SALINE IRRIGATORS

Scientific research has shown that irrigating the nostrils with saline (salt water) from a device such as a Water Pik can help with hay fever.

Suppliers include: Allergy Clean Environments, Allergy Control Products, The Allergy Store, National Allergy Supply

FACE MASKS

Face masks, which filter air going into the nose and mouth, can be helpful in certain situations, when you are exposed to a high level of allergen for a short period. The mask must fit tightly against your nose and face, forming a seal at all the edges. A beard or mustache may prevent a good seal being formed.

If you experience any difficulty in breathing, you should remove the mask immediately.

Occasions When Masks Can Be Useful

You might want to wear a mask at certain times of year, or in certain places, to protect against various items in the air, as follows.

Natural allergens and irritants in outdoor air

- pollen

- pollen fragments

- volatile chemicals produced by plants (occasionally a source of trouble if they act as irritants)

- mold spores in the air

- mold spores being released in large amounts (e.g. from a compost heap, rotting wood, or crop plants during harvesting)

- other allergens, such as insect particles (rare causes of allergy)

Pollutants in outdoor air that might aggravate hay fever symptoms, or trigger an asthma attack

- sulfur dioxide (from factories and power stations)

- acidic droplets in the air (from factories and power stations)

- ozone (from sunlight + vehicle exhaust)

- nitrogen oxides (from vehicle exhaust)

- diesel particles (from buses, trucks, and other diesel engines)

- volatile hydrocarbon molecules (from gasoline, etc.)

Natural allergens in indoor air

- pollen stirred up during ordinary housework

- pollen coming into the house when the windows are open

- mold spores stirred up during ordinary housework

- mold spores coming into the house when the windows are open

- mold spores being released in large amounts by renovation work, redecorating, or a major cleanup operation in a damp (or previously damp) house

- mold spores being released in large amounts from stored hay, bird droppings, bird nesting material, mushroom compost, or rotten timbers

- dust-mite droppings stirred up during ordinary housework

- dust-mite droppings stirred up during a major cleanup operation, replacement of a carpet, or removal of an old sofa or mattress, for example

- cat, dog, or feather allergens stirred up during ordinary housework

- cat, dog, or feather allergens stirred up during a major cleaning operation, replacement of a carpet, or removal of an old sofa or armchair, for example

- other allergens (e.g., insect particles) stirred up during a major cleaning operation

- animal allergens found in urine (laboratory workers only)

- wood dust or other allergens encountered at work (but if you have asthma due to these allergens, a mask is not the answer: you should not be working anywhere near the affecting allergen because you risk developing severe and irreversible asthma.

Pollutants in indoor air that might irritate the airways

- paint fumes during decorating

- solvent fumes following protective wood treatment

Finding the Right Mask for the Job

There are two basic types of mask: those that have a dust filter only and those that combine a dust filter with an activated carbon filter. (Powered respirator helmets, used for special applications, are dealt with on page 308.)

Activated Carbon Masks

Activated carbon masks filter out certain gases and volatile chemicals that cannot be removed by dust masks because they are not particles. They are used primarily to protect against synthetic pollutants such as paint fumes, ozone, and sulfur dioxide, but should also take out natural volatile substances produced by certain plants, such as pines and oil-seed rape.

To make a face mask, a thin pad of fabric or a piece of foam rubber is impregnated with particles of activated carbon.

The ability of activated carbon to attract and hold chemicals will decline with use because the surfaces become coated with the chemicals already filtered from the air. According to some manufacturers, its powers can be regenerated by washing with detergent, which they claim removes the chemicals that are bound to the carbon. Other manufacturers dispute this claim. Replacement carbon filters are sold for some of the masks.

Activated carbon is also a component of certain masks for industrial use, which do have to conform to standards. One of these could be used to protect against pollutants.

Activated carbon will take out various chemicals from the air, including:

- sulfur dioxide (from factories and power stations)

- acidic droplets in the air (from factories and power stations)

- ozone (from sunlight + vehicle exhaust)

- volatile hydrocarbon molecules (from gasoline, etc.)

- volatile substances from plants (e.g., birch trees, pines, oil-seed rape)

- solvent vapor from paint

- solvent vapor following protective wood treatment

Some antipollution masks take out nitrogen oxides as well. Activated carbon alone cannot take out these gases, but the carbon can be treated so that some nitrogen dioxide is absorbed.

Very few masks contain a pad of activated carbon material alone, but a few do. Although the activated carbon may take out some dust particles, it is not designed for this purpose, so it will have limited action against pollen and diesel particulates, for example. There is also a strong possibility that some activated carbon particles will become detached from the fabric or foam that carries them, and thus be inhaled. Since activated carbon can act as an IgE-specific adjuvant (see page 43) in just the same way as diesel particulates, inhaling carbon particles is not a good idea. Any mask where the activated carbon pad is directly against the nose and mouth could represent a hazard, and should therefore be avoided. There should be a dust filter between the activated carbon material and the face.

Dust Masks

Dust masks will take out particles from the air, but it is crucial to know the smallest size removed; the simplest dust masks remove only fairly large particles. A claim that a dust mask or antipollution mask removes "95 percent of particulates" is meaningless unless the size of those particulates is given.

Dust masks that are manufactured and sold for the protection of workers have to meet certain standards based on the smallest particle size they will filter out efficiently. Buying a mask from a supplier dealing with industrial protection equipment (such as AO Safety or Ohio Glove & Safety) is a good idea because you can ask for the technical specifications and will have a clear idea of what you are buying.

Masks sold *only* for protection from allergens or traffic pollutants are not governed by any compulsory standards. One of the antipollution masks, made by 3M, is based on dust masks designed for industrial use and complies with the standards applied to them.

Nuisance Dust Masks

Nuisance dust masks filter out only relatively large particles, usually those larger than 5 microns. There are no compulsory standards set for the efficiency with which they remove these particles. The manufacturers are allowed to state that such masks filter out pollen, and of course they do—but not those pollen fragments smaller than 5 microns in size.

Using appendix 2, check the size of the particles from which you need protection. If the particles are larger than 5 microns, a nuisance dust mask will be adequate. If some or all of the particles are smaller than 5 microns, you may need a mask that complies with standards. However, since nuisance dust masks are cheap and readily available, it is worth trying them to see if they reduce your symptoms.

Suppliers include: AO Safety, Allergy Clean Environments, Allergy Control Products, The Breathing Club, Ohio Glove & Safety, National Allergy Supply

POWERED RESPIRATORS

These are used mainly by laboratory workers who are exposed to high levels of allergen from mice or rats (see page 218). They may also be of value to farmworkers or plant breeders with hay fever. Air is filtered by a battery-powered unit strapped to the waist (see page 122).

Suppliers include: AO Safety, Ohio Glove & Safety

PROTECTIVE EYEWEAR

If you get red, itchy, watery eyes in the hay fever season, protective glasses or goggles, worn outdoors, can bring a huge improvement.

Plastic goggles are widely available in do-it-yourself shops and are very cheap. You can also add your own shields to an existing pair of glasses or sunglasses (see page 120) or buy clip-on side shields from companies such as AO Safety.

More sophisticated protective eyewear, designed to look like ordinary glasses or like ultra-cool shades, is now available. Some designs are very attractive indeed.

Choose a pair that gives as much coverage as possible at the side and above the lens. A few designs also give coverage below the lens.

AIR FILTERS AND AIR CLEANERS

The terminology can be confusing here: This section deals with freestanding electrically powered devices that take air in and remove particles and (sometimes) other impurities. These devices are usually called **air cleaners** or **air purifiers.**

Most air cleaners rely on a filter plus a fan that draws in air and pushes it through the filter. Some people use the term **air filter** to mean this kind of electrically powered device. But most manufacturers restrict the meaning of "air filter" to the filter itself, not the unit as a whole. The term "air filter" is also used for filter pads that can be added to the hot-air vents of your existing heating system or to the outlets of a ventilation system. A few air cleaners rely on water, rather than a filter, to take out particles and impurities from the air—these are sometimes called **air washers.**

Making sense of the sales literature on different brands of air cleaners and assessing their relative merits is far from easy. The information given below is intended to help you understand the claims made and compare one device with another.

The small, table-top devices that claim to remove pollen are most unlikely to be powerful enough to make any impact on the air in an average room. Any device that is for sale without technical information on air throughput (see page 309) and filtration efficiency should be rejected. With any air cleaner, you need to ask some pertinent questions of the supplier or manufacturer and, if possible, try out the device at home before you buy.

How Air Filters and Cleaners Work

As with masks, an air filter or cleaner may remove either particles, or gases and volatile chemicals, or both. Most deal with both.

The removal of gases and volatile chemicals (such as paint fumes) is a very different matter from removing dust and other particles. Gases and volatiles must be removed with something that attracts and holds them chemically, a "chemical sponge" such as **activated carbon** (see page 306). Some newer products use a combination of activated carbon and **zeolite,** a mi6eral that absorbs and retains certain chemical molecules.

In the case of particles, there are two basic approaches to removing them. One is to use a fibrous filter that takes them out by a sieving action; **HEPA filters** work in this way and offer the maximum efficiency among sieving filters. The other approach is to give the particles an electrical charge and then attract them to a plate that carries the opposite charge; devices employing this method are called **electrostatic precipitators, electronic air cleaners,** or **electrostatic air cleaners.**

A hybrid method also exists, using a fibrous filter in which the fibers carry an electrical charge. The particles in the air apparently have sufficient natural charge to attract them to the fibers of the filter, and this supplements the sievelike effect of the filter. These are known variously as **charged media filters, precharged electrostatic filters, electrostatic microfilters,** or **electrets.**

HEPA Filters

High Efficiency Particulate Air (HEPA) filters must remove particles of 0.3 micron diameter with an efficiency of at least 99.97 percent—a stringent requirement indeed.

Once in use, the efficiency of a HEPA filter actually increases because the particles caught reduce the size of the channels through which other particles can flow. However, there is a downside to this: the **air throughput** or **airflow** (the amount of air processed each minute) declines because of the increased resistance. The specification for HEPA filters stipulates that this should not drop more than a certain amount.

These filters have a limited life—the filter has to be replaced when it is so full of particles that the air throughput drops considerably.

The filter may last as long as five years or it may last only a year. In part, this depends on the presence (and efficiency) of **prefilters,** which take out larger particles so that they do not clog up the HEPA filter. The more prefilters there are, the longer the HEPA filter should last. Manufacturers generally quote the cost of replacement HEPA filters alongside the cost of the air cleaner device because they are so expensive, and customers need to see at the outset what they are getting into. Be wary of manufacturers that don't include this information.

Other Sievelike Filters

Some air cleaners use sievelike filters that are not up to HEPA standard but are still good enough to help those with allergies. (These are sometimes referred to as **panel filters, extended surface filters,** or **"HEPA-type filters."**) If there are no figures given in the sales literature supplied, you should ask for the filtration efficiency at 0.3 micron or 0.5 micron.

Very simple sievelike filters are used in small, table-top air cleaners. They are unlikely to state their filtering efficiency, but tests have shown that it is about 75 percent at 20 microns—the size of pollen grains. This filtration rate might help some hay fever sufferers, but the fans in these machines are too weak to achieve the air throughput needed for cleaning the air in a normal room.

Electrostatic Precipitators

These have an electrode that discharges ions into the incoming air, thus giving the particles an electrical charge. A fan draws the air toward collecting plates, which carry the opposite electrical charge. The charged particles are attracted toward the plates and stick to them.

When first running, electrostatic precipitators have a very high efficiency, even for very small particles. Tobacco smoke particles, for example, will be removed with 80 to 90 percent efficiency. However, within a few days the efficiency begins to drop because the particles already deposited on the plates interfere with their ability to attract and hold more particles. The plates therefore have to be cleaned regularly to maintain performace.

If considering an electrostatic precipitator, you should ask how often the plates need to be cleaned and how much their efficiency drops in the interval between cleaning. Also find out how difficult it is to remove the plates and how much scrubbing is needed to get them clean.

Electrostatic precipitators inevitably produce small amounts of ozone because they ionize the oxygen in the air. Ozone can cause irritation of the airways (see page 70), but with newer devices this is said not to be a problem because the amount produced is very small. However, should you experience any irritation or find that you are coughing more than usual, ozone may be the explanation. Experiment with not using the air cleaner for a while and see if your symptoms change.

Charged Media Filters

Also known by a variety of other names (see page 309), these filters are relatively new and have not yet been tested by researchers looking at their effects on allergy patients. According to one manufacturer, the efficiency of its filtration medium is 99 percent at 1 micron and 93 percent at 0.3 micron. While not as good as a HEPA air cleaner, this efficiency may be sufficient for many allergy sufferers. In general, these devices are less expensive than HEPA air cleaners, but the filter medium has to be replaced more often.

Air Ionizers

Air ionizers have an effect very similar to that of an electrostatic precipitator, except that walls and other surfaces in the home act as the collecting plates. Their effects as air cleaners are discussed on pages 315–316.

Air Washers

Not widely sold yet, these rely on a completely different approach, with no filter involved. A set of fast-spinning plates pass through a tank of water. Particles in the air stick to the plates (simply as a result of water tension—no electrostatic effects are involved here). As the plates pass through the water, the particles are washed off.

Ceiling Fan Filters

These are small filter pads that you stick onto the blades of your ceiling fan. It is claimed that they remove allergens from the air, and they are sold by at least one big allergy supply company. We have inquired about research data showing that these pads actually work, but no data exist. It seems unlikely to us that the stick-on filters would in fact work because all filters create some resistance to the flow of air through them, and given this resistance, most of the air hitting the ceiling fan will flow around the outside of the filter rather than through it.

Which Type of Device Is Best?

If you want your filter to remove irritant gases and volatile chemicals from the air or to eliminate bad smells, you need to buy one with an activated carbon filter, as well as a particle filter.

For particle filtration most researchers favor HEPA filters over electrostatic precipitators because their efficiency tends to increase with use, rather than declining, and less maintenance is involved. An electrostatic precipitator also has the disadvantage that, if an electrical fault develops that prevents the collecting plates from becoming charged, the device stops working entirely, yet the fan can still be running so the machine seems to be functioning. Charged media filters do not have this drawback, as the charge is intrinsic to the fibers of the filter. They are also easier to maintain. This type of device may come to rival HEPA-based devices in the future, but still needs to be tested more fully.

Ensuring the Air Cleaner Is Up to the Job

Once you have established that the filter will efficiently take out particles of the size required, there is another important measurement to look at: **air throughput** or **airflow.** This may be stated in cubic meters per minute (cmm), cubic meters per hour (cmh), or cubic feet per minute (cfm). If you are trying to make sense of brochures and leaflets on air filters obtained from manufacturers, look out for these abbreviations. Occasionally, air throughput is stated in yet another way: liters per second. Table 3 gives conversions among these three different units, allowing you to compare the throughput of different brands of air cleaner.

Work out the minimum air throughput that you need as follows. Measure the length, breadth, and height of the room in which you want to use the filter. If several rooms are to be treated and you therefore want to buy a portable device for moving around the house, measure the largest of the rooms. (Remember to consider ceiling height in assessing which is the largest.)

Multiply the three figures: length x breadth x ceiling height. This gives the volume of air in a room. For example, a room that is 5 meters long by 6 meters wide, with a ceiling height of 3 meters, will have an air volume of 90 cubic meters.

Divide the air volume in the room by the air throughput of an air cleaner, and you can discover how often that device will clean all the air in the room.

For example, if you buy a device with an air throughput of 1.5 cubic meters per minute (cmm), it will take 90 divided by 1.5 to process all the air in the room—that is, 60 minutes—so the air in the room will be cleaned every hour. This is considered the absolute minimum rate and is not ideal. (Far higher rates of air exchange are achieved in an old-fashioned house without draft-proofing, for example.) The recommended rate is to clean the air in a room four times an hour. Thus, a device with an air throughput of 6 cmm is needed for a room of 90 cubic meters. (However, the air in the room will not be completely cleared of particles every 15 minutes because there is bound to be some mixing between cleaned and dirty air.)

Table 3: Air Throughput Conversions

The air throughput figures given here are typical values for the widely available brands of air filters and cleaners.

cubic meters per minute (cmm)	cubic meters per hour (cmh)	cubic feet per minute (cfm)	liters per second
0.67	40	23.7	11
1.0	60	35	16
1.5	90	53	25
2.5	150	88	42
2.8	168	99	47
3.3	200	118	55
4.3	255	150	71
5.0	300	175	80
5.9	349	208	97
6.6	400	236	110
8.5	510	302	142
16.6	1000	600	278
21.7	1300	760	360
34	2050	1200	570

If buying a HEPA device, choose one with an air throughput figure slightly above that required, since this tends to drop as the filter becomes dirty.

Some manufacturers and suppliers give a figure for the size of room to which an air cleaner is suited, rather than revealing the air throughput. They may refer to this as the capacity of the device. Ask how this room size figure is calculated—that is, how many air changes per hour the device gives in a room of that size.

If the room size is quoted in terms of area (square feet, for example), you also need to ask what ceiling height they've assumed for the purposes of their calculation. If your ceilings are higher, the performance of the filter will not be as good as that quoted.

Another figure that may be given is the clean air delivery rate. This is a measure of how much the rate of removal of particles by the air cleaner exceeds that occurring due to natural settling of particles (see page 203).

Allergen Disturbance by Fans

All air cleaners rely on a fan to move air through them, and the fans themselves create a disturbance in the air. The more powerful the fan, the more the air is disturbed. If there is a large reservoir of allergen particles on the floor or on other surfaces, the air movements created by the fan will make some of these particles airborne, partially offsetting the effects of the air cleaner. This is particularly likely with small particles such as those produced by cats. To get the best effects from your filter, therefore, you need to reduce the amount of allergen in the carpets and furniture by thorough cleaning measures (see Jerry's story on pages 202–207 for those needed for cat allergens).

If it is difficult to reduce the reservoir of allergens, there are other measures you can take. Placing the device off the floor will reduce the amount of allergen disturbed from the carpet. Two air cleaners running simultaneously, each with an air throughput of, say, 2.5 cmm will have the same cleaning effect on the air as one air cleaner with a throughput of 5 cmm, but will not cause as much disturbance of allergens because the fans are less powerful.

Other Features

Several air cleaners have an additional feature of some kind.

Dehumidifier

If you are sensitive to both pollens and dust mites, or pollens and mold spores, a combined air cleaner and dehumidifier may well be your best choice, since it will allow you to keep the windows closed without suffering the consequences in condensation and damp. For more details on dehumidifiers, including those that also filter the air, see pages 317–18.

Humidifier

Anything that increases the humidity of the air is not recommended for most houses (see page 200).

Air Ionizer

When ionizers are added to air cleaners, they may improve their air-cleaning performance to some extent. In the case of air filters with a low air throughput, this may be valuable. However, this is not the reason for adding them to high-powered filtering devices. In such cases, they are added because ions are claimed to have a direct benefit on health.

Fragrance Diffuser

These are not recommended for anyone with asthma or rhinitis, as continuous exposure to the fragrance may irritate the airways. The use of the fragrance diffuser is usually optional, even if one is fitted.

Questions to Ask about Air Cleaners

- Does it contain an activated carbon filter?

- What type of system is used for removing particles from the air?

- With what efficiency are particles of 0.3 micron or 0.5 micron removed?

- What is the air throughput when operating at its highest speed?

- Is the device designed to be portable?

- Is the device available for a free trial period, or on a money-back basis, or can it be rented so that its effectiveness can be assessed before buying?

- What are the running costs in terms of electricity used?

For Electrostatic Precipitators:

- How often do the plates need cleaning, and how difficult are they to clean?

- With what efficiency are particles removed a month after cleaning? And after two months?

For All Other Types of Air Cleaner:

- How often do the filters need replacing, and how much do they cost?

Suppliers include: Allergy Control Products, National Allergy Supply

AIR-CONDITIONING

As well as cooling the air, air-conditioning systems will take out more than 90 percent of the pollen grains (see page 116). The air also becomes drier, which helps to decrease the number of dust mites.

FILTRATION UNITS FOR
EXISTING AIR-CONDITIONING SYSTEMS

These are available, but note that air-conditioning itself reduces the pollen count in the air considerably, and that adding a filter produces only a small additional improvement (see page 116). However, such filters maybe of benefit for some people.
Suppliers include: The Allergy Store, Allergy Supply Company, Allergy Control Products

FILTERS FOR EXISTING HEATING DUCTS
OR VENTILATION SYSTEMS

Some modern buildings have central heating systems that provide warm air by running it through air ducts. These can be fitted with filters that effectively reduce the pollen and mold spore counts in the air. Filters are also useful in the ventilation systems of large office blocks, where the air travels in through air ducts. These will probably have some type of filter already, but the filtration performance can usually be improved.

Suppliers include: The Allergy Store, Allergy Supply Company, Allergy Control Products, National Allergy Supply

FILTERS AND IONIZERS FOR CARS

There are relatively few products available, and none has been independently tested, so it is difficult to say how much help they might give.

Any filtration or ionization system within a car will work only if the windows are closed. There is little doubt that a car with built-in air-conditioning will provide a cooler and more comfortable solution to the problem of pollen when driving.

Removal of Pollen

An air cleaner will remove pollen within the car as long as the air throughput (see page 309) is adequate to change the air in the car four times an hour or more.

An air ionizer should also remove some pollen grains from the air in the car. As with domestic ionizers, a direct benefit from the ions on the well-being of driver and passengers is claimed, but their effectiveness is a matter of debate. Car ionizers plug into the cigarette lighter socket.

Dust filters that are taped over the air intake on the vehicle will take out pollen entering the car by this route. However, the pollen that was in the car to begin with will remain. To what extent this settles from the air when the car is in motion with windows closed is unknown.

A combination of dust filters taped over the air intake and an ionizer or filter within the car may be the most effective way of reducing the pollen and pollution load. It does not, however, solve the problem of heat building up within the car.

Removal of Pollutants from Traffic

To remove gases and fumes, activated carbon (see page 306) is required.

Diesel particles require a dust filter (see page 308), preferably one that can deal with particles smaller than a micron. They might also be removed by an air ionizer.

Suppliers include: National Allergy Supply

AIR IONIZERS

The cleaning effect of ionizers is beyond dispute: the dirt that accumulates on the wall behind them is testimony to their effectiveness. They are, in fact, like electrostatic precipitators, but instead of having collecting plates, they use the walls and other surfaces. Unlike electrostatic precipitators, however, they have no fan, so air is not circulated around the room. This means that the cleaning power tends to decline as you move farther away from the ionizer, but this can be overcome by having two or more ionizers operating in the room.

Coping with the mess created by an ionizer is something that has concerned many purchasers, particularly those using the device to combat cigarette smoke. A sticky brown deposit collects close to the ionizer and can be very difficult to clean. Some users have found that taping a large piece of paper to the wall behind the ionizer is the solution, or hanging a curtain behind it, which can be washed regularly.

A few of the newer ionizer models now incorporate a "Faraday cage" and a charged medium filter, which help to reduce the amount of dirt deposited.

Despite the drawbacks, an ionizer may be a good solution to allergen-loaded air in certain circumstances. Ionizers are inexpensive to buy and very cheap to run since they use hardly any electricity. They are also quieter than air filters and cleaners. For an elderly person, or someone on a low income, where keeping the decor looking nice is not the top priority, an ionizer could be useful in cleaning the air. Unlike an air cleaner, an ionizer will not disturb settled allergens from the carpet and other surfaces because it has no fan.

Ozone is produced in small amounts by ionizers, but the levels are usually within safety limits. Some of the cheaper models may produce ozone in troublesome amounts, however. Should you experience any irritation of the airways, or an increase in coughing, this could be due to ozone. Try moving the ionizer farther away from you if it is very close to your bed or armchair. If the symptoms persist, stop using the ionizer.

Choosing an Ionizer

The most important figure to be quoted for an ionizer is the cleaning range. Most achieve 20 feet (6 meters), but some can manage more on a higher setting, up to 30 feet (9 meters) on the maximum setting.

The ion concentration at a given distance from the ionizer is often quoted. This should be over 100,000 ions per cubic centimeter (cc) at 3.3 feet (1 meter) away, and over 1,000 ions per cubic centimeter at 16.5 feet (5 meters) away.

Is the Ionizer Working?

A survey by the consumer magazine *Which?* (March 1992) found that some of the ionizers tested produced no ions at all. If there is no dirt deposited on surfaces near the ionizer, then it is probably not working.

The effects of the ionizer in cleaning the air will also be much reduced by objects being placed too close to it, particularly television sets. The ionizer should be positioned at the very front of a shelf, or the front edge of any other surface, as long as it is not metallic. The needles should be cleaned with a matchstick every three to four weeks.

DEHUMIDIFIERS

Dehumidifiers are useful for anyone with allergy to mold spores or dust mites. To be effective, a dehumidifier must reduce the relative humidity of the air to 45 percent, which is the target for most ordinary dehumidifiers. The aim is to reduce the overall humidity of the house, and thus stop the growth of molds and put a brake on dust-mite growth and reproduction. The effect is a long-term one: you probably won't experience any immediate benefits. You need to combine a dehumidifier with other anti-mite strategies, such as vigorous vacuuming with a specialized cleaner to remove dust-mite allergens, or use of an air cleaner to remove mold spores if mold allergy is your problem.

Alternatively, you can view the dehumidifier as a follow-up treatment after buying new armchairs and carpets or using superheated steam to kill mites in your carpets (see pages 325–27), or heat-treating your armchairs in a Diathermic Envelope (see page 325). The dehumidifier is a way of ensuring that dust mites don't make a quick comeback after such purges.

Despite the fact that it is a dehumidifier, the Banamite Dehumidifier is a fundamentally different kind of product, designed to kill all dust mites in a relatively short period (a matter of days or weeks). This powerful device reduces the relative humidity of the air to a very low level, just 25 percent.

In these very dry conditions, the dust mites just can't survive. It is best to use this device when the room is unoccupied (for example, in a bedroom during the daytime). The door should be closed for maximum effect. At bedtime turn off the dehumidifier and leave the door to the room open for 30 minutes. This will restore the humidity to a normal level, making it comfortable for human occupants. This dehumidifier also incorporates an electrostatic microfilter to remove particles such as dust-mite droppings, mold spores, and pollen from the air.

All dehumidifiers work by cooling the air, using the same technology as a refrigerator. Water condenses out of the air as it is cooled, and is collected in a tank from which it cannot evaporate again. The dry, cool air is blown out of the device and is heated up by contact with the warmer air in the room.

Choosing a Dehumidifier

Dehumidifiers are rated according to the amount of water they can remove from the air in a 24-hour period, but these figures cannot be compared unless the temperature and humidity of the air are quoted; the amount of water removed varies as these figures vary. Ask for the removal rate at 70°F (21°C) and 70 percent relative humidity, as these are fairly typical conditions.

Ideally, a dehumidifier should have a built-in control that regulates it according to the humidity of the air, switching off the device when the air gets sufficiently dry.

Check how large the water tank is in relation to the amount of water the device can remove each day. It should be large enough to allow you to empty the tank just once a day. Good machines have an automatic cut-out to turn off the device when the

tank is almost full. The next best option is a warning light that tells you when the
tank is nearly full.

Suppliers include: Allergy Buyers Club is a good source for basic dehumidifiers;
Medivac, a British company, makes the Banamite Dehumidifier.

Ordinary electrical stores may sell dehumidifiers, but these are likely to be low-
powered machines that won't help much with allergies. Don't buy any dehumidifier
that doesn't come with some technical information on performance.

ALLERGEN-PROOF BEDDING AND COVERS

Fitting allergen-proof covers (sometimes called encasements) to the mattress, comforter, and pillows is the single most effective measure for anyone with dust-mite
allergy. You should, if at all possible, begin with a new mattress and bedding, so that
there are no dust mites to start with trapped inside the covers (see page 178).

There are a great many different products to choose from when it comes to bedding, and you need to be well informed. First, don't be taken in by vague terms such
as "antiallergenic," "nonallergenic," and "hypoallergenic." This may just mean that
the pillow contains polyester fiber or foam filling rather than feathers, which makes
little difference if you are allergic to dust mites and not allergic to feathers. In fact,
foam pillows tend to breed more dust mites than feather pillows, because the fabric
cover is less tightly woven and lets in the dust mites more easily.

Allergen-Proof Covers

If buying covers, remember that they need to form a barrier against dust-mite droppings, which are pretty small—just 10 to 30 microns in diameter. (A micron is a thousandth of a millimeter.) The mites themselves are considerably larger, though still too
small to be seen.

The allergen-proof covers are acting like giant filters or sieves, keeping the allergenic droppings inside. Ordinary pillow slips and comforter covers let the allergens
through because the spaces between the threads are larger than the droppings.

Controversy exists about whether the covers also need to protect against tiny
fragments of droppings. Some dust-mite experts believe that the droppings crumble
away when dry to create particles that may be as small as half a micron (0.5 mm).
Other experts disagree about the existence of these fragments or think they are too
few to matter.

This controversy has important implications for allergen-proof bedding covers.
Keeping a half-micron particle at bay is quite a feat, and the bedding covers designed
with this in mind have very small openings indeed. Air cannot easily flow through
the material, especially with covers that utilize a a microporous membrane (see below). This membrane is made of some kind of plastic material, with only the tiniest of
pores in it, so when you put your head on the pillow, the casing tends to billow up
around you and then slowly deflates. This can feel uncomfortable. The flow of moisture through the covers may also be a problem—perspiration cannot evaporate quickly,
so you may feel sticky and hot in bed.

If dust-mite droppings don't fragment, then the pores in a microporous membrane (or the gaps between the threads in a woven fabric) can be much larger—though still smaller than the gaps in regular fabric.

This controversy has not been resolved yet, but you can find out the latest information by going to the Allergy-Intolerance Web site at www.allergy-intolerance.com.

A research study at the University of Virginia, published in 1999, suggests that fragments are not a significant source of allergen. The research team found that mattress/bedding covers with pores of about 6 microns (6 mm) exclude almost all the dust-mite allergen while allowing adequate airflow. The covers that gave good results for both allergen containment and airflow were:

- Wondertex (made by GSI)

- Pristine (manufactured by Precision Fabrics Group, Inc., and available from Allergy Buyers Club and Allergy Control Products)

- Medibed (available from The Breathing Company)

- Softek (available from National Allergy Supply)

- Microfiber (available from Priorities; note that other covers from this company did not give such good airflow—see list below—and make sure you buy the right kind)

The following fabrics were good barriers against dust-mite allergen, but gave poor airflow. They will do the job for you, but you might find them less comfortable to use:

- 3M Propore

- ACb Elite cotton/polyester and Elite stretch

- Allergy-free environment: Ultra and terry cloth

- Aller/Guard: standard polyester/cotton, premium polyester/blend, and terry cloth

- Satin Soft

- Cotton Guard

- Priorities: stretch knit, polyester/cotton, and cotton terry

A summary of points to check before you buy:

- Mattress covers for long-term use should enclose the whole mattress, not just the top and sides. The seams should be well made and durable, with fine stitching.

- Check how the covers are fastened once in place. The fastening needs to be good, because the covers should form a complete seal around the mattress, pillow, or comforter, so that mites cannot enter and dropping particles cannot leave. Covers that just fold around a mattress and do not fasten together are unlikely to work.

- If the covers have a zipper, check that this does not provide an access route for mites. Some manufacturers supply a roll of special adhesive tape to block the tiny holes between the teeth of the zipper: this helps considerably in keeping mites out and allergen in. Where this is not supplied, you can seal the zip with any strong fabric tape—hardware stores usually sell various kinds for repairing tents, etc. You can also buy tape designed for this purpose from National Allergy Supply. This tape seal should be renewed every three months.

- Ask for a sample of the fabric used, so that you can check how soft and pliable it is. Some of the fabrics are quite stiff, and you may find them uncomfortable or hear them rustling when you roll over.

- Also check the sample to see how strong the fabric is—will it tear easily?

- Ask how long the covers are guaranteed for.

- Ask what type of material it is. Generally speaking, the synthetics known as **polyolefins** are less durable than other types of synthetic fabric and membranes, and they feel more papery.

- Ask how the covers should be cleaned: Can they be washed if necessary? At what temperature? (Only 131°F and above is sure to kill mites.)

- Are the covers safe for babies and young children? The ones made from a synthetic fabric, or with a plastic membrane, carry a risk of suffocation. Always check this point with the manufacturer.

There are six basic types of cover:

1. Covers made of a plastic such as polyethylene or PVC, which are completely impermeable. The cheapest option, and nothing can get through them, but that, unfortunately, includes water vapor (see pages 176–177).

2. Covers of the "microporous" or "semipermeable" kind. These are made either of a fairly soft synthetic fabric with tiny pores to let water vapor through, or cotton with a plastic membrane added, the membrane having tiny pores. (The latter may be referred to as a "laminated natural fabric.") The crucial question to ask is: How big are the pores? To form a barrier to droppings without restricting airflow, you need pores of about 6 microns. Up to 10 microns might be safe but, as the University of Virginia research team (see above) points out, the pores could get bigger as the cover is used and laundered. It recommends playing safe and buying a cover with a pore size of about 6 microns.

   If you are very sensitive to dust mites, you might benefit from covers with smaller pores. And if you are hoping to contain cat allergen rather than dust-mite allergen, then go for a smaller pore size—2 microns or less.

These covers, if fitted to comforters, can make the sleeper feel warmer than before, so if you are buying a new comforter, it may be advisable to go for a thinner one. There may be a risk of suffocation if these covers are used for young children.

3. A few covers are made from a material with a plastic membrane added, but without any pores. The membrane used is a special kind that can absorb moisture and transmit it to the other side of the fabric by a chemical process. These covers are very strong, and while they are more expensive, they do come with a guarantee. There may be a risk of suffocation if these covers are used for young children—check with the manufacturer. It is possible that they will make the comforter feel warmer, as the microporous covers do.

4. A new type of anti-mite cover is made from closely woven cotton or a polyester/cotton mixture. They have the advantage of feeling like ordinary pillowcases and comforter covers. Some of these did well in the University of Virginia tests.

The smallest pores (about half a micron) are found in covers made from very high-quality cotton (often called Egyptian cotton, though it isn't made in Egypt) that is boiled after being woven. This shrinks the cloth and makes the pores extremely small. These covers can be washed at very high temperatures and come with a lifetime guarantee. They can also withstand dry heat, which means you can use an electric blanket to dry out the bed thoroughly during the day. Because they are made of pure cotton, they are also suitable for people who are sensitive to synthetic fabrics and plastics. Be sure that you are buying covers designed specifically for anti-mite purposes: not all Egyptian cotton is made to this high standard.

5. A new type of cover uses electrostatic charge to hold the allergen particles while letting air through. This type of cover doesn't appear to be on sale in the United States and Canada at present.

6. Some covers work on a completely different principle, being treated with a pesticide (an acaricide) that kills the mites. Although the chemical used has been tested for safety, the long-term effects of daily close contact simply cannot be predicted. Many doctors feel uneasy about their patients sleeping in direct contact with pesticide-treated cloth night after night. Think very carefully before buying this type of cover.

Mattresses and Pillows with Built-in Covers

If you are going to buy a new mattress and pillow anyway, these are an attractive option. Most of the questions listed above are relevant to these products as well. Talk to the manufacturer about how you should go about controlling the dust mite levels on the outer surface (since you cannot take the covers off and wash them).

Suppliers include: Allergy Control Products, National Allergy Supply

Partial Mattress Covers for Traveling

If you travel a lot and are badly affected by mattresses when away from home, you could also buy a cover that just fits over the top and sides of the mattress (with an elasticized edge, like a shower cap). These are cheaper than full mattress covers and can be fitted very quickly. They do decrease the amounts of allergen breathed in, but mite allergens will still fall out underneath and eventually get into the sleeper's airways, so they are not recommended for long-term use at home. While removing the bedding and fitting the mattress cover, wear a mask to keep allergens out of your airways. Keep it on and leave the room for an hour or so, to let disturbed allergen settle, before retiring for the night.

Suppliers include: Allergy Control Products

Washable Pillows and Comforters

If you have a large washing machine and a tumble dryer, these may be a good alternative to allergen-proof covers. They should be able to withstand washing at 140°F or higher. One advantage of these products is that there is no risk of suffocation for young children, whereas some of the covers may carry this risk.

Suppliers include: Allergy Control Products, National Allergy Supply

Washable Blankets

If they can be washed at 140°F or higher, these are very useful as underblankets or as an alternative to a comforter.

Suppliers include: Allergy Control Products, National Allergy Supply

Custom-made Allergen-Proof Covers

Certain allergy supply companies allow you to order custom-fitted mite covers for any size cushion or mattress. These can be useful if, for example, you decide on a new futon-style sofa and armchairs (see page 185–186) for the living room.

Suppliers include: Allergy Control Products

VACUUM CLEANERS

High-retention vacuum cleaners are useful for people with dust-mite allergy, in combination with other anti-mite measures, such as bedding covers. These vacuum cleaners may also be valuable to people with cat allergy and, perhaps, to those with hay fever if they are being affected by pollen fragments (see page 115). The crucial test is whether you suffer increased symptoms during vacuuming or after someone else has vacuumed the house.

Ordinary vacuum cleaners spray allergen particles into the air. This increases the amount of allergen inhaled. There can be three times as much mite allergen in the air after vacuuming as before, even with a top-brand vacuum cleaner. The amount and size of the particles emitted vary considerably from one manufacturer to another, but all ordinary vacuum cleaners let out enough to affect someone who is sensitized to dust-mite allergen.

Vacuum cleaners designed for those with dust-mite allergy generally employ a HEPA filter (see page 309) to filter the exhaust. Most of this section is about HEPA vacuum cleaners, but first we will deal with the other options.

Some newer vacuum cleaners employ water to filter the exhaust. These machines are very heavy, because of the water. Their big advantage is that there is no bag to empty—the waste water can be disposed of with much less risk to the allergy sufferer than fly-away dust.

Centralized vacuum cleaning systems (see below) are probably the very best option, if you can afford one.

Wet vacuuming systems are not recommended (see pages 325–27). (Superheated steam cleaners *are* recommended—see pages 325–27 —but these don't generally include a vacuum cleaning facility. They just produce steam, and you have to vacuum as a separate operation.)

For now, most people will be buying a HEPA vacuum cleaner, so it is important to look at the performance of these machines.

Almost all the claims made for HEPA vacuum cleaners (claims about how much dust is extracted from the emitted air) are based on the effectiveness of the HEPA filter itself, not the machine as a whole. Unfortunately, there are reasons for thinking that, in some machines at least, dust may evade the HEPA filter. This can happen, for example, if the seal around the filter is not airtight. Some scientists studying allergy prevention have found that in some HEPA vacuum cleaners, a lot of dusty air goes around the edges, rather than through the filter.

Unfiltered air can also escape from the joints of the vacuum cleaner if these become distorted slightly while the cleaner is in use. This may happen with some plastic casings when subjected to heat and high working pressures from the machine's motor.

When manufacturers quote the filtration rate for their vacuum cleaner, they are simply talking about the HEPA filter, and this may give no real indication of the amount of dust escaping from the machine. A slightly better test is to assess the dust particles in the exhaust stream from the vacuum cleaner (as done in some published tests of vacuum cleaners) but this does not measure the amount of *allergen* emitted, nor take into account leakage from the joints of the machine when the motor gets hot.

The best testing method is to look at the level of *allergen* in the air after vacuuming a room: this tests the emissions from the machine as a whole, and by looking at the allergen, rather than at dust particles, it measures what actually causes allergy symptoms and asthma attacks.

Only one type of antiallergy vacuum cleaner, the Medivac, has been rigorously tested in this way and the test results published. A scientific trial conducted at Wythenshawe Hospital in Manchester, England, has shown that there is no increase in the amount of mite allergen in the air after using this machine, whereas there is three times as much allergen in the air after using a standard (non-HEPA) vacuum cleaner. The Medivac has a metal body, which prevents the joints from becoming distorted and leaky. It relies on a very high-quality HEPA filter, which is protected from clogging by a prefilter.

Other HEPA vacuum cleaners, in which the filters have been tested but not the whole machine, may be adequate for many allergy sufferers. Indeed, people with allergies frequently report feeling better after using them. If one of these machines works well for you or your allergic child, then stick with it. But if you still experience allergy symptoms after vacuuming, you might want to consider the Medivac.

Be on your guard when buying a vacuum cleaner because several companies producing ordinary vacuum cleaners have now begun to make claims about the dust-retaining power of their machines in an attempt to attract allergy sufferers. A claim that a vacuum "retains 99.9 percent of dust" is useless unless the particle size to which the claim relates is given. It may well be relevant only for particles more than a micron in size, in which case smaller allergenic particles will be emitted. Specialized vacuum cleaners, designed for those with allergy, should retain over 99 percent of particles of 0.3 micron in size.

There is no such thing as a cheap HEPA vacuum cleaner. These machines are considerably more expensive than a normal vacuum cleaner because they have to be made to much higher specifications, and the motor has to be more powerful to overcome the air resistance created by the HEPA filter.

Suppliers include: Most allergy supply companies offer one or more vacuum cleaners, but for a wider range of different brands, and the best prices, a specialist dealer such as ABCvacuum.com is recommended.

The Medivac can be ordered via the Medivac Web site. For use in the United States and Canada it needs a voltage converter (transformer), available from www.DirectMerchandiseUSA.com or www.geocities.com/voltage_converter.

Central Vacuum Systems

These built-in vacuum systems are a good but expensive option. A system can be installed in new houses or into existing houses as long as they have cavity walls. A high-power vacuum unit is installed in the garage, basement, or other storage area, and concealed pipes lead to each room in the house. There is an inlet hole (fairly inconspicuous) in each room, and you plug your flexible vacuum hose into one of these. The dust is sucked up efficiently and taken directly out of the room through the pipes and into the central vacuum unit. It should be foolproof. Someone who is not allergic should be responsible for emptying the centralized collection unit when necessary. If this isn't possible, wear a really good dust mask.

Suppliers include: ABCvacuum.com, Cyclo Vac, American Systems Service Center Ltd. ServiceMaster is also planning to sell a system of this kind in the near future.

Filters for Ordinary Vacuum Cleaners

These fit over the exhaust of a conventional vacuum cleaner. They will reduce the amount of dust allergen thrown out, but certainly won't eliminate it. However, these can be useful as a cheap short-term measure while you save up for a proper vacuum cleaner.

Suppliers include: Allergy Control Products

Wet Vacuuming Devices

You may find that some allergy companies are still marketing a wet vacuuming system with a special anti-mite shampoo. Although good results are claimed for this treatment, one study showed that it was no better than intensive dry vacuum cleaning. Another found that there was an increase in mite populations in the carpet after the treatment, probably because of the increase in humidity and the selective removal of other mites that normally prey on *Dermatophagoides*. The general conclusion is that wet vacuuming cannot be recommended at present.

DUSTING CLOTHS

There are dusting clothes available that carry an electrostatic charge, similar to that of a charged media filter (see pages 309 and 310). These cloths attract and hold the dust so that very little becomes airborne during dusting. (A similar effect can be obtained by wet dusting, but the electrostatic cloth is less bother.)

Suppliers include: Allergy Supply Company, The Breathing Company, National Allergy Supply

ACARICIDE TREATMENTS FOR CARPETS AND FURNITURE

The pros and cons of using acaricides are discussed on pages 183–85. We would caution against any treatments containing pyrethroids or permethrin. Check exactly what the treatment contains before you buy (and remember that pyrethroids can quite legitimately be labeled "natural"). Treatments based on benzyl benzoate or disodium octaborate tetrahydrate (sold under the brand name Dustmitex) are less worrying, but we would be concerned about you using them regularly on a long-term basis if you have small children. (Again, the word "natural" is being used in the marketing for disodium octaborate tetrahydrate, implying that it is therefore totally safe—this, of course, is naive; see page 185 for the symptoms caused by overexposure to this substance.) There are many other ways to tackle dust mites now. These may involve more financial outlay in the short term, but they are good investments, and over the long run the cost will probably be about the same.

Sprays such as tannic acid that inactivate allergen but don't kill mites are dealt with on page 326.

Suppliers include: For Dustmitex: Allergy Control Products, The Ecology Works, Allergy Clean Environments, National Allergy Supply

SUPERHEATED STEAM CLEANERS

Superheated steam not only kills mites; it also inactivates Der p1, a key dust-mite allergen. This finding has been put to work in the development of steam cleaners specifically designed to combat dust mites.

Two super-heated steam cleaners have been tested against dust mites—the Medivap and the Polti Vaporetto. Both were tested by independent scientists.

The Polti Vaporetto was tested by The Medical Entomology Centre in Cambridge, England, in 1995, and the results can be found at www.polti.ca. Three minutes of cleaning on a square meter of carpet reduced the number of mites in the carpet by 96.8 percent.

This sounds good, but bear in mind that there were still mites left—119 live mites in one carpet square. Mites breed fast, and in ideal conditions those 119 mites could multiply rapidly, producing a lot of allergic droppings in the process.

The Medivap was tested at the University of Glasgow in Scotland, and the results published in *Clinical and Experimental Allergy* in 1995. The Medivap killed all the mites in eight carpet squares. A rigorous test was used to ensure that there really were no live mites left in the carpet.

Both machines had the same effect on the amount of Der p1 allergen, reducing it by over 85 percent.

The length of cleaning needed to produce these results was 3 minutes per square meter (1 square yard) for the Polti Vaporetto and 2.5 minutes per square meter for the Medivap. Take note of this if you are thinking of buying a superheated steam cleaner—an average-sized living room (15 feet by 15 feet) would need to be cleaned for an hour with the Medivap, and longer with the Vaporetto, to be sure of achieving these results. But when you did the job with the Medivap you would know that all the mites were dead, and the chore would not need repeating for at least a month. (In the laboratory, the carpets remained mite-free, but in a real-life situation, new mites will arrive, stowaways on people's clothing, so the numbers will very gradually build up again—unless you use other ongoing measures, such as a dehumidifier; see page 317.

Both of these machines use high pressure to produce abnormally hot steam—the temperature of the steam is well above the usual boiling point of water (which is 212°F or 100°C). It has to be at this high temperature to still be good and hot by the time it reaches the base of the carpet pile (which is where the dust mites lurk) and to keep that zone hot long enough to kill the mites.

The Medivap heats the water to 302°F (150°C) in the tank, and delivers steam that is at 251.6°F (122°C). The Vaporetto heats water to above 300°F (149°C) and delivers steam that is at 248°F (120°C).

Several other products are now being marketed for mite allergy. None of these devices appears to have been tested directly on dust mites. They include:

- The Ladybug and the Tidyvap, which quote "steam temperatures" of 296–298°F (146–148°F). Inquiries have revealed that these are actually the temperatures within the boiler. According to the supplier's data, the temperature of the steam as it comes out of the nozzle is 180 to 200 °F (82–93°C)—which means it is not actually steam at all. This just won't be good enough to kill a significant number of mites.

- The Delongi Vapor Steam Cleaner, which claims to heat the water to over 248°F. Assuming this is the boiler temperature rather than the steam delivery temperature (the suppliers have not been able to clarify this point for us), this device definitely wouldn't be up to the job.

- The Supervapore Cleaning System claims to "hold up to two hours of high-pressure steam heated to 240°F." Again, this sounds like the boiler temperature, not the steam delivery temperature. Even if it is the steam delivery temperature, it is too low to kill all the mites.

Keep these technical points about temperatures in mind when looking at other devices that call themselves "steam cleaners." Unfortunately, many devices are now being sold that are described as steam cleaners but are nothing of the kind. This is what Consumer Search, the acclaimed independent product review company, has to say about the steam cleaners that are widely sold: "Their names notwithstanding, consumer carpet cleaners don't clean with steam. They spray a hot-water/detergent solution onto the carpet, agitate the carpet fibers with powered brushes, and then extract the solution and dirt with suction." (See www.consumersearch.comhouse_and_home/steam_cleaners.) In other words, they are nothing more than a hot-water washing or wet vacuuming system.

A machine that produces steam but not superheated steam may kill some of the mites, but the fact that the steam cools quickly once it hits the carpet limits its effectiveness. Such a device is unlikely to have much effect on the mite allergens in your carpet, and leaves behind far more moisture than superheated steam. The surviving mites will thrive and multiply, and you will soon be back to square one.

Thus, a so-called steam cleaner that doesn't produce superheated steam *could actually make the dust-mite problem worse.*

Commercial operators who offer to visit your home and carry out a "steam treatment" on your carpets are usually offering just wet-vacuuming or a treatment with ordinary steam (rather than superheated steam). They will not help much with your allergies and will probably boost the numbers of dust mites in the long run.

Suppliers include: The Medivap can be found on the Medivac Web site. There are various local distributors for the Polti Vaporetto—check the Polti Web site at www.polti.ca for your nearest distributor.

HEAT TREATMENT FOR BEDS AND FURNITURE

There is now a special process that goes where no dust-mite treatment has gone before: right inside beds and furniture. It kills the mites by using prolonged high temperatures, first enclosing the bed or furniture in an enormous plastic bag (called a Diathermic Envelope) and then pumping in hot air. The Diathermic Envelope keeps the temperature high and ensures that the heat gets deep inside the upholstery. As well as killing the mites, it inactivates one of the two main allergens, Der p1.

If you have living room furniture that you love too much to part with, or a high-quality bed/mattress that would be costly to replace, then this may be the answer.

This treatment is quite expensive, so you probably wouldn't want to repeat it too regularly. It makes sense to combine this with other ongoing measures to keep down mite numbers, such as improved ventilation and an allergen-proof mattress cover.

This treatment was invented in Britain, where it is increasingly popular with allergy sufferers. There are hopes that it will become available in the United States and Canada in mid-2002: check the Allergy-Intolerance Web site at www.allergy-intolerance.com for news of this.

Supplier: ServiceMaster

TANNIC ACID SPRAYS

These are sprays that denature (see the box on page 181) the dust-mite allergen and are probably effective against other allergens too. *They do not kill mites.* As well as denaturing the allergen, the tannic acid makes it less sticky so that it is taken up more readily by a vacuum cleaner. The tannic acid spray itself dries to a powder within about three hours. This powder can likewise be removed by thorough vacuuming.

By destroying the reservoir of allergen in carpets and upholstery, the tannic acid spray has an effect that lasts for two to three months, even though the mites themselves are still alive and the tannic acid does not have any ongoing effect on the allergens they produce.

Tannic acid is sold in a spray form under the brand name Allersearch ADS. It is also available in Allersearch X-MITE, which consists of "non-abrasive , sponge-like particles" that contain a detergent along with the tannic acid.

Don't confuse these products with Allersearch Allergy Wash, which is simply a detergent (see "Laundry Additives" below).

Suppliers include: Allergy Control Products, Allergy Clean Environments, The Allergy Store, National Allergy Supply

OTHER SPRAYS THAT INACTIVATE ALLERGEN

Rather than denature the allergen, sprays containing polysaccharide (starch) just stick the allergen particles together, making big lumps that are too large to become airborne and be inhaled. They are thought to be safe, but no studies on the effects of long-term use have been carried out.

Numerous sprays that claim to "deactivate" allergens are on the market now, and many are bashful about their contents, listing only "natural" or "plant-derived" ingredients on the label. Ask the retailer to provide more information.

LAUNDRY ADDITIVES

A useful aid in the fight against dust mites is a laundry additive containing benzyl benzoate (brand name De-mite), which kills dust mites in your clothes, draperies, and bedding, even when washing at low temperatures (washing at temperatures below 131°F would normally allow the mites to survive). The benzyl benzoate is removed from your clothes during the rinse cycle, so there are no worries about toxicity.

Watch out, however, for laundry additives being marketed for allergies that simply claim to "remove all allergens" from your clothes. These are basically just detergent, and they offer you nothing more than an ordinary detergent offers. All allergens are removed by washing with ordinary detergent—at whatever temperature. You don't need a special laundry product for this.

Another laundry product being promoted for allergies claims to denature allergens in your clothes. Denaturing allergens (inactivating them by altering them chemically) is a useful approach in the case of carpets and furniture (see box on page 181). But with clothing—where ordinary washing, at whatever temperature, will wash away all the allergens anyway—denaturing is utterly irrelevant.

There is no value in special laundry additives unless they kill mites.

Suppliers include: For De-mite: The Allergy Store, The Breathing Company, National Allergy Supply

SPRAYS AND SOLUTIONS FOR MOLD

There is a solution available for cleaning molds from bathroom tiles, vinyl baths and bathmats, garbage cans, and surfaces being prepared for painting. It contains a form of bleach and has a fairly strong smell, but is more effective in removing black mold than domestic bleach.

A spray that prevents mildew regrowth on shower curtains as well as hard surfaces such as tiles and wood is also sold. This contains a fungicide.

Suppliers include: Allergy Control Products, National Allergy Supply

TREATMENTS FOR PETS

There is a product marketed for pets that is applied to the animal's coat and is claimed to reduce the amount of pet allergen in the air. This product was tested by a group of scientists at the Henry Ford Hospital in Detroit, and the results published in the *Journal of Allergy and Clinical Immunology* in 1995. Using the product once a week, according to the manufacturer's instructions, for a period of 8 weeks, the scientists found that there was no reduction in the amount of cat allergen in the air. Another study was carried out by the manufacturers of the product and published on their Web site but not in a scientific journal. This study measured only the amount of cat allergen in settled dust and in the towels used to treat the cats. The researchers were unable to measure cat allergen in the air, which is the thing that actually matters to allergy sufferers. This seems to be a less rigorous study than the one carried out by the Detroit scientists. While it suggests that there was less allergen in the towels used on the cats and in the settled dust, this doesn't necessarily mean that the amount in the air would be reduced. Another research study would be useful here.

INDOOR POLLUTION AND "SICK BUILDING SYNDROME"

Two companies now offer consultancy and treatment services for offices that are afflicted by "Sick Building Syndrome." They are Rentokil W & V Consultancy Services and Healthy Buildings International.

For indoor pollution, the best treatment is to eliminate the sources of pollutants. If formaldehyde is suspected as a problem, there is a formaldehyde-monitoring badge, made by 3M, that can show how much formaldehyde you are exposed to every day.

MANUFACTURERS
AND SUPPLIERS

ABC Vacuum Warehouse
6720 Burnet Rd.,
Austin, TX 78757
Tel: 800-285-8145
E-mail: discount@abcvacuum.com
Web site: www.ABCVacuum.com
Sells a comprehensive range of vacuum cleaners, including centralized vacuum systems.

Allergy Buyers Club
161 North St.
Newtonville, MA 02460
Tel: 888-236-7231
Fax: 617-332-0292
E-mail: saleshelp1@allergybuyersclub.com
Web site: www.allergybuyersclub.com

Allergy Clean Environments
3500 Jefferson, Suite 103
Austin, TX 78731
Tel (at the Austin store): 512-323-5522
Toll-free for orders: 800-882-4110
E-mail: sales@allergyclean.com
Web site: www.allergyclean.com
This company can sell via the Internet, but operates nonvirtual stores in Texas—in addition to the one in Austin, there are stores in Fort Worth, Bedford, Richardson, and Dallas. Check the Web site for details.

Allergy Control Products
96 Danbury Rd.
Ridgefield, CT 06877
Tel: 800-422-3878
Fax: 203-431-8963
E-mail: info@allergycontrol.com
Web site: www.allergycontrol.com

The Allergy Store
1841 SW 94th Ave.
Miami, FL 33165
Tel: 888-337-5665
305-223-5710 (local calls)
Fax: 305-220-3334
E-mail: sales@allergystore.net
Web site: www.allergystore.net

Allergy Supply Company
11994 Star Ct.
Herndon, VA 20171
Tel: 800-323-6744
703-391-2011(within Washington, DC)
Fax orders: 800-681-5454
E-mail: allergy@allergysupply.com
Web site: www.allergysupply.com
A reputable medical company. It sells a limited range of products but all are good (e.g., Enviracaire air cleaners).

American Allergy Supply
P.O. Box 722022
Houston, TX 77272-2022
Tel: 800-321-1096
E-mail: American@netropolis.net
Web site: www.americanallergy.com

AO Safety
Web site: www.aosafetysrx.com/frames
Sells some attractive safety glasses and goggles, which will keep pollen out of your eyes. For hay fever sufferers who normally wear glasses for near- or farsightedness, this company can make up safety specs with prescription lenses or sell you some inexpensive clip-on side shields for your existing prescription glasses. The web site can direct you to your nearest distributor.

The Breathing Company
P.O. Box 898
Soquel, CA 95073
Tel: 877-475-8647
831-475-4300 (local calls)
Fax: 831-475-4300
E-Mail: info@thebreathingcompany.com
Web site: www.thebreathingcompany.com

Cyclo Vac International
Trovac Industries
3 rue Marcel Ayotte
Blainville
Quebec J7C 5L7
Canada
Tel: 888-77CYCLO or 800-361-9553
450-434-2233 (local calls)
Fax: 450-434-6111
Web site: www.cyclovac.com
Supplies built-in centralized vacuum systems for houses.

The Ecology Works
P.O. Box 9067
San Rafael, CA 94912
Tel: 888-353-2649
415-459-3903 (local calls)
Fax: 415-459-3924
E-mail: ali@silcon.com
Web site: www.dustmitex.com

Dolisos
3014 Rigel Ave.
Las Vegas, NV 89102
Tel: 800-365-4767
Homeopathic supplier that offers regional allergy mixes for use in homeopathic desensitization treatments.

Medivac Healthcare Ltd
Wilmslow House
Grove Way
Wilmslow
Cheshire SK9 5AG
United Kingdom
Tel: 011 44 1625 539401
Fax: 011 44 1625 539507
E-mail: medivacuk@aol.com
Web site: www.medivac.co.uk
This company produces the Medivac vacuum cleaner, the Medivap steam cleaner, and the Banamite Dehumidifier, all designed specifically to combat dust mites, made to exceptionally high standards, and independently tested in reputable scientific laboratories to show that they really do work. There is an electronic dust monitor that fits onto the Medivac machine to show when vacuuming is complete.

All the machines run on UK voltage, and to use them in North America you will need a voltage converter (transformer), available from www.DirectMerchandiseUSA.com or www.geocities.com/voltage_converter

National Allergy Supply
1620 Satellite Blvd., Suite D
Duluth, GA 30097
Tel: 800-522-1448
Fax: 770-623-5568
E-mail: info@natlallergy.com
Web site: www.natlallergy.com

Ohio Glove & Safety, Inc.
Tel: 800-686-1459
330-989-1344 (local calls)
Fax: 330-898-7812
E-mail: Sales@ohioglove.com
Web site: www.ohioglove.com/
    disposable-respirators3.htm
Sells some stylish safety glasses and goggles
to keep pollen out of the eyes. Also sells a
good range of quality dust masks, plus
masks that will take out gases and
volatiles as well as dust. It also stocks more
sophisticated respirators for those with
severe allergy problems.

Vimco, Inc.
1519 Mars-Evans City Rd.
Evans City, PA 16033
Tel: 724-538-5050
Fax: 724-538-9801
Web site: www.vimcoinc.com
Homeopathic supplier offers "allersodes"
—grass and weed mixes for use in ho-
meopathic desensitization therapy.

Appendix 4
MEDICINAL DRUGS

This appendix covers the drugs commonly used in hay fever and asthma.

Drugs are referred to in two ways—by their proper (generic) name and by the trade names given them by manufacturers. The same drug may be marketed under a number of different trade names if it is produced by different manufacturers. Some medicines contain a mixture of two or more drugs. Drugs are described here under their generic names, which are given in italics (e.g., *acrivastine*). The trade names are shown with a capital letter (e.g., Actidil).

This list of drugs is reasonably comprehensive, but new drugs are introduced all the time, so a medicine you are prescribed may not be mentioned here if it is fairly new on the market.

How to Use the Lists
Beside each drug is a code number that shows what type of drug it is, referring to the following:

1 Mast-cell stabilizers (see page 86)
2 Antihistamines (see page 87)
3 Sympathomimetic nose sprays and drops (see page 94)
2/3 Antihistamine and sympathomimetic combined in tablet or liquid form (see page 96)
4 Corticosteroids (see page 98)
5 Antileukotriene drugs (see page 104)
6 Anticholinergics (see page 230)

Generic names
acrivastine 2
alclometasone 4
atropine 6
azatadine 2
azelastine 2
beclomethasone 4
betamethasone 4
brompheniramine 2, 2/3
budesonide 4
butethamate 6
cetirizine 2

chlorpheniramine 2, 2/3
clemastine 2
clobetasol 4
clobetasone 4
cromolyn 1
cyproheptadine 2
desonide 4
desoxymethasone 4
dexamethasone 4
diphenhydramine 2, 2/3
diflucortolone 4
fexofenadine 2

fluclorolone 4
flunisolide 4
fluocinolone 4
fluocortolone 4
fluorometholone 4
flurandrenolone 4
fluticasone 4
halcinonide 4
hydrocortisone 4
hydroxyzine 2
ipratropium 6
ketotifen 2
levocabastine 2
loratadine 2
medrysone 4
methylprednisolone 4
mizolastine 2
mometasone 4
naphazoline 3
nedocromil, nedocromil sodium 1
oxitropium 6
oxymetozoline 3
phenindamine 2
pheniramine 2, 2/3
phenylephrine 3, 2/3
phenylpropanolamine 2/3
prednisolone 4
promethazine 2
pseudoephedrine 3, 2/3
rimexolone 4
sodium cromoglycate 1
tetrahydrozoline 3
triamcinolone 4
trimeprazine 2
triprolidine 2, 2/3
xylometazoline 3

Trade names

This is not, and cannot be, an exhaustive list. Some of the older drugs (those no longer covered by a patent) are produced by many different pharmaceutical companies, and are therefore sold under a great variety of brand names. New brands are introduced all the time.

Actidil 2
Actifed 2/3
AeroBid 4
Afrin 3
AK Dex 4
AK-Pred 4
Alconefrin 3
Allegra 2
Aller-Chlor 2
Allerdryl 2
Allermax 2
Anergan 2
Apo-Hydroxyzine 2
Astelin 2
Atarax 2
Beconase 4
Beconase AQ Nasal 4
Betnesol 4
Chlor-Pro 2
Claritin 2
Claritin RediTabs 2
Congesteze 2/3
Contac Allergy 12-Hour 2
Decadron Opthalmic Suspension 4
Decadron Phosphate 4
Decadron Phosphate Turbinaire 4
Dexa-Rhinaspray 4
Dimotane 2
Dimotane Plus 2/3
Dristan Nasal Spray 3
Dristan Allergy 2/3
Econopred 4
Eumovate 4
Flarex 4
Flixonase 4
Flonase 4
Fluor-Op 4
FML 4
FML Forte 4
FML Liquifilm 4
Genasal 3

Hayfebrol 2/3

Haymine 2/3

HMS 4

Inflamase Forte 4

Inflamase Mild Opthalmic 4

Intal

Lasma 58

Livostin 2

Maxidex 4

Metreton 4

Minims 4

Mizollen 2

Multipax 2

Myidyl 2

Nalcrom 1

Nasacort 4

Nasacort AQ 4

Nasalcrom 1

Nasalide 4

Nasonex 4

Neosynephrine 3

Nolahist 2

Nostrilla 3

Opticrom 1

Optimine 2

Otrivine-Antistin 2, 3

Otrivine 3

Oxivent 5C

Periactin 2

Phenazine 2

Phenergan 2

Phenetron 2

Pred Forte 4

Pred-Mild 4

Predsol 4

Privine 3

Prothazine 2

Rhinocort 4

Rhinocort Aqua 4

Rynacrom, Rynacrom Compound 1

Semprex 2

Sinarest 3

Sinex 3

Sudafed Plus 2/3

Syntaris 4

Tavist 2

Teldrin 2

Temaril 2

Tilade 1

Tyzine 3

Vancenase Nasal 4

Veltane 2

Vexol 4

Vibrocil 2/3 (+ an antibiotic)

Vista-Methasone 4

Vistaryl 2

Vistazine 2

Zaditen 2

Zyrtek 2 ✓

Appendix 5
Getting Additional Help

POLLEN COUNTS AND FORECASTS

A good service should give pollen counts (from the previous day), pollen forecasts for the coming day, and the general outlook for the next three days. The best services cover different types of pollen separately and give counts for mold spores.

You can check out your local newspaper to see if it offers good pollen information, but the easiest place to look is the Internet. The two Web sites below allow you to search for local information, but a search engine may point you to other options.

www.pollen.com. Gives a four-day forecast and lists predominant pollens.

www.allernet.com. A site maintained by the National Pollen Network that provides information about local conditions and offers allergy forecasts. Lists levels for grass, tree, and weed pollens as well as molds.

PATIENT SUPPORT GROUPS AND CAMPAIGNING ORGANIZATIONS

Asthma and Allergy Foundation of America (AAFA)
1233 20th St. NW, Suite 402
Washington, DC 20036
Tel: 202-466-7643
Toll-free help line: 800-7-ASTHMA (727-8462)
Fax: 202-466-8940
Web site: www.aafa.org

Allergy/Asthma Information Association (AAIA)
Tel: 800-611-7011
Web site: www.aaia.org
A Canadian patient support group.

PROFESSIONAL MEDICAL ASSOCIATIONS

These can be helpful if you need to find a well-qualified allergist.

Canadian Society of Allergy and Clinical Immunology
Web site: www.csaci.medical.org

American Academy of Allergy, Asthma, and Immunology
Web site: www.aaaai.org

BREAST-FEEDING SUPPORT AND ADVICE

La Leche League International
1400 N. Meacham Rd.
Schaumburg, IL 60168-4079
Tel: 847-519-7730 (U.S.)
Tel: 800-665-4342 (Canada)
Web site: www.lalecheleague.org
Offers mother-to-mother help and encouragement to mothers who want to breast-feed their children. There are local groups in all 50 U.S. states as well as many other countries. Its Web site can help you find a local group.

Motherwear
320 Riverside Dr.
Northampton, MA 01062
Tel: 800-950-2500
Web site: www.motherwear.com
Motherwear offers tops, dresses, night-wear, swimsuits, bras, breast pumps, and other items for nursing mothers.

ADVICE ON ALLERGY PRODUCTS

For detailed advice on products marketed for allergy and intolerance sufferers, go to the Allergy-Intolerance Web site at www.allergy-intolerance.com.

ADVICE AND SUPPLY SERVICES FOR DOCTORS ONLY

This organization cannot deal with inquiries from the general public—please ask your doctor to contact them.

Dome Hollister Stier
P.O. Box 3145
Terminal Annexe
North 3525 Regal St.
Spokane, WA 99220
Tel: 509-489-5656
Supplies a very wide range of individual allergens for skin-prick testing.

FURTHER READING

For detailed information on asthma, food allergies, and food intolerance, please refer to the following books, both by Jonathan Brostoff, M.D., and Linda Gamlin:

Asthma: The Complete Guide to Integrative Therapies (Healing Arts Press, 2000)

Food Allergies and Food Intolerance: The Complete Guide to Their Identification and Treatment (Healing Arts Press, 2000)

You can order these titles directly from Healing Arts Press by calling 800-246-8648 or on the Web at www.InnerTraditions.com.

Appendix 6
AIR POLLUTION

The main sources of pollution are summarized here, and suggestions for avoiding or combating them are given at the end of the appendix.

VEHICLE EXHAUST

Pollution from traffic is steadily increasing and will continue to do so as the volume of traffic continues to increase.

Of the many pollutants formed by vehicles, carbon dioxide, carbon monoxide, and lead are not considered important in allergy, although they may affect health in other ways. Other pollutants that are relevant to allergic problems include diesel particulates and nitrogen dioxide. Volatile organic compounds are also important because they play a role in producing ozone, which acts as an irritant to the airways. See chapter 4, "Suspect Number Four: Air Pollution," for details.

Nitrogen Oxides

Nitric oxide (chemical formula: NO) is produced by the burning of gasoline. Having left the exhaust pipe, it combines with oxygen in the air to form nitrogen dioxide (NO_2). The latter is a reddish brown gas that you can actually see in the air when smog forms over busy urban areas, particularly if you are looking down on the city from a hillside or a tall building. However, there can also be significant levels of nitrogen dioxide in homes with gas stoves (see page 338). Nitrogen dioxide is an irritant in its own right, but also plays a part in producing ozone (see below).

Volatile Organic Compounds

Gasoline evaporates when cars are filled at a gas station and whenever any is spilled on the road. Oil also evaporates when it is spilled or when it leaks from engines. These are major sources of **volatile organic compounds,** or **VOCs.** (There are other sources, however, including fluids used for dry cleaning, solvents used in products such as glue and paint, spray paints used on cars, and industrial processes. Natural VOCs are described below.)

VOCs can be harmful in themselves—some are carcinogens, for example. They can also play a role in the formation of ground-level ozone (see below).

Ground-level Ozone

Useful though it may be in the stratosphere, at ground level ozone is a menace, a serious irritant to the airways.

Ozone is produced not directly by vehicles, but through a complex interaction of nitrogen dioxide, VOCs, sunlight, and the natural oxygen in the air. The worst time for ozone formation is in summer. This interaction creates the **photochemical smogs** that now plague Los Angeles, Athens, and Mexico City. Photochemical smogs can become very acidic in certain situations, which adds to the irritant effects of ozone and nitrogen dioxide.

Because nitric oxide in exhaust fumes can also break down ozone, the highest levels of ozone are often found in the countryside downwind of a big city, which receives a stream of ozone-rich air from the urban traffic but lacks the nitric oxide concentrations needed to break down ozone again.

In addition to man-made VOCs, there are naturally occurring VOCs produced by plants (see page 117). Trees, in particular, produce large amounts of these. When combined with nitrogen dioxide from traffic, they may contribute to the reactions of photochemical smogs and the consequent formation of ozone, but their contribution is minimal compared to synthetic pollutants. In the countryside, some natural VOCs can help to break down ozone.

Diesel Particulates

When properly maintained and finely tuned, diesel engines are actually less polluting than gas engines. However, lack of tuning makes diesel engines produce large amounts of particulates (soot particles) carrying various chemicals. Poorly maintained diesel engines also produce sulfur dioxide, an irritant to the airways. Nitrogen oxides are produced in approximately the same amounts from diesel as from non-diesel engines, but there are more **polycyclic aromatic hydrocarbons (PAHs),** some of which may be irritants or carcinogens.

DOMESTIC HEATING AND POWER STATIONS

Unless very high temperatures are used, burning any fuel produces smoke—that is, a mixture of carbon particles and gases. There are generally more particulates from coal than from oil or gas. Wood-burning stoves can also produce carbon particles, plus PAHs (see previous section).

Coal contains variable amounts of sulfur, more in the poorer grades of coal. This forms **sulfur dioxide** (SO_2) when burned, a gas that is highly irritating to the bronchi.

This type of pollution has been much reduced; however, there are still problems with sulfur dioxide pollution and sulfuric acid mists in some areas. Those near coal-fired power stations or heavy industry are likely to be the most affected.

CIGARETTE SMOKE

Cigarette smoke is a major form of pollution for many people. It includes small carbon particulates, PAHs, (see above), and a cocktail of other chemicals. Cigarette smoke is carcinogenic, even to those who simply inhale other people's smoke ("passive smokers"). It is also an irritant, but one that affects some people much more severely than others. Passive smoking is known to increase the risk of asthma.

BURNING YARD WASTE

The smoke from a bonfire or burn pile contains a similar assortment of damaging chemicals as that from a cigarette, including irritants and carcinogens. If plastic or foam rubber is added to the blaze, even more powerful irritants can be produced. The widespread idea that this form of pollution causes no harm is mistaken.

INDOOR POLLUTION

For many people, the air in the home can be more polluted than that which they breathe outdoors. Tight draft-proofing in modern houses leads to poor ventilation, and if pollutants are then generated they can build up to high levels.

Tobacco smoke is one major source of pollution in the home. Another is the kitchen, where burning fats and oils create a fine blue smoke that can be highly irritating to the airways. If the cooking is done on a gas stove, some nitrogen dioxide is generated (see page 57), which can build up to significant levels if ventilation is poor.

Formaldehyde is produced by various items in the home (see page 215) and can act as an irritant. Recent studies have shown that high levels in the air encourage the development of allergies. Solvents from paint and household chemicals are frequently allowed to evaporate into the air within the home. Air fresheners and aerosol sprays add to the rich cocktail of synthetic chemicals in the air. Plastic wallpapers and flooring "outgas" various chemicals. Research from Finland shows that children whose homes contain such items are more allergy-prone.

ACTION ON POLLUTION

Reducing Your Own Exposure

Reducing your exposure to cigarette smoke is relatively easy if you are determined about it. This applies whether you are an active or a passive smoker. In the past decade various aids to giving up smoking have been developed. Ask any pharmacist about these products.

Kitchens with gas stoves should have some additional ventilation installed, such as a small extractor fan. Alternatively, just open the window a little when cooking. Keep ovens clean to reduce the smoke generated when they are turned on. Frying should always be done over a gentle heat, and the oil or fat watched carefully so that it does not begin to smoke.

Indoor pollution from formaldehyde can be combated by painting or varnishing all items made of particleboard or plywood. See pages 214–215 for other items that may give off formaldehyde. If you cannot get rid of these, store them in a well-ventilated room, garage, or loft space. Air the house and create better ventilation. An air cleaner containing activated carbon may be useful for a while (see page 307).

Various volatile substances (see page 117) can irritate the nose, and if anything seems to make you react, it should be removed or sealed in an airtight container. Some common irritants include felt-tip pens, air fresheners, and aerosols. Most things that are sold in aerosols can be found in some other type of container, or a substitute can be used. A house can be kept clean with a few simple items: dish-washing liquid, scouring powder, and toilet cleaner. Unscented versions are preferable. Clear out all other cleaning materials, mineral spirits, turps, meths, dry-cleaning fluids, polish, bleach, mothballs, and disinfectant—and the rags used to apply any of these.

Once you have reduced the level of "pleasant" artificial odors in the house, you may begin to notice other smells. (Air fresheners actually deaden the sense of smell.) If any plastic items seem to have a strong unpleasant smell, try to replace them. Clean thoroughly to tackle other nasty household odors. Should any smells prove resistant to cleaning efforts, an air cleaner containing activated carbon (see appendix 3) will eliminate them, although this is not a cheap solution to the problem.

Outdoor pollution is obviously more difficult to avoid. When levels of pollutants are high, keep away from traffic-laden streets, particularly in the afternoon and during the evening rush hour, when pollution peaks. Don't undertake any strenuous outdoor exercise in the afternoon during these high-pollution periods. Stay indoors if your throat feels sore or your eyes are stinging in the outdoor air. Consider using an antipollution mask (see appendix 3). Those with asthma should take particular care and increase their preventer medication if symptoms get worse.

Unfortunately, reducing our intake of traffic fumes often means traveling by car rather than walking or cycling, so we are helping to perpetuate the problem. In the long run the pollution issue has to be tackled by legislation, better public transport, and improved traffic planning, but the political will to do this is currently lacking.

The need for burn piles can be avoided by turning leaves and other waste into compost or bringing it to your community's yard waste facility, if one exists. An alternative option is to wrap such material in plastic bags and put them in the garbage. In some communities there is a special collection time for bagged yard waste each spring. Never light a burn pile on a damp or misty day, and discourage neighbors from doing so.

Appendix 7
FOODS THAT MAY
RELEASE SULFUR DIOXIDE

Sulfur dioxide is a gas that can irritate the airways of asthmatics and provoke an asthma attack. Some preservatives give off this gas in small amounts, and it is inhaled during eating. There is no need to avoid these preservatives unless you are sure they trigger attacks.

Most dried fruits are treated with sulfur dioxide and give off the gas when chewed. Dried fruit that has not been treated will usually be labeled "unsulfured."

The following preservatives give off sulfur dioxide:

sodium sulfite
sodium hydrogen sulfite
sodium metabisulfite
potassium metabisulfite
calcium sulfite

These preservatives are widely used in wine, beer, and cider. Homemade wine is no exception: Campden tablets, sold to winemakers, contain potassium metabisulfite.

One "hidden source" of sulfur dioxide is restaurant, take-out, and cafeteria food. French fries used in the catering trade have usually been dipped in a metabisulfite solution and give off significant amounts of sulfur dioxide. Prepared salads, avocado dip, shrimp, prawns, and lobster are also likely to have been treated with these preservatives and sometimes cause problems.

Fruit salad, glacé cherries, fruit juices, fruit pie fillings, dried vegetables and soup, fruit drinks, fruit jellies, and custard are other possible sources of sulfur dioxide in the catering trade. It is not worthwhile avoiding these foods unless you know they trigger your asthma attacks.

Packaged foods often contain sulfites and metabisulfites, but these are easier to avoid as they are declared on the label.

SCIENTIFIC NAMES OF PLANTS

The common names of plants vary from one part of the world to another, so for clear communication it is better to use the scientific names.

These are the scientific names for the plants included in the main body of the text. *The list is only intended to show which plant we refer to by a particular common name:* some of the common names listed may be used for different species by other authors.

Common name	Scientific name	Notes
alder	*Alnus* spp.	
alfalfa	*Medicago sativa*	
amaranth	Amaranthaceae family	
ash	*Fraxinus excelsior*	
aspens	*Populus tremula* (Britain); *P. tremuloides* (North America)	
aster	*Aster* spp.	
bald "cypress"	*Taxodium distichum*	Not a true cypress but a relative of the redwood.
barley	*Hordeum distichon, H. vulgare*	
bean	*Phaseolus* spp.	
begonia	*Begonia* spp.	
birch	*Betula* spp.	
bog myrtle	*Myrica gale*	
box elder	*Acer negundo*	Also called Manitoba maple or ash-leaved maple.
brittle bush	*Encelia* spp.	
buttercup	*Ranunculus* spp.	
cabbage	*Brassica oleracea*	
cabbage family	Cruciferae or Brassicaceae	
carrot	*Daucus carota*	
carrot family	Umbelliferae or Apiaceae	
cedar	*Cedrus* spp.	Note that Japanese red cedar is not a true cedar, but a relative of the redwood.

Common name	Scientific name	Notes
"cedar"	any member of the Cupressaceae referred to as a cedar; includes species of *Thuja, Juniperus*, and *Chaemaecyparis*	
chamomile	*Matricaria chamomilla, Chamaemelum nobile,* and other species	The species implicated in the cross-reaction described on p. 166 was *M. chamomilla;* the plant used for chamomile lawns is *C. nobile.*
cherry	*Prunus avium, P. cerasus*	
chicory	*Cichorium* spp.	
chrysanthemum	*Chrysanthemum* spp.	
clover	*Melilotus* spp.	
coltsfoot	*Tussilago* spp.	
corn	*Zea mays*	
couch grass	*Agropyron repens*	
cyclamen	*Cyclamen* spp.	
cypress	*Cupressus* spp. and *Chamaecyparis* spp.	These are the true cypresses. Other trees and shrubs in the same family (Cupressaceae) commonly cross-react.
dahlia	*Dahlia* hybrids	
dandelion	*Taraxacum* spp.	
dock	*Rumex* spp.	Note that *Rumex* also includes a variety of species known as sorrels. These will undoubtedly cross-react with docks.
Easter lily	*Lilium* spp.	
eastern white pine	*Pinus strobus*	Also called white pine or Weymouth pine.
elder, elderberry	*Sambucus nigra*	
false oat grass	*Arrhenatherum elatius*	
fir	*Abies* spp.	
goldenrod	*Solidago* spp.	
giant ragweed	*Ambrosia trifida*	
Lamb's-quarters,	Chenopodiaceae, goosefoot family	
grass	Gramineae or Poaceae family	

Common name	Scientific name	Notes
hazel	*Corylus* spp.	
heather	*Calluna* spp. and *Erica* spp.	
heather family	Ericaceae	
honeysuckle	*Lonicera* spp.	
hornbeam	*Carpinus* spp.	In the United States, *Carpinus* is called ironwood and hornbeam means *Ostrya* spp.
horse chestnut	*Aesculus* spp.	
hydrangea	*Hydrangea* spp.	
ironweed	*Vernonia* spp.	
Japanese red cedar	*Cryptomeria japonica*	Not a true cedar.
juniper	*Juniperus* spp.	
knapweed	*Centaurea* spp.	
lily	*Lilium* spp. and *Gloriosa rothschildiana*	
lucerne	*Medicago sativa*	
marigold	*Tagetes* spp.	
meadow fescue	*Festuca pratensis*	
millet	*Panicum miliaceum*	
mimosa	any species of *Albizia* or *Acacia* or *Mimosa* known as mimosa	
mugwort or sagebrush	*Artemisia vulgaris*	There are many other *Artemisia* spp. known as wormwood, tarragon, southernwood, etc.; these probably all cross-react with mugwort/sagebrush.
nettle	*Urtica* spp.	
oat	*Avena sativa*	
oil-seed rape	*Brassica napus*	
olive	*Olea europaea*	
orange	various *Citrus* spp., but principally *C. sinensis*	
osier	*Salix viminalis* and other *Salix* spp.	
peach	*Prunus persica*	

Common name	Scientific name	Notes
pellitory-of-the-wall	*Parietaria judaica*	Can be taken to include all other *Parietaria* spp., since they will cross-react.
pigweed	*Amaranthus* spp.	Name can be used for various other plants as well.
pine	*Pinus* spp.	"Australian pine" *(Casuarina)* is not a true pine.
plantain	*Plantago* spp.	
plum	*Prunus domestica* and other *Prunus* spp.	
pond "cypress"	*Taxodium ascendens*	Not a true cypress but a relative of the redwood.
poplar	*Populus* spp.	
privet	*Ligustrum ovalifolium* (used for hedging) and *L. vulgare* (wild privet)	
pussy willow	*Salix caprea* and other *Salix* spp.	
rabbit brush	*Chrysothamnus* spp.	
ragweed	*Ambrosia* spp.	
ragwort	*Senecio* spp.	
redwood	*Sequoia* and *Sequoiadendron*	
rice	*Oryza sativa*	
rose	*Rosa* spp. and hybrids	
rose family	*Rosaceae*	
rosinweed	*Grindelia* spp.	
rye	*Secale cereale*	
ryegrass	*Lolium perenne*	
sallow	*Salix cinerea, S. caprea*	
Santa Maria feverfew	*Parthenium hysterophorus*	
sedge	Cyperaceae family	Reeds also belong to this family.
she-oak	*Casuarina* spp.	Also called "Australian pine" and beefwood.
sneezeweed	*Helenium* spp.	
sorghum	*Sorghum vulgare*	

Common name	Scientific name	Notes
spruce	*Picea* spp.	
sugarcane	*Saccharum officinarum*	
sunflower	*Helianthus annuus*	
swamp "cypress"	*Taxodium distichum*	
sweet gale	*Myrica gale*	
sweet pea	*Lathyrus* spp.	
thistle	*Cirsium* spp., *Sonchus* spp.	
timothy	*Phleum pretense*	
wheat	*Triticum aestivum, T. durum, T. dicoccum*	
white cypress	*Callitris columellaris*	Also called Murray pine. Not a true pine but a native Australian conifer.
wild oat	*Avena fatua*	
willow	*Salix* spp.	
yew	*Taxus* spp.	
zinnia	*Zinnia* spp.	

INDEX

ABOUT THE AUTHORS

Jonathan Brostoff, M.D., is a physician in charge of the Allergy Clinic at the Middlesex Hospital in London and Reader in Clinical Immunology at University College London Medical School. After training as a general physician, he became interested in inhalant and food allergy. He has spent many years studying the way the immune system works and how it produces allergic diseases such as hay fever, asthma, eczema, and food allergy. He is currently engaged in programs of research in these areas. Dr Brostoff is recognized as a leading international authority on allergy and is coauthor of several principal textbooks on this subject.

Linda Gamlin trained as a biochemist and worked in scientific research for several years before turning to scientific writing. She specializes in writing about allergic diseases, the effects of diet and the environment on health, psychosomatic medicine, and evolutionary biology. In 1994 she won the Rhone-Poulenc Science Book Prize, and in 1995 the Golden Trilobite Award of the American Paleontology Society. She writes for medical journals, newspapers, and a range of magazines. This is her fifth book on popular health matters.